Using the Clinical Laboratory in Medical Decision-Making

Using the Clinical Laboratory in Medical Decision-Making

Edited by

George D. Lundberg, MD

Vice-President for Scientific Information
Editor, *The Journal of the American
Medical Association*
American Medical Association
Chicago

American Society of Clinical Pathologists Press
Chicago

Library of Congress Cataloging in Publication Data

Lundberg, George D.
  Using the clinical laboratory in medical decision-making.

  Includes index.
  1. Medicine, Clinical—Decision making.
2. Medical laboratories—Utilization. 3. Diagnosis,
Laboratory. I. Title. [DNLM: 1. Diagnosis,
Laboratory—Collected works. 2. Laboratories—
Organization and administration—Collected works.
QY 4 L962]
RC48.L8 1983   616.07′5   83-2801
ISBN 0-89189-164-1

First Reprinting, March 1984
Second Reprinting, October 1984

Contents

v

—— Preface ——

In 1973, Bob Moser became the 12th editor of *The Journal of the American Medical Association (JAMA)*. Shortly thereafter, he formed the first formal Editorial Board in the 90-year history of the Journal and invited me to be the pathologist on that Board. He suggested that I begin a series on the laboratory, emphasizing any aspect I chose. About that time I heard Larry Weed give one of his spectacular presentations on the problem-oriented medical record in Los Angeles. I was tremendously impressed and soon visited with Dr. Weed in Vermont, securing creative ideas about how he believed physicians should behave in their practice.

I had completed six of my ten years in the Section of Laboratories and Pathology at the Los Angeles County–University of Southern California Medical Center, where we were building the largest and most productive hospital laboratory in the world. This laboratory growth was motivated primarily by our self-defense against hundreds of physicians in training, medical students, and staff physicians. These physicians recently had emerged from nearly a decade of actual ration stamps and other restrictions on the performance of laboratory tests and seemed to be going wild ordering laboratory tests as the technology of clinical laboratory medicine exploded.

Obviously, we became deeply involved in management at that time and wrote "Managing the Patient Focused Laboratory" to share experiences in running laboratories. In regard to laboratory use, we believed there must be a better way than what we were observing. So we developed a division of interpretive clinical pathology, worked with many advisory medical staff committees, changed laboratory request slips to guide ordering patterns, abolished bad tests, established innovative panels, created a panic value system, organized the entire laboratory based on turn-around time, and freely used in-house and out-house laboratories interchangeably to meet patient needs and physician demands. But even all that wasn't enough.

We discovered then, and in subsequent seminars in different states and countries, that the reasons physicians order laboratory tests are very many. The reasons include the following: (1) confirmation of clinical opinion, (2) diagnosis, (3) establishing a base line, (4) monitoring, (5) completing a data base, (6) fraud and kickbacks, (7) public relations, (8) curiosity, (9) insecurities, (10) hospital policy, (11) screening, (12) legal requirements, (13) medical-legal needs, (14) documentation, (15) peer pressure, (16) patient pressure, (17) recent-literature pressure, (18) a previous abnormal result, (19) questionable accuracy of previous test, (20) unavailability of prior result, (21) prognosis, (22) habit, (23) buying time, (24) CYA, (25) hunting or fishing expeditions, (26) personal education, (27) research, (28) personal reassurance, (29) personal or institutional profit, (30) demonstration for an attending physician, (31) frustration at nothing else to do, and (32) availability and the fact that they are easy to do.

The physicians at our institution came from most medical schools in the United States, and they arrived knowing very little about how to use the laboratory correctly, merely following rote learning or the habits of older physicians. Most senior professors cared little about guiding proper laboratory use.

It became apparent that the only way we could influence the thousands of physicians practicing in our own institution was to influence physicians at large. Since *JAMA* is the most widely circulated clinical journal in the world, it seemed the ideal vehicle for wielding this influence. Therefore, we set about to attempt to guide physicians in practice to use the laboratory correctly for most common problems for which laboratory use is prominent and to interpret the results properly. Those were the basic reasons for creating our "Toward Optimal Laboratory Use" (TOLU) series in *JAMA*, and they have always been the goals of the series.

All the chapters in this book were published previously in the TOLU series in *JAMA* between 1975 and 1982. They were rigorously peer-reviewed prior to original publication and have stood the test of total readership review since then. In every instance, they have been revised and updated by the authors as needed and again peer-reviewed by ASCP. So they are 1983 fresh.

This book is aimed primarily at practicing clinicians, especially those in direct patient care. The book also should be helpful to pathologists who guide clinicians in using the laboratory correctly. Medical students and postgraduate physicians in training may profit appreciably from understanding the principles espoused here and applying the suggested practices.

In 1981, Patricia B. Lorimer, then Director of the ASCP Press, approached me about putting the TOLU series into a book and letting ASCP publish it. We asked the AMA for permission, and that was generously granted.

Many other people were very helpful as the series originated. At USC, Phil Manning provided many early suggestions, and Nancy Warner made time available for me. Terry Southgate had the editorial responsibility at the AMA for the entire series. Susan LeDoux in Sacramento administered much of the later programs. The ASCP Press staff is due particular thanks for their recent work.

Using the laboratory properly is rarely simple although many of our chapters may appear straightforward. There are some caveats and omissions. Many are stated in Chapter 1, and the reader is referred there for disclaimers. While this book deals definitively with predictive value theory and algorithms and hints at decision analysis, it does not apply cluster analysis, biologic time series models, or the various forms of discriminant analysis. These will be subjects of later articles in the TOLU series as it continues to evolve. Nothing is perfect. Algorithms are only one way to go. Yet, the nature of human activities in problem solving is such that decisions naturally flow in sequence. Because of the limitations of time and space, events must occur in a stepwise manner. Often, subsequent steps depend upon the results of preceding events. All purposeful human behavior flows from one decision point to the next. Algorithms in fact do work displaying decisions.

We hope that your next decision will be to read Chapter 1 and get on with the book.

I wish you good results and no open loops.

George D. Lundberg, MD

Contributors

Elias Amador, MD, Professor and Chairman, Department of Pathology, Drew Postgraduate Medical School, University of California, and Martin Luther King, Jr General Hospital, Los Angeles

Richard L. Atkinson, MD, Assistant Professor of Medicine, Division of Endocrine-Metabolism, Department of Internal Medicine, University of Virginia School of Medicine, Charlottesville

Raymond C. Bartlett, MD, Director, Division of Microbiology, Department of Pathology, Hartford Hospital; Professor, University of Connecticut School of Medicine (Laboratory Medicine), Hartford

George S. Benson, MD, Associate Professor, Division of Urology, Department of Surgery, University of Texas Medical School, Houston

Stephen P. Boyers, MD, Assistant Professor, Division of Reproductive Endocrinology, Department of Obstetrics and Gynecology, Harbor-UCLA Medical Center, UCLA School of Medicine, Torrance, California

George A. Bray, MD, Professor, Division of Diabetes and Clinical Nutrition, Department of Medicine, University of Southern California, Los Angeles

Eileen D. Brewer, MD, Assistant Professor, Department of Pediatrics, University of Texas Medical School, Houston

Joseph E. Buttery, PhD, Principal Hospital Scientist, Department of Clinical Chemistry, The Queen Elizabeth Hospital, Adelaide, South Australia

Ofelia J. Centeno, MD, Associate Pathologist, Department of Pathology, Holy Cross Hospital, Detroit

William T. Dahms, MD, Assistant Professor of Pediatrics, Department of Pediatrics, Case Western Reserve School of Medicine, Rainbow Babies and Children's Hospital, Cleveland

Herbert L. DuPont, MD, Professor and Director, Program in Infectious Diseases and Clinical Microbiology, University of Texas Medical School, Houston

Edward R. Eichner, MD, Professor of Medicine, and Chief, Section of Hematology, Department of Medicine, College of Medicine, University of Oklahoma Health Sciences Center, Oklahoma City

John M. Eisenberg, MD, Sol Katz Associate Professor of General Medicine; Chief, Section of General Medicine, Department of Medicine, University of Pennsylvania School of Medicine; Senior Fellow, Leonard Davis Institute of Health Sciences, University of Pennsylvania, Philadelphia

Yehudi M. Felman, MD, Director, Bureau of Venereal Disease Control, City Health Department, New York

Murry G. Fischer, MD, Attending Surgeon, Beth Israel Medical Center; Associate Clinical Professor of Surgery, Department of Surgery, Mount Sinai School of Medicine, City University of New York, New York

Esther F. Freier, MS, Professor and Co-Director, Division of Clinical Chemistry, Department of Laboratory Medicine and Pathology, University of Minnesota Medical School, Minneapolis

James F. Fries, MD, Associate Professor of Medicine, Division of Immunology, Department of Medicine, Stanford University School of Medicine, Stanford, California

Robert S. Galen, MD, Chairman, Department of Biochemistry, The Cleveland Clinic, Cleveland

S. Raymond Gambino, MD, President, Eastern Laboratory Division, MetPath, Inc; Adjunct Professor of Pathology, Columbia University College of Physicians and Surgeons, New York

Alvin M. Gelb, MD, Chief, Division of Gastroenterology, Department of Medicine, Beth Israel Medical Center; Associate Clinical Professor of Medicine, Division of Gastroenterology, Department of Medicine, Mount Sinai School of Medicine, Mount Sinai Medical Center, New York

Sheldon Greenfield, MD, Associate Professor of Medicine and Public Health, Division of General Internal Medicine, Department of Medicine, University of California, Los Angeles

Frank L. Greenway, MD, Assistant Clinical Professor, Division of Endocrinology, Department of Medicine, University of California School of Medicine, Los Angeles

Robert R. Holland, MD, Resident, Department of Medicine, University of Vermont, Burlington

J. Willis Hurst, MD, Candler Professor of Medicine (Cardiology), and Chairman, Department of Medicine, Emory University School of Medicine; Chief of Medicine, Emory University Hospital, Atlanta

Henry A. Jordan, MD, Director, Institute for Behavioral Education, King of Prussia, Pennsylvania; Clinical Associate Professor, Department of Psychiatry, University of Pennsylvania School of Medicine, Philadelphia

M. Colin Jordan, MD, Chief, Infectious Diseases, Veterans Administration Medical Center, Martinez, California; Associate Professor of Medicine, University of California, Davis, School of Medicine, Davis

Spencer B. King III, MD, Professor of Medicine (Cardiology), Emory University School of Medicine; Director, Cardiovascular Laboratory, Emory University Hospital, Atlanta

Harvey C. Knowles, Jr, MD, Professor of Medicine, Division of Endocrinology/Metabolism, Department of Internal Medicine, University of Cincinnati College of Medicine, Cincinnati

Anthony L. Komaroff, MD, Associate Professor of Medicine, and Medical Director, Laboratory for the Analysis of Medical Practices, Division of General Medicine and Primary Care, Department of Medicine, Harvard University Medical School, Boston

Arthur F. Krieg, MD, Chief, Division of Clinical Pathology, Pennsylvania State University School of Medicine, Milton S. Hershey Medical Center, Hershey, Pennsylvania

Calvin M. Kunin, MD, Professor and Chairman, Department of Medicine, Ohio State University College of Medicine, Columbus

Terrence J. Lee, MD, Clinical Assistant Professor of Medicine, Department of Medicine, University of North Carolina School of Medicine, Chapel Hill; Asheville Infectious Disease Consulting Pathologist, Asheville, North Carolina

George D. Lundberg, MD, Vice-President for Scientific Information, and Editor, *JAMA*, American Medical Association, Chicago

Aaron Lupovitch, MD, Director, Department of Pathology, Holy Cross Hospital, Detroit; Clinical Associate Professor, Department of Pathology, Wayne State University College of Medicine, Detroit

Robert F. Maronde, MD, Professor of Medicine, and Head, Section of Clinical Pharmacology, Department of Medicine, University of Southern California School of Medicine, Los Angeles

Donald M. Mitchell, MD, Professor, Division of Rheumatology, Department of Medicine, University of Saskatchewan College of Medicine, Saskatoon, Saskatchewan, Canada

Mark E. Molitch, MD, Associate Professor of Medicine, Division of Endocrinology and Metabolism, Department of Medicine, Tufts University School of Medicine; Associate Director, Clinical Study Unit, New England Medical Center, Boston

J. Donald Ostrow, MD, Sprague Professor of Medicine, Section of Gastroenterology, Department of Medicine, Northwestern University Medical School; Chief, Section of Gastroenterology, Department of Medical Service, Veterans Administration Lakeside Medical Center, Chicago

Peter R. Pannall, MBBCH, FRCPath, FRCPA, Director in Clinical Chemistry, Department of Clinical Chemistry, The Queen Elizabeth Hospital, Adelaide, South Australia

Zdena Pavlova, MD, Hematopathologist and Assistant Professor of Clinical Pathology, Division of Pediatric Pathology, Department of Pathology, University of Southern California School of Medicine, Los Angeles County-University of Southern California Medical Center, Los Angeles

Robert K. Quinnell, MD, Director, Fairfax Family Practice Center, Department of Family Practice, Medical College of Virginia, Virginia Commonwealth University, Richmond

Samuel Raymond, MD, Associate Professor of Pathology, Pepper Laboratory, Department of Pathology, University of Pennsylvania School of Medicine, Philadelphia

Nicholas B. Riccardi, PhD, Department of Biology, Fordham University, Bronx, New York; Bureau of Venereal Disease Control, Department of Health, New York

Terry K. Satterwhite, MD, Associate Professor of Medicine, Program in Infectious Diseases and Clinical Microbiology, University of Texas Medical School, Houston

Ethan A. H. Sims, MD, Professor of Medicine Emeritus, Metabolic Unit, Department of Medicine, University of Vermont College of Medicine, Burlington

Laurence P. Skendzel, MD, Director of Laboratories, Munson Medical Center, Traverse City, Michigan

Jack W. Smith, Jr, MD, Assistant Professor, Division of Chemistry, Department of Pathology, Ohio State University College of Medicine, Columbus

Molly Marriott Solares, RN, Nursing Care Specialist, Division of Endocrinology, Department of Medicine, Harbor-UCLA Medical Center; Endocrine-Diabetes Coordinator, Harbor General Hospital, Torrance, California

Stuart V. Sostrin, MD, Director of Laboratories, Panorama Community Hospital, Panorama City, California; Clinical Assistant Professor, Department of Pathology, University of Southern California, Los Angeles

P. Frederick Sparling, MD, Professor and Chairman, Department of Bacteriology and Immunology, University of North Carolina School of Medicine, Chapel Hill

Carl E. Speicher, MD, Professor and Director, Clinical Laboratories, Department of Pathology, Ohio State University College of Medicine, Columbus

Ronald S. Swerdloff, MD, Professor and Chief, Division of Endocrinology, Department of Medicine, Harbor-UCLA Medical Center, UCLA School of Medicine, Torrance, California

M. Michael Thaler, MD, Professor of Pediatrics, Division of Pediatric Gastroenterology and Nutrition, Department of Pediatrics, University of California, San Francisco

Donald M. Vickery, MD, President, The Center for Consumer Health Education, Inc, Vienna, Virginia; Assistant Professor, Department of Community and Family Medicine, Georgetown University School of Medicine, Washington, DC

Gerhard E. Voigt, MD, Professor of Forensic Medicine, Department of Forensic Medicine, University of Lund, Sweden

Ralph O. Wallerstein, MD, Clinical Professor, Departments of Medicine and Laboratory Medicine, University of California, San Francisco

Leonard A. Weingarten, MD, Assistant Clinical Professor of Medicine, Department of Medicine, Mount Sinai School of Medicine; Associate Attending Physician in Medicine, Beth Israel Medical Center, New York

Bradley G. Wertman, MD, Pathologist, Department of Pathology, Medical Center Del Oro Hospital, Houston

Charles L. Whitfield, MD, Associate Professor of Medicine and Family Medicine, Alcohol and Drug Abuse Program, University of Maryland School of Medicine, Baltimore

Sankey V. Williams, MD, Assistant Professor of Medicine, Henry J. Kaiser Family Foundation Faculty Scholar in General Medicine, Section of General Medicine, Department of Medicine, University of Pennsylvania School of Medicine; Associate

Director for Medical Affairs, Senior Fellow, Leonard Davis Institute for Health Sciences, University of Pennsylvania, Philadelphia

Edward T. Wong, MD, Associate Professor of Pathology, Department of Pathology, University of Southern California School of Medicine; Head, Interpretive Clinical Pathology Unit, Section of Laboratories and Pathology, Los Angeles County-University of Southern California Medical Center, Los Angeles

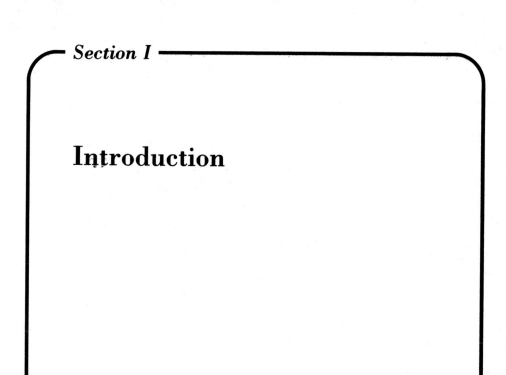

Section I

Introduction

Chapter 1

The Modern Clinical Laboratory

George D. Lundberg, MD

The huge variety and volume of available laboratory tests confronts the physician with a major dilemma. What tests should be ordered on what patients? When, how, how often, at what cost, grouped or individually, and in what sequence? What is the interpretation of the results and what steps then should be taken?

The frequency with which a laboratory test may be ordered varies from none to constant monitoring of all variables. What should be done? What constitutes good laboratory medicine? Should the physician order one of each available laboratory test on each patient once a lifetime, once a year, once an hour, or never? Many forces influence these decisions. Among them are availability of laboratory service, policies of technical instrument and reagent manufacturers, what the physician knows about the medical need for the test, and economic considerations, such as cost and who makes the profit or takes the loss. Laboratory tests should not be ordered without a plan for using the information gained. What will be done if the test result is normal? High? Low?

The Data Base

Weed[1] has proposed that physicians should focus on problem solving by seeking and identifying specific patient problems and pursuing each to its logical conclusion, based on defined goals. He proposes that one should define and obtain an initial comprehensive data base and proceed from there. Every encounter between a patient and a health-provider establishes a data base of some sort, but this data base may be infinitely variable. It may result in the identification of *no* problems. More likely, it will identify one problem or more, some simple, others complex. Some problems require no laboratory use. Others are solved principally by the use of the laboratory. Some problems are even produced (first observed) through a laboratory test. Many are approached best by combining clinical observations and laboratory tests plus observations of clinical course, therapeutic response, and the like.

The purpose of this book is to identify a reasonable, defendable approach to the use of the laboratory in identification and solution of important common problems. There are hundreds of types of laboratory determinations capable of identifying and following the progress of many significant diseases. Further new useful tests will be devised. But the issue at hand is to apply existing knowledge expeditiously and beneficially by rearranging and integrating existing forces. The goal should be to perform every appropriate laboratory test well and economically and to perform none that are not properly indicated.

Master List of Problems

In developing a plan for this book, the most common problems or diagnoses have been obtained from general practitioners' offices and community hospitals. This list of problems or diagnoses was reduced to those in which there is heavy involvement of the laboratory in proceeding toward the solution. Chapters addressing these problems constitute most of this book.

Algorithms

Feinstein[2] has termed the development of suitable algorithms for the strategy of diagnostic work-ups "a critical challenge in modern medicine." "Algorithm" is a word common to computer activities, and refers to a plan of strategy for solving a problem. Algorithms may be displayed best in flow charts that diagrammatically symbolize each act of reasoning in the strategy. Flow charts depicting branching logic may be called decision trees. Discussion of each problem in this book will be accompanied by a branching-logic, decision-tree display with use of the algorithm; a narrative explanation of the problem will also be included.

Decision tables were developed by US industry about 15 years ago as an alternative to flow charts or narratives in guiding manufacturing steps. They communicate decision-making processes by compactly representing elements such as conditions and actions and the logic that links conditions to actions. In some instances in this book, the algorithmic approach to problems will be presented by decision tables in addition to, or instead of, flow charts.[3]

The purpose of this book includes demonstration of disciplined method and process in problem-solving, as well as presentation of definitive approaches and information. The clinical judgment of a skilled physician may make strict application of the algorithmic approach in many human situations unnecessary.

Yet physicians principally should be skilled observers logically proceeding through disciplined method toward correct solutions. Algorithms are effective, as long as their limitations are understood, and their rigidity blended with use of good clinical judgment, when appropriate.

Issues and Discipline

Every organized effort is a subsystem within a set of interactive systems.[4] Systems must include purpose, direction, plans, goals, and feedback loops. All loops must be closed. Each step can be audited. Specific goals of strategy are critical and are reviewed and reinforced. Patients are not divisible by discipline, nor is this book. The mingling of sequences of history, physical examination, laboratory tests, and therapeutic trials is shown.

We understand that definitive, complete, interdisciplinary decision-tree problem-solving will require electronic, rather than paper-pencil, modes of display. This is beyond the scope of this book. However, it is practical to construct and display the high points in the approach to important and common problems coupled with explanatory narrative depicting process as well as facts. This book should serve as a reasonable prelude to definitive computer formats, programs, and displays to include not only the logic of each branch decision and its resultant action, but also predicted frequencies of association of branch points and predicted percentages of each branch choice in relation to all other data elements.

We are not proposing a precipitous rush to the laboratory for help in every clinical problem. Rather, we champion an integrated, interdisciplinary approach blending clinical observations and judgment with laboratory use. Laboratory performance can be judged by the indexes of its products—data. Laboratory utilization performance is far more difficult to judge. Standards have not been established, but are urgently needed. The final questions include these: Were the laboratory tests appropriate? Were they beneficial? Were they economical? Were all loops closed? Was *every* laboratory test maximally useful?

References

1. Weed LL: *Medical Records, Medical Education, and Patient Care*. Cleveland, the Press of Case Western Reserve University, 1971.
2. Feinstein AR: An analysis of diagnostic reasoning: III. The construction of clinical algorithms. *Yale J Biol Med* 1974;45:5–32.
3. Pollack SL, Hicks HT, Harrison WJ: *Decision Tables: Theory and Practice*. New York, Wiley-Interscience, 1971.
4. Lundberg GD: *Managing the Patient Focused Laboratory*. Oradell, NJ, Medical Economics Publishing Co, 1975.

Chapter 2

Health and Normality

Elias Amador, MD

In order to diagnose any disease, a standard of reference is required. This standard is the state of health or normality. The term "health" is said to be the "general condition of the body or mind with reference to soundness or vigor, and to freedom from disease or ailment" (*Random House Dictionary of the English Language*, unabridged edition, 1966). When we say that a person is in good health, we mean that this person may indulge in physical and mental activities without distress, and is free from diseases that may threaten his or her well-being or life.[1] Similarly, the orthodox medical definition of normal "denotes the absence of infection, disease, or malformation, or the absence of experimental, or therapeutic manipulations" (*Webster's New International Dictionary of the English Language*, second edition, unabridged, 1960).

With these definitions, we may expand the concept of normality to include and describe each of the classes of characters of the body, which taken together allow us to judge from objective and subjective data that a person is indeed healthy. In order to serve our medical purposes, the concept or general idea of normality must (1) include qualitative, quantitative, and molecular characters; (2) be applicable in clinical practice; and (3) be objectively verifiable by others, ie, should be reproducible.

For these reasons, it is convenient to treat normality as a *concept* (in the sense proposed by Wittgenstein[2]) consisting of multiple, similar ideas in the same way multiple threads intertwine to form a cord. Wittgenstein also recognizes that a word can have a multiplicity of different meanings or uses. The use of "concept" as a family of ideas or meanings also has the advantage that its contents may change in step with advances in knowledge. An example is the concept of the cell as the vital unit, as useful today as it was in the first half of the 19th century, despite the fact that its ideological content has changed much since the times of Schwann and Virchow.

Qualitative Normality

The description of normal bodily characters, and of disease processes, is in large part qualitative and subjective.[3] The subjective approach commonly used in biology results from the speed of the human brain to perceive whole constellations and configurations of characters, to compare them in an almost wholly nonquantitative way, and to weigh them by means of its own previous experience.[4]

When we judge multiple qualitative characters in an organ or in a disease process, we tend to group the characters by their affinitives in order to form with them a mental image or matrix.[3-5] For example, in dealing with such entities as an organ or limb, the observer first determines if it is present or absent; then if present, the observer describes its placement, form, color, proportion of its parts, texture, characteristics of its vessels, ducts, and nerves. For each organ, tissue, or cell, it is possible to formulate a matrix or table of important characters that will allow a detailed comparison of a test organ with the comparable characters that are considered to indicate normality. It is also possible to describe qualitative characters in a dynamic fashion, through a description of the way in which they vary and adapt to physiologic changes with time. These characters (as well as quantitative and molecular characters) thus serve to indicate in a coherent fashion that the portion of the organism under consideration is or is not normal. Therefore, the observer employs the criterion of _coherence_ to reach a judgment of normality. Moreover, qualitative characters can be described and codified in an objective fashion so that the observations and judgments based on them can be made in a reproducible fashion. "Truth tables" based on Bayes theorem and the assignment of numbers to "weigh" each character in order to construct tables such as those used in numerical taxonomy allow an effective definition of the normality of groups of qualitative characters.[3, 5]

Quantitative Normality

The normal values for the concentration of the many chemical constituents and of the number of cells in a given volume of the body fluids, for the organ weights, and measurements of parts of the body are quantitative characters. Commonly, the limits of these normal values are given as the mean ± 2 standard deviations. This practice implies that the distribution of values compatible with health follows a bell-shaped, or Gaussian, frequency distribution. The application of this Gaussian curve to describe biologic variables was popularized by the English naturalist Sir Francis Galton, cousin of Charles Darwin. Galton showed through analyses of natural events, as well as through the construction of ingenious mechanical devices, that random changes imposed on an initially homogeneous population produce deviations with a Gaussian frequency distribution[6] (Figure 2–1).

Nowadays, a value compatible with health is called "normal," a term

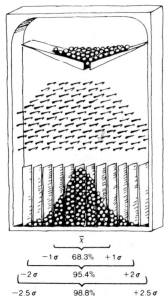

Figure 2–1. Probability device devised by Galton to demonstrate that Gaussian frequency distribution results from random action of many factors on individuals of homogeneous population. Spheres contained in funnel (upper third of figure) fall through narrow orifice with uniform direction and speed. During their fall, the spheres acquire an erratic movement as they bounce against the nails (middle third) and fall in random fashion into each one of the series of cavities or class intervals (bottom third). Resulting distribution is bell-shaped, and may be described completely by mean and standard deviation ($\bar{\chi}$, σ). Percentage of population included between certain distances to each side of mean is indicated by numbers at base of figure.

that has led to confusion because of its biologic and statistical uses. The two usages, "normal" indicating health and "normal" indicating Gaussian, are not synonymous, for the frequency distribution of test values for healthy persons often is not Gaussian.[7] Also, the fact that a group of test results has a Gaussian frequency distribution does not mean that the test results necessarily were obtained from healthy persons.[8]

Quantitative variables lend themselves to statistical analysis, with useful results if and when biologic considerations are kept in mind and the experimental design is done with care. In a previous review,[1] I have discussed the statistical methods that are most appropriate for the characterization of quantitative normal values, and also the way in which one may select normal subjects. Briefly, when a preliminary graphic analysis with normal probability paper indicates that the values appear to follow Gaussian distribution, one then determines if this is an arithmetic or logarithmic Gaussian distribution, if it is symmetrical or skewed, if its degree of peakedness (kurtosis) is compatible with the Gaussian curve, and if the areas under each segment of the observed frequency distribution agree, as shown by the χ^2 test for goodness of fit, with the expected Gaussian values.

If these tests indicate that the normal values follow a Gaussian curve distribution, then we may describe this distribution with the mean and the standard deviation, and we may select the probability values that are most appropriate for the test being studied (Figure 2–1). Usually the 95.4% probability limits given by the mean ±2 standard deviations are used. A sample size of 36 provides a good parametric estimate of the population mean and standard deviation, because the confidence with which these values can be estimated increases only asymptotically with increasingly larger sample sizes.

When the frequency distribution of the observed test results is not Gaussian, it is possible to analyze and describe its probability limits through nonparametric statistical methods.[7, 9] For each group, ie, men or women, the smallest adequate sample size is about 120 persons when nonparametric methods are used.

The study of any quantitative character also requires its correlation with other variables such as age, sex, body weight, race, and in women the presence or absence of menstruation or pregnancy. These variables should also be correlated statistically for those characters that can change with the time of day, with eating, or with marked emotional or physical activity.[1, 10]

The long-term stability of the values of bodily constituents of normal subjects has been studied by several authors, and by and large, the data appear to indicate that these values do remain relatively constant. However, a detailed analytic and statistical examination of long-term quantitative stability of bodily components is complex, and is the subject of current studies.[11]

The ready availability of large numbers of test results obtained from patient samples, as contrasted to those obtained from healthy subjects, together with the ease of statistical analysis performed by graphic or electronic means, has led certain authors to study the possibility of deriving normal ranges through the study of patients' test results.[12] The frequency distribution of a large group of patients' test results has a peak or mode that is more or less near to the mean of the normal range, but with a tail that is markedly skewed towards the values more frequently observed in disease.[13] On the basis of this observation, several workers have assumed that the most frequently appearing values will be normal and have a Gaussian frequency distribution, and that the mode will equal the mean of healthy results.[8] These workers have then proposed a variety of indirect statistical methods to estimate the normal range. For an indirect method to be acceptable, it must (1) yield means and standard deviations similar to those of the healthy population, (2) take into account the proportion of abnormal values in any given sample, (3) indicate the type of frequency distribution followed by the normal values, and (4) be shown to yield reliable estimates of the normal range for the majority of commonly used laboratory tests. Although an accurate indirect method appears desirable because it would be easy to perform routinely, none of the published methods appears to fulfill these criteria of reliability.[7, 8]

Molecular Normality

The dramatic advances in biochemistry over the past 20 years have provided a detailed physiochemical characterization of many normal and abnormal macromolecules, especially proteins. Molecular abnormalities may be intrinsic to the body (and many of them are probably genetic) or they may be extrinsic. When certain foreign molecules such as carbon monoxide and cyanide enter the body, their presence constitutes a quantitative abnormality, since their dose may be variable, and a molecular abnormality, since they constitute a threat to health and life.

In the case of intrinsic abnormalities, well-substantiated examples are still few, but the basic principle has been demonstrated clearly in the case of hemoglobin S, for which the genetic, biologic, and clinical details are well known. We can now exploit the advantages offered by molecular definitions of health and disease; besides providing us with molecular standards, such new developments also satisfy the prediction made by Rudolph Virchow in 1855, who said that

while we require that cellular pathology be the basis of the medical viewpoint . . . in the last analysis all disease can be reduced to passive or active alterations of major or minor groups of vital elements, whose functional capacity is altered in accordance with the state of their molecular composition.[14]

The identification of the molecular nature of the many cellular alterations obviously has to be based on a detailed comparison of the composition and structure of normal vs abnormal molecules. Well-characterized proteins provide us with molecular standards of normality, which allow us to describe with exactitude the variations, at times pathologic, that result from changes in the nucleotides of the gene. These changes may lead to the synthesis of proteins whose abnormality may be silent throughout life, may remain silent until some conditioning factor brings out their clinical manifestations, or the protein may be sufficiently altered to produce overt clinical disease.

Silent protein abnormalities include hemoglobins that have one amino acid substitution, but produce no red blood cell or clinical abnormality. An example of protein abnormalities that may produce disease under certain conditions is that of the genetically abnormal plasma pseudocholinesterases, which ordinarily are asymptomatic, but which can, when muscle-relaxant drugs such as succinylcholine are administered, lead to prolonged apnea.

In the third category are proteins whose genetic abnormality, ie, an amino acid substitution, leads to severe derangements in the structure and function of the molecule. Hemoglobin S is now a classic example. Conversely, hemoglobin F in the human fetus and hemoglobin A in the human adult are molecular standards of normality, against which variations of composition, structure, and function of all other human hemoglobins may be compared.

Another genetic standard of normality that it is now feasible to establish is the number and structure of human chromosomes. Chromosomal aberrations produce diseases so dramatic and well known that it is superfluous to mention them here. Although the majority of the population probably possess a normal genetic complement, a statistical majority is not necessary from a biologic viewpoint in order to define normality. We may say that a molecule or a gene is normal if and when it is compatible with well-being, activity, longevity, and reproduction of the individual, and hence with the survival of the species. Conversely, molecules and genes can be considered to be abnormal when they interfere with these biologic imperatives.

References

1. Amador E: Normal ranges, in Stefanini M (ed): _Advances in Clinical Pathology_. New York, Grune & Stratton Inc, vol 5, pp 59–83, 1973.
2. Wittgenstein L: _Philosophical Investigations_. New York, The Macmillan Co, Publishers, 1958, p 32.
3. Lodwick GS: _The Bones and Joints: An Atlas of Tumor Radiology_. Chicago, Year Book Medical Publishers, Inc, 1971, pp 3–79.
4. Cain AJ: Taxonomic concepts. _Ibis_ 1959;101:302–318.
5. Sokal HA, Sneath HA: _Principles of Numerical Taxonomy_. San Francisco, WH Freeman and Co, 1963.
6. Pearson K: _The Life, Letters and Labours of Francis Galton_. Cambridge, England, Cambridge University Press, 1930, vol 3a, pp 8–12.
7. Elveback LR, Guillier CL, Keating F: Health, normality and the ghost of Gauss. _JAMA_ 1970;211:69–75.
8. Amador E, Hsi BP: Indirect methods for estimating the normal range. _Am J Clin Pathol_ 1969;52:538–546.
9. Reed AH, Henry RJ, Mason WB, et al: Influence of statistical method used on the results of estimating the normal range. _Clin Chem_ 1971;17:275–284.
10. Wurtman RJ, Rose CM, Chou C, et al: Daily rhythms in the concentration of various amino acids in human plasma. _N Engl J Med_ 1968;279:171–175.
11. Williams GZ, Young DS, Cotlove E: Biological and analytical components of variation in long term studies of serum constituents in normal subjects. _Clin Chem_ 1970;16:1016–1032.
12. Becktel JM: Simplified estimation of normal ranges from routine laboratory data. _Clin Chem Acta_ 1970;28:119–125.
13. Owen JA, Campbell DG: Comparison of plasma electrolyte and urea values in healthy persons and in hospital patients. _Clin Chem Acta_ 1968;22:611–618.
14. Virchow R: Cellular pathologic. _Virchow's Archiv_ 1855;8:3–39.

Chapter 3

Decision Tables

Robert R. Holland, MD

A constructive approach to the information explosion can be seen in the work of Calvin Kunin, MD, on urinary tract infections (UTIs). The first edition of his book *Detection, Prevention, and Management of Urinary Tract Infections* is 200 pages long and represents the findings of 240 articles; the second edition represents 500 articles and is 300 pages long. Realizing that it would be impossible under the time constraints of practice for everyone to either read or remember accurately the content of his book or the original articles, Dr. Kunin has reduced the content to seven pages, including three flow charts, in Chapter 9. This was done with the expectation that the information he presents could then be used in the day-to-day practice of medicine for all patients regardless of time constraints, rather than just existing lifelessly between bookcovers.

This communication presents decision tables as an alternative to flow charts for the presentation of medical knowledge so that its use in the day-to-day practice of medicine may be facilitated. Decision tables were independently developed in the late 1950s by two companies (General Electric and Sutherland) because the complexity of their manufacturing processes had exceeded their ability to understand or describe them with the standard techniques of narrative description or flow charts. The literature of decision tables is replete with stories of how this tool succeeded where the older techniques failed. Decision tables are able to clearly communicate decision-making processes because they compactly represent all the elements of the process: conditions (variables), actions (conclusions), and the logic linking conditions to actions.[1]

How to Use Decision Tables

The fundamental element of the decision table is the decision rule. This is a statement that prescribes the set of conditions that must be satisfied in order

From: Decision Tables. Their Use for the Presentation of Clinical Algorithms. *JAMA* 1975;233:455–457. Copyright 1975 by the American Medical Association.

that an action or a series of actions be executed. A decision table is the structure for describing a set of related decision rules. To illustrate, consider the following ancient Persian poem:

He who knows not and knows not that he knows not is a fool—shun him.
He who knows not and knows that he knows not can be taught—teach him.
He who knows and knows not that he knows is asleep—wake him.
He who knows and knows that he knows is a prophet—follow him.

The poet never knew that he could have written it as follows[2]:

He knows		N		Y	
He knows that he knows not	N		Y	. . .	
He knows that he knows				N	Y
Shun him	X				
Teach him			X		
Wake him				X	
Follow him					X

All the items above the horizontal double line are condition boxes. Those below are action boxes. Each box to the left of the vertical double line is called a stub; each box to the right is called an entry. Above the horizontal double line, the combination of a stub and an entry forms a condition; below the horizontal double line, a stub and an entry forms an action. In the condition area, above the horizontal double line:

"Y" means that the condition is present.
"N" means that the condition is absent.
". . ." means that the condition is immaterial.

In the action area, "X" means that the action is to be executed if all the conditions of the rule are satisfied.[1]

In the example decision table only "yes" and "no" have been used as entries in the condition boxes. It is possible to put several conditions rather than just "yes" or "no" in a condition row. For example, a condition row may appear as:

Age, yr 0–25 25–50 50–75 >75.
This is called an extended-entry condition row.

Decision Tables for Urinary Tract Infection

Decision Tables 3–1 through 3–4 given here represent the decision rules from Kunin's flow chart for dealing with the patient with symptoms of UTI who is

Table 3—1.
Tests to Rule Out Urinary Tract Infection.

Too weak or confused to void, or obese female, or obstructed male	Y		N	
Bladder distended	Y	N	. . .	
Age			Infant	Others
Catheterization		X		
Bladder aspiration	X			
Clean voided urine				X
Strap on or catch			X	
Microscopic examination and quantitative culture	X	X	X	X

first seen in an office practice. (The flow chart does not conform to the standard rules for building flow charts for content to be computerized. If it were modified to reach that standard, it would become more complex and would require more paper for its representation. Kunin has attempted to simplify the flow charts in order to make them more usable.)

Findings and Comment

These decision tables are a direct translation of the logic from the flow chart; the only differences are the structure and the deletion of some narrative that was not necessary for the decision-making process, such as the procedure for collecting a specimen, the alternative culture, and microscopic examination techniques. This information is best put in narrative form separate from the flow chart or decision table, and then referred to when necessary.

The listing of all the conditions and actions in one column for a single decision allows an overview of the decision to be easily obtained. This makes gaps in the logic more apparent than when the logic is buried in narrative description or a flow chart. Questions that are not answered by the flow chart that become obvious on studying the decision tables are (1) What additional information is required on an infant with a UTI? (2) When should cystoscopy be done on men with a UTI? (3) What should be done with recurrences that are not frequent or closely spaced?

It will be noted that there are four separate decision tables: "Tests to Rule Out UTI," "Interpretation of Tests and Additional Information Required if UTI Present," "Treatment and Follow-up of Initial Infection," and "Treatment and Follow-up of Recurrent Infection." This logical division is not readily apparent from the flow chart.

Table 3–2.
Interpretation of Tests and Additional Information Required if Urinary Tract Infection Present.

Sex/Age	Infant			Boy		Man		Woman	
Test result (microscopic examination and culture)	Positive microscopic examination	Positive culture	Both negative	Either positive	Both negative	Either positive	Both negative	Either positive	Both negative
Initiate therapy		X		X		X		X	
Obtain sensitivity test results				X		X		X	
IVP: correct any abnormalities						X			
IVP and cystourethrogram: correct any abnormalities				X					
Confirm with suprapubic tap	X								
If symptoms persist, repeat culture			X		X		X		X

IVP = intravenous pyelogram.

Table 3–3. Treatment and Follow-up of Initial Infection.			
Sensitivity test results available	Y	N	
Highly symptomatic		Y	N
Treat blindly with drug not recently used		X	
Treat 10–14 days with least toxic, least expensive antimicrobial	X		
Follow-up cultures: desirable 2–3 days after initiation of therapy, essential 1–2 wk after therapy and then every 1 mo, 3 times, then every 3 mo, 3 times	X	X	
Await sensitivity test results			X

In both the flow chart and decision table there are several phrases whose meaning is not clear: closely spaced recurrences, frequent recurrences, search for a prostatic focus, periodic cultures, and suppressive therapy. Given the present state of knowledge about UTI, it may be that a more precise definition of these terms is not possible. However, if we allow the definition of these terms to vary over time and between patients, we will lose the opportunity to improve medical knowledge. By accurately defining these terms we will be able to draw meaningful conclusions from the observation over time of the consequences of our decisions.

Although it is readily apparent from the decision table which factors are to be considered and what actions are to be taken, it is not so obvious on exactly what basis those factors or conditions were chosen or for which environment and resources they were intended. We may all be willing to assume that the conditions and actions have sufficient scientific basis to serve as a first approximation for all of us. What we cannot assume is that all practitioners will have the resources to reliably implement all the conditions and actions—particularly the roentgenogram, culture, and sensitivity test requirements. Practitioners with a large load and limited resources have at least three choices: First, to accept the tables as they are and refer more patients to technologically advanced facilities, letting the patients be responsible for the necessary travel and expense. Second, to conclude that many patients could not do that and to make a determined effort to enlarge their facilities (by being more aggressive with new techniques of management and use of personnel, seeking government and community support for clearly articulated needs). Or finally, practitioners can modify the tables in a precise manner, consulting with experts (such as Kunin), and comparing results to those of others who use more elaborate and expensive conditions and actions. Practitioners may be able to demonstrate that through more limited but realistic actions (decision rules) for their environment and load, they can deliver uniformly better care for their community than can be achieved by utilizing the decision rules meant for a wealthy few. One thing seems clear: No population of people can be well served

Table 3—4.
Treatment and Follow-up of Recurrent Infection.

Time relationship of positive culture to course of therapy	While on therapy	After course of therapy				
IVP previously done		N	Y			
Recurrence is closely spaced or recurrences are frequent			N	Y		
Sex and urinary tract status				Female without correctable abnormality	Male without obvious structural or neurological lesion	
Prior course of trimethoprim-sulfamethoxazole					Y	N
Treat with an alternative agent	X					
Obtain IVP and correct any abnormality		X				
Use decision table for initial treatment		X	?*			
Bedtime dose of nitrofurantoin or trimethroprim-sulfamethoxazole for several months				X		
Search for a prostatic focus						X
Treat with trimethroprim-sulfamethoxazole suppression						X
Periodic cultures				X	X	X
Nitrofurantoin or trimethoprim-sulfamethoxazole suppression					X	

IVP = intravenous pyelogram.
*The flow chart does not indicate the appropriate action. It is assumed that the infection is to be treated as an initial infection.

in the long run if practitioners of limited resources or academic people of great resources respond by using no defined conditions or actions at all, improvising as they go without a rigorous feedback loop to themselves or the people they serve. The excuse of limited resources, research, or the "art of medicine" should not be permitted. This is not to deny the remarkable achievements of a few individuals at the intuitive level for certain problems, but there does not appear to be justification for continuously acting in this manner. This is not to deny insights, but to demand their proof.

The Role of Decision Tables in Comprehensive Care

Decision tables aid in the analysis and planning for a single problem, but this is only a small part of total care. Comprehensive care requires the following considerations:

1. Each problem should be placed in the context of the patient's environment, other problems, and the goals and plans for dealing with the other problems; this requires that patient data be effectively organized.

2. The best care that the current state of medicine can offer must be considered for all problems. This requires access to the appropriate, current medical information at the time it is needed in patient care and removal of the restrictions of reliance on human memory and vague textbook references.

3. All information on a single patient from multiple doctors, clinics, hospitals, and offices must be available for each encounter; this requires coordination in the use of medical data.

An approach under consideration to enable comprehensive care is the Computerized Problem-Oriented Medical Record (CPOMR), which links computers to a defined system of medical action.[3] It was in this context that decision tables were found to be a useful way of organizing modules of information before their integration into a computerized medical information system. Once in electronic form, the requirements for comprehensive care are met, and in addition both the process and outcome of medical care may be monitored to establish positive feedback loops for improving the quality of care.

Because the paper form of the decision table cannot be automatically coupled to total care and because it does not allow the establishment of positive feedback loops or updating as easily as the electronic form, its role in medical care should be that of a temporary expedient to be used only with full consideration of these limitations in each instance.

This work would not have been possible without association with and critical evaluation by all members of PROMIS Laboratory. Calvin M. Kunin, MD, gave permission for use of his work with urinary tract infections in the text of the chapter.

References

1. Pollack SL, Hicks HT, Harrison WJ: *Decision Tables: Theory and Practice*. New York, Wiley-Interscience, 1971.
2. Humby E: *Programs from Decisions Tables*. New York, American Elsevier Pub Co, 1973.
3. Hurst JW, Walker HK (eds): *The Problem Oriented System*. Medcom Press, 1972, pp 199–274.

Problems Observed Clinically

Chapter 4

Hypertension

Robert F. Maronde, MD

Diagnostic Work-up

Actuarial data cannot be used to predict the morbidity and mortality of individual patients with uncomplicated hypertension. As physicians, our decisions are based on statistical probabilities for *groups* of patients. A diastolic pressure of 90 mm Hg is associated with an increase in mortality of two to three times the normal (Figure 4–1).[1] This diastolic level is selected arbitrarily as being "hypertensive."

A decrease in mortality from hypertension has been demonstrated since the advent of drug therapy (Figure 4–2)[2]; results of controlled studies have also established a decrease in morbidity.[3,4]

Falsely high blood-pressure readings may be obtained if the bladder inside of a blood pressure cuff does not cover 75% of the arm circumference. In patients with large arms, the standard cuff can be used on the forearm, or a thigh cuff on the arm.[5]

The detailed algorithm (Figure 4–3) can function as an aid in resolving diagnostic questions about hypertension in the *individual* patient.

Systolic Levels

Systolic hypertension is as closely related as diastolic pressure to the increased morbidity and mortality associated with hypertension.[6] In elderly patients, systolic hypertension is often the result of atherosclerotic changes, with resultant inelasticity of the aorta. The mean pressure, however, which determines the degree of tissue perfusion, may be normal. The question then arises as to

From: The Hypertensive Patient. An Algorithm for Diagnostic Workup. *JAMA* 1975;233:997-1000. The Hypertensive Patient. An Algorithm for Treatment. *JAMA* 1975;233:990-992. Copyright 1975 by the American Medical Association.

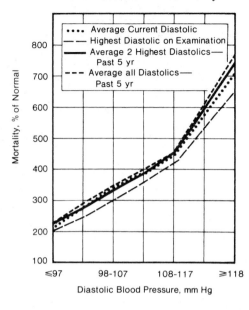

Figure 4—1. Mortality ratio associated with diastolic blood pressure levels. (From Bolt, Bell, Harnes.[1] Used by permission.)

whether the increased morbidity and mortality is the result of the atherosclerosis or of the systolic blood pressure level. Lowering of the systolic pressure would decrease the mean blood pressure and possibly the tissue perfusion to a level that could prove harmful. Until we have evidence that antihypertensive treatment is beneficial in such patients, caution should be exercised in treating them.

Diastolic Pressure Over 135 mm Hg

A diastolic pressure of more than 135 to 150 mm Hg may be associated with arterial endothelial proliferation and medial arteriolar hemorrhagic necrosis, particularly in the kidneys (malignant nephrosclerosis). Ischemia and death of tissue results. Irreversible renal damage may develop within a few days. Lowering of the blood pressure reverses the arterial and arteriolar changes and prevents these ischemic changes.

Parenteral antihypertensive therapy should be instituted promptly.[7] If the serum creatinine level is elevated to 5 mg/dL (442 μmol/L) or more, lowering of the diastolic pressure below levels of 110 mm Hg may precipitate clinical uremia.

Chronic renal disease is the most common cause of secondary hypertension. A serum creatinine value of 1.3 mg/dL (114.9 μmol/L) that is persistent and not associated with a "prerenal" cause such as congestive heart failure, shock, or dehydration is indicative of renal disease. Lowering of the blood pressure usually may result in further elevation of the serum creatinine value.

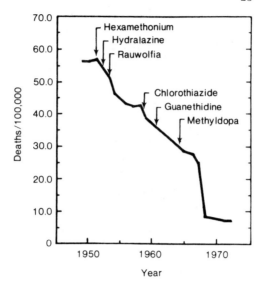

Figure 4—2. Declining death rate from hypertension since the advent of drug therapy for hypertension. (From Silverman and Lee.[2] © 1974 University of California Press. Used by permission.)

Unusual Causes of Hypertension

Primary Hyperaldosteronism. Patients with this condition represent approximately 1% of the hypertensive population in a referral hospital clinic.[8] It may be even more uncommon in the hypertensive population at large. On the other hand, secondary hyperaldosteronism is common in patients with malignant hypertension. Treatment of patients with malignant hypertension should not be delayed while a work-up for an aldosterone-producing tumor is completed. Primary hyperaldosteronism may best be diagnosed by plasma aldosterone and plasma renin activity concentrations. In primary hyperaldosteronism, the respective ratio is >30.1.[9]

Pheochromocytoma. This is a rare cause of hypertension (one in 1,000 hypertensive patients).[10] Thus, measurements of catecholamine levels or related determinations are probably not indicated on a routine basis. Rather, supporting clinical evidence should be considered before ordering the tests.

Contraceptive Oral Medications. These agents will produce hypertension that is, however, reversible within three months after use of the agents is discontinued. Limited evidence suggests that this type of hypertension may be mediated by the renin-angiotensin-aldosterone system.

Coarctation of the Aorta. This is an infrequent cause of hypertension. Palpation of the femoral, popliteal, or dorsalis pedes pulses is a good screening test. If any of the pulses is diminished, indirect thigh blood pressures should be measured with a thigh cuff. If coarctation exists, the leg pressure will be lower than the arm pressure. In questionable cases, direct femoral artery pressures should be measured.

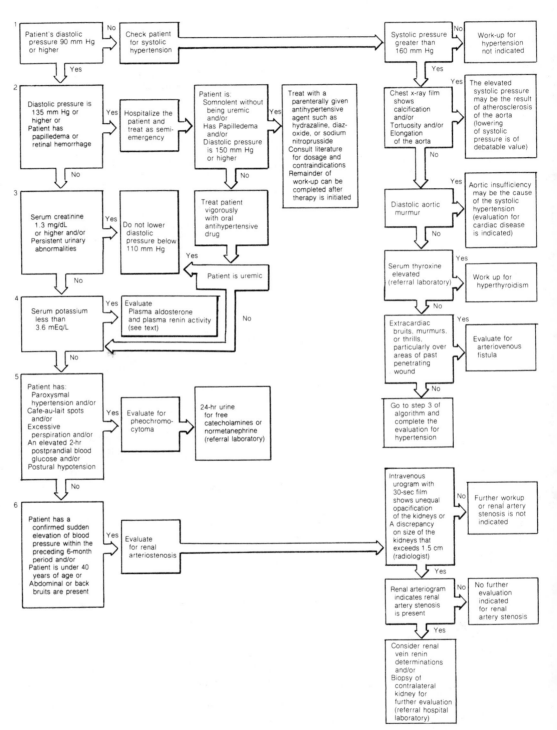

Figure 4–3. Hypertensive patient algorithmic flow chart. (Urinalysis; white blood cell count; determinations of serum creatinine, potassium, bicarbonate, glucose, and uric acid levels; electrocardiogram; and chest x-ray film are considered as routine procedures for all patients.)

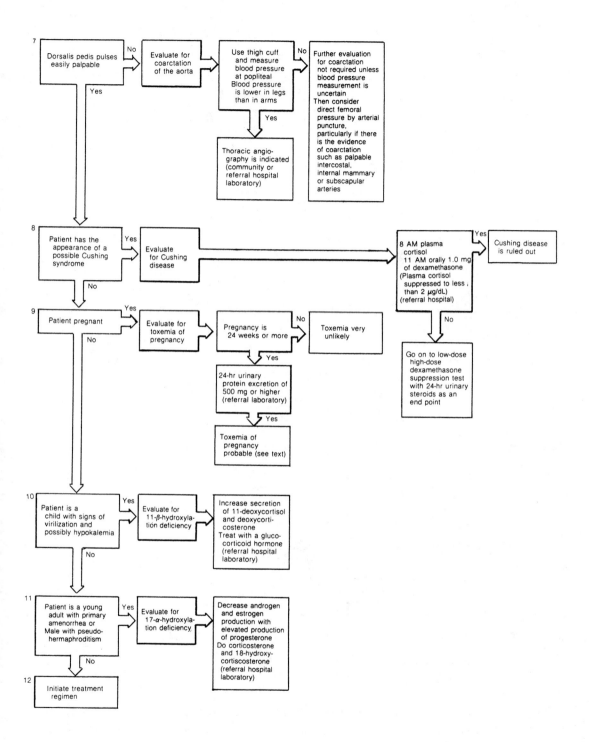

7 | Dorsalis pedis pulses easily palpable — No → Evaluate for coarctation of the aorta → Use thigh cuff and measure blood pressure at popliteal Blood pressure is lower in legs than in arms — No → Further evaluation for coarctation not required unless blood pressure measurement is uncertain Then consider direct femoral pressure by arterial puncture, particularly if there is the evidence of coarctation such as palpable intercostal, internal mammary or subscapular arteries

Yes (down from box 7)

Use thigh cuff... — Yes → Thoracic angiography is indicated (community or referral hospital laboratory)

8 | Patient has the appearance of a possible Cushing syndrome — Yes → Evaluate for Cushing disease → 8 AM plasma cortisol 11 AM orally 1.0 mg of dexamethasone (Plasma cortisol suppressed to less than 2 μg/dL) (referral hospital) — Yes → Cushing disease is ruled out

No

8 AM plasma cortisol... — No → Go on to low-dose high-dose dexamethasone suppression test with 24-hr urinary steroids as an end point

9 | Patient pregnant — Yes → Evaluate for toxemia of pregnancy → Pregnancy is 24 weeks or more — No → Toxemia very unlikely

No

Pregnancy is 24 weeks or more — Yes → 24-hr urinary protein excretion of 500 mg or higher (referral laboratory) — Yes → Toxemia of pregnancy probable (see text)

10 | Patient is a child with signs of virilization and possibly hypokalemia — Yes → Evaluate for 11-β-hydroxylation deficiency → Increase secretion of 11-deoxycortisol and deoxycorticosterone Treat with a glucocorticoid hormone (referral hospital laboratory)

No

11 | Patient is a young adult with primary amenorrhea or Male with pseudohermaphroditism — Yes → Evaluate for 17-α-hydroxylation deficiency → Decrease androgen and estrogen production with elevated production of progesterone Do corticosterone and 18-hydroxycorticosterone (referral hospital laboratory)

No

12 | Initiate treatment regimen

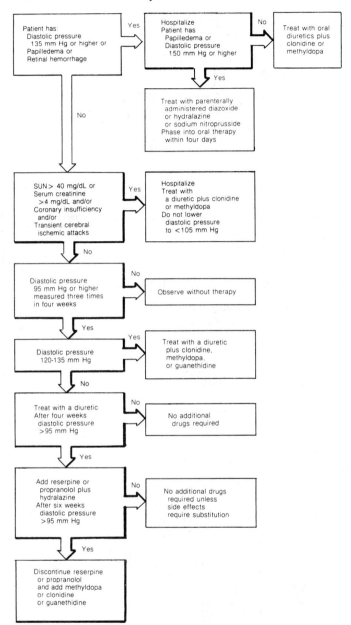

Figure 4—4. Algorithm for treatment of hypertensive patient.

Renal Artery Stenosis. Stenosis of this artery is not as common as it was once thought to be. In our medical center the incidence is less than 1% of the hypertensive population. Surgery has resulted in "cures" in a very few patients. Drug therapy usually is effective.

Cushing Syndrome. The hypertension associated with this disorder, should be treated by correcting the cause, if feasible. Primary Cushing disease is uncommon. However, Cushing syndrome as a result of steroid administration is relatively frequent. In secondary cases, administration of the steroid every other day may successfully deal with the problem. If drug treatment of hypertension is required, however, it should be instituted.

Toxemia of Pregnancy. Hypertensive women who are pregnant may have a drop in blood pressure in the first trimester and then a rise to levels that might be interpreted as toxemia of pregnancy. However, in true toxemia, a close check of the patient's urine will show proteinuria before hypertension develops.

Hydroxylation Deficiencies. Finally, hypertension secondary to 17-α-hydroxylation deficiency and to 11-β-hydroxylation deficiency are extremely rare entities. These diagnoses should be established by an endocrinologist in a referral hospital.[11]

Treatment

The goal of the physician in the treatment of the hypertensive patient should be to achieve a blood pressure as near normal as possible with minimal adverse drug effects. Therapeutic compliance by the patient is inversely related to the severity of reactions attributed to medication. Patients frequently will not volunteer such information. Questioning in some detail by the physician may be required to assess correctly the degree of patient compliance. See Figure 4–4 for an algorithm for treatment.

Indications for Hospitalization

Diastolic Pressure of 135 mm Hg. Patients with a diastolic pressure of 135 mm Hg or higher, or patients with retinal hemorrhages or papilledema, should be hospitalized and treated promptly. If papilledema is present or if the diastolic pressure is sustained at levels of 150 mm Hg or higher, parenteral therapy with diazoxide, hydralazine hydrochloride, or sodium nitroprusside should be instituted. Diazoxide should be given in a bolus intravenously. Hydralazine and sodium nitroprusside are given by constant intravenous infusion. The dose of hydralazine hydrochloride is 0.1 to 0.4 mg/min given in a non-glucose-containing fluid. The product brochures should be read carefully before these drugs are administered. Diazoxide is contraindicated in patients with congestive heart failure and stroke. Hydralazine is contraindicated in patients with angina or acute myocardial infarction.

Oral therapy should be started as soon as possible with a diuretic plus clonidine hydrochloride or methyldopa. Hypokalemia due to secondary hyperaldosteronism is common in these patients. It is not a contraindication for diuretic therapy. Triamterene or spironolactone may be given with the diuretic if excessive potassium loss is evident.

There is no evidence that one diuretic is more effective than another as an antihypertensive drug. In fact, a comparison of furosemide with hydrochlorothiazide indicates that hydrochlorothiazide may be more effective.[12] Claims that one diuretic may cause less potassium loss than another are nonfactual when applied to the nonedematous hypertensive patient.

Clonidine is a rapid-acting antihypertensive drug. The initial dosage is 0.1 mg twice a day. This may be increased by daily increments of 0.2 mg/day to the maximum recommended dosage of 2.4 mg/day.

The initial dosage of methyldopa is 250 mg twice a day. It can be increased at daily intervals by 500 mg/day. The maximum recommended dosage is 3 g.

Dosage should be regulated by the level of the standing blood pressure to prevent postural hypotension. If the supine pressure is excessively elevated compared to the standing pressure, the legs at the head of the bed should be elevated by 10 cm (4 in.) to accentuate gravitational venous pooling of blood.

Elevated Serum Urea Nitrogen or Serum Creatinine Levels. If the serum urea nitrogen (SUN) level is elevated above 40 mg/dL (14.28 mmol/L), or the serum creatinine concentration to above 4 mg/dL (353.6 μmol/L), the patient should be treated initially while in the hospital. Lowering of the blood pressure may reduce renal blood flow and result in further elevation of the SUN or creatinine levels. Clinical uremia may be precipitated.

Use of a diuretic as an antihypertensive is usually not contraindicated in the presence of impaired renal function. Diuretics will reduce the dosage requirement of methyldopa or clonidine. The incidence of dose-related side effects, particularly postural hypotension, will thereby be decreased. In general, these patients should not have the standing diastolic blood pressure lowered below 105 mm Hg.

Coronary Insufficiency or Transient Cerebral Ischemic Attacks. Lowering of the blood pressure may reduce the coronary or cerebral blood flow in patients with symptomatic atherosclerotic disease. Excessive blood pressure lowering should be avoided because of the danger of myocardial infarction or stroke. A diuretic plus clonidine or methyldopa should be administered while the patient is hospitalized and the dosage stabilized in the hospital by using the standing diastolic pressure as a guide.

Outpatient Treatment

Diastolic Pressure of 120 to 135 mm Hg. If the diastolic pressure is 120 to 135 mm Hg, outpatient therapy should be started with a diuretic plus clonidine or methyldopa or guanethidine sulfate. The initial dose of guanethidine sulfate is 10 mg/day. This may be increased by 10-mg increments every fourth day to the maximum recommended dosage of 150 mg/day. The dosage regimens for clonidine and methyldopa have been presented previously.

Diastolic Pressure of 95 to 120 mm Hg. If diastolic elevation of pressure is substantiated by three measurements over a four- to six-week period, or if it is obvious that target organ disease, such as hypertensive heart disease, is present, therapy may be started. The first drug should be a diuretic. At least 15% of patients will have a satisfactory blood pressure response with a diuretic alone.[13]

After four to six weeks, if the blood pressure response is not satisfactory, 0.1 to 0.25 mg/day of reserpine may be added. The reports associating reserpine with breast cancer[14-16] did not take into account the increased incidence of breast cancer in the postmenopausal, hypertensive woman.[17] Control populations used for comparison in these studies were not selected from hypertensive populations. Therefore, the association of cancer with reserpine may be the result of a bias introduced by the study design.

Seventy percent to 80% of patients will have a satisfactory blood pressure response to a diuretic plus reserpine, and the incidence of side effects, including depression, is no more and possibly less than with a diuretic plus methyldopa.[18] The occurrence of severe depression with a dosage of 0.1 to 0.25 mg of reserpine per day is, in my experience, very uncommon.

Propranolol hydrochloride may be used in place of reserpine. The reports that propranolol lowers blood pressure by the reduction of renin secretion have been questioned.[19] Propranolol does negate the effect of the reflex sympathetic overactivity associated with hydralazine therapy and thereby prevents reflex tachycardia. It would be expected that reserpine would have the same effect.[20] The initial dosage of propranolol hydrochloride is 10 mg orally twice a day, increased to a suggested maximum of 80 mg four times a day. Cardiac failure may be a side effect.

Hydralazine, if added to a regimen of diuretic plus reserpine or a diuretic plus propranolol, will increase the number of controlled cases by approximately 10%. The effectiveness of hydralazine prescribed without reserpine or propranolol is impaired because of the reflex autonomic sympathetic overactivity that may occur.

If the patient does not respond to the regimen of a diuretic plus reserpine or propranolol and hydralazine, the reserpine or propranolol should be discontinued and the diuretic continued. Either clonidine or methyldopa or guanethidine therapy should be instituted in conjunction with the diuretic therapy. The dosage regimen for these drugs has already been presented.

Parvis Shokrizade helped in the layout, format, and design of the algorithms.

References

1. Bolt W, Bell MF, Harnes JR: A Study of Mortality in Moderate and Severe Hypertension. New York, *Transactions of the Association of Life Insurance Medical Directors* 1957;41:61–100.

2. Silverman M, Lee PR: *Pills, Profits, and Politics*. Berkeley, Calif, University of California Press, 1974, p 10.

3. Freis E: Effects of treatment on morbidity in hypertension, Report of Veterans Administration Cooperative Study Group. *JAMA* 1967;202:1028–1037.

4. Freis E: Effects of treatment on morbidity in hypertension, Report of Veterans Administration Cooperative Study Group. *JAMA* 1970;213:1143–1152.

5. Karvonen MJ, Teliviro LJ, Jarvinen JK: Sphygmomanometer cuff size and the accuracy of indirect measurement of blood pressure. *Am J Cardiol* 1964;13:688–693.

6. Kannel WB, Castelli WP, McNamara PM, et al: Role of blood pressure in the development of congestive heart failure: The Framingham Study. *N Engl J Med* 1972;287:787–789.

7. Maronde RF: Drug therapy in essential hypertension. *Heart Bull* 1967;8:12–15, 20.

8. Horton R: Aldosterone: Review of its physiology and diagnostic aspects of primary aldosteronism. *Metabolism* 1973;22:1525–1548.

9. Mitchell JR; Taylor AA; Pool JL, et al: Renin-aldosterone propiling in hypertension. *Ann Intern Med* 1977;87:596–612.

10. Crout JR: Pheochromocytoma. Read before the 22nd Annual Postgraduate Assembly of the Endocrine Society, St. Louis, September, 1970.

11. Biglieri EG Jr, Stockigt SR, Schambelan M: Adrenal mineral-corticoids causing hypertension. *Am J Med* 1972;52:623–632.

12. Anderson J, Godfrey BE, Hill DM, et al: A comparison of the effect of hydrochlorothiazide and of furosemide in the treatment of hypertensive patients. *Quart J Med* 1971;60:541–560.

13. Maronde RF, Haywood SL: Drug therapy of hypertension. *Calif Med* 1962;97:206–208.

14. Reserpine and breast cancer, Boston Collaborative Drug Surveillance Program. *Lancet* 1974;2:669–671.

15. Armstrong B, Stevens N, Doll R: Retrospective study of the association between use of rauwolfia derivatives and breast cancer in English women. *Lancet* 1974;2:672–674.

16. Heinonen OP, Shapiro S, Tuominen L, et al: Reserpine use in relation to breast cancer. *Lancet* 1974;2:675–677.

17. de Waard F, Baanders-van Halewijn EA, Huizinga S: The bimodal age distribution of patients with mammary carcinoma. *Cancer* 1964;17:141–151.

18. Smith WM, Bachman B, Galante SG, et al: Cooperative clinical trial of α-methydopa: III. Double-blind control comparison of α-methyldopa and chlorothiazide, and chlorothiazide and rauwolfia. *Ann Intern Med* 1966;65:657–671.

19. Velasco M, O'Malley R, Robie N, et al: Differential effects of propranolol on heart rate and plasma renin activity in patients treated with minoxidil. *Clin Pharmacol Ther* 1974;16:1031–1038.

20. Zocent R, Gilmore E, Koch-Weser J: Treatment of essential hypertension with combined vasodilation and β-adrenergic blockade. *N Engl J Med* 1972;286:617–622.

Chapter 5

Jaundice in the Newborn

M. Michael Thaler, MD

Jaundice in the newborn and young infant differs in several important respects from jaundice in older patients. First, almost uniquely in the newborn, bilirubin may be a cause of disease as well as its consequence. The potential toxicity of the unconjugated pigment lends urgency to diagnostic deliberations. Second, the first two months after birth are a period of continuous maturational and adaptive change, which alters the character and manifestations of disease processes. Third, many inherited disorders manifest themselves during the newborn period. It is important to measure without delay the severity of unconjugated hyperbilirubinemia in newborns, since high concentrations of the unconjugated pigment may cause brain damage. The causes of conjugated hyperbilirubinemia should also be investigated promptly, but do not usually constitute emergencies.

Studies have been made of bilirubin metabolism,[1] causes of unconjugated neonatal bilirubinemia (physiologic, hemolytic, and hereditary),[2] and conditions associated with conjugated hyperbilirubinemia (cholestatic jaundice) in infancy.[3] This communication reports the use of algorithms in the differential diagnosis of jaundice in newborns and young infants.

Classification of Jaundice

The first step in dealing with infantile jaundice is to establish its type and severity. This is accomplished with a single procedure, the fractional diazo reaction on serum, which measures the total bilirubin level and the conjugated (direct-reacting) fraction (Figure 5–1). Unconjugated hyperbilirubinemia is present when less than 15% of the total bilirubin is of the direct-reacting type. Conjugated hyperbilirubinemia is present when more than 30% of the total bilirubin is of the

From: Jaundice in the Newborn. Algorithmic Diagnosis of Conjugated and Unconjugated Hyperbilirubinemia. *JAMA* 1977;237:58–62. Copyright 1977 by the American Medical Association.

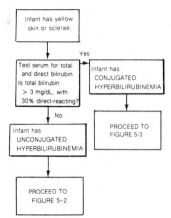

Figure 5–1. Classification of jaundice.

direct-reacting type. Unconjugated hyperbilirubinemia in the newborn is considered severe and potentially dangerous when the total serum bilirubin level exceeds 10 mg/dL (171 μmol/L), especially in premature or ill babies.

Conjugated hyperbilirubinemia may reflect parenchymal disease, biliary obstruction, or both. However, a direct-reacting serum bilirubin level of less than 4 mg/dL (68.4 μmol/L) is unlikely to be due to complete biliary obstruction. The process of establishing the cause of unconjugated and conjugated hyperbilirubinemia in infants is described in Figures 5–2 and 5–3, respectively.

Unconjugated Hyperbilirubinemia

According to adult standards, all infants are hyperbilirubinemic during the first week after birth, and most are transiently jaundiced. This "physiologic jaundice" usually peaks between the third and fifth day (later in premature babies) and declines thereafter.

Birth to Two Days of Age. Jaundice at this time is a danger signal that must be investigated as soon as it is recognized. Babies with erythroblastosis may be jaundiced at birth, because their cord blood may contain elevated bilirubin concentrations. The diagnosis and management of hemolytic disease of the newborn has developed into a highly standardized routine. However, the key determination remains the direct Coombs' test, which is used to detect blood type incompatibility.

Three to Seven Days of Age. Jaundice due to hemolysis may persist or may occasionally have its onset at this time. However, the overwhelming majority of jaundiced infants have physiologic hyperbilirubinemia, which may be complicated by prematurity, hypoxic states, acidosis, or hypoglycemia.

One to Eight Weeks of Age. Several congenital hematologic disorders (red cell enzymopathies, spherocytosis, aplastic or hypoplastic anemia), hypothyroidism, and perinatal complications (hemorrhage, sepsis) may be manifested by

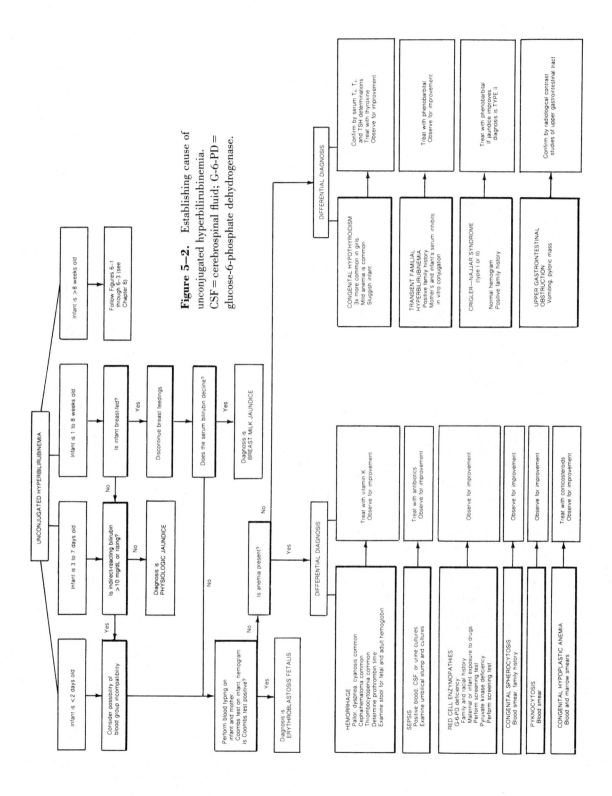

Figure 5–2. Establishing cause of unconjugated hyperbilirubinemia. CSF = cerebrospinal fluid; G-6-PD = glucose-6-phosphate dehydrogenase.

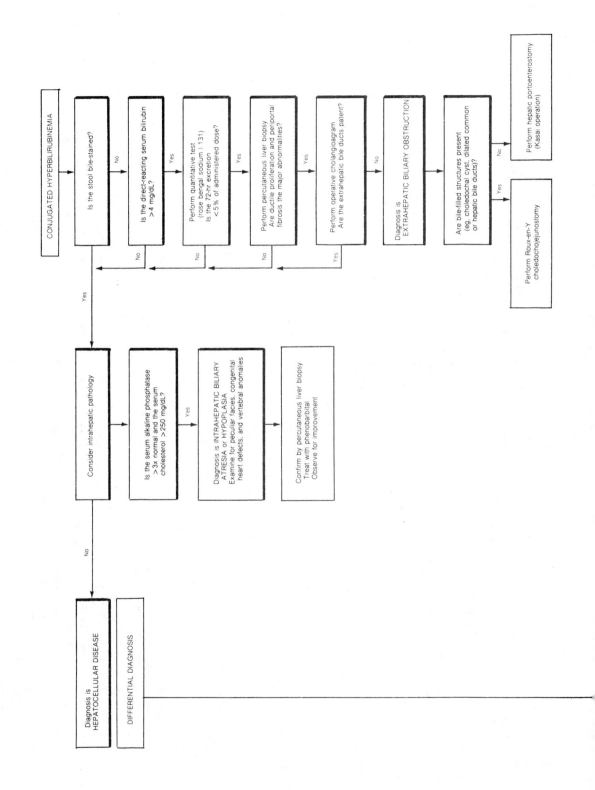

CONJUGATED HYPERBILIRUBINEMIA

Is the stool bile-stained?

No → Is the direct-reacting serum bilirubin >4 mg/dL?

Yes → Perform quantitative test (rose bengal sodium I 131) Is the 72-hr excretion <5% of administered dose?

Yes → Perform percutaneous liver biopsy Are ductile proliferation and periportal fibrosis the major abnormalities?

Yes → Perform operative cholangiogram Are the extrahepatic bile ducts patent?

No → Diagnosis is EXTRAHEPATIC BILIARY OBSTRUCTION

→ Are bile-filled structures present (eg, choledochal cyst, dilated common or hepatic bile ducts)?

No → Perform hepatic portoenterostomy (Kasal operation)

Yes → Perform Roux-en-Y choledochojejunostomy

Yes (from stool bile-stained) → Consider intrahepatic pathology

→ Is the serum alkaline phosphatase >3x normal and the serum cholesterol >250 mg/dL?

Yes → Diagnosis is INTRAHEPATIC BILIARY ATRESIA or HYPOPLASIA Examine for peculiar facies, congenital heart defects, and vertebral anomalies

→ Confirm by percutaneous liver biopsy Treat with phenobarbital Observe for improvement

No → Diagnosis is HEPATOCELLULAR DISEASE

DIFFERENTIAL DIAGNOSIS

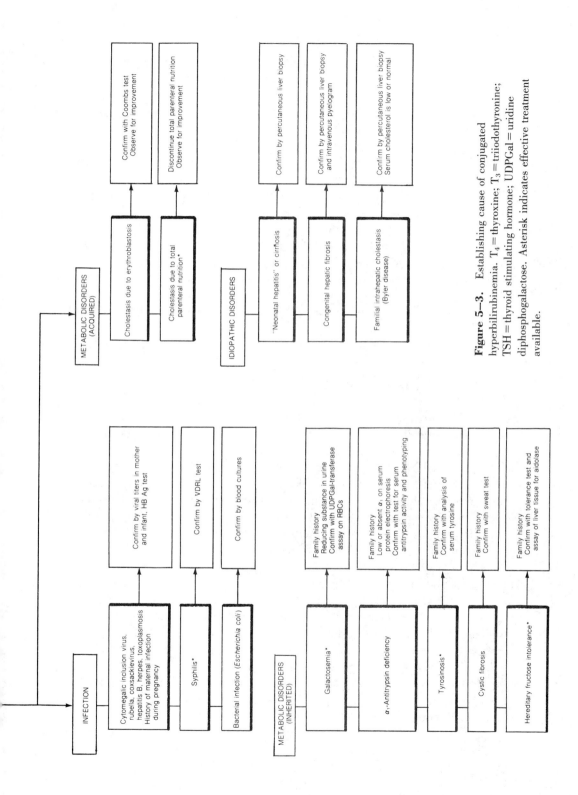

Figure 5–3. Establishing cause of conjugated hyperbilirubinemia. T_4 = thyroxine; T_3 = triiodothyronine; TSH = thyroid stimulating hormone; UDPGal = uridine diphosphogalactose. Asterisk indicates effective treatment available.

jaundice at this age. In breast-fed infants, unconjugated hyperbilirubinemia may develop; this may be due to interference with bilirubin conjugation by substances in human milk (fatty acids, lipases, steroids). "Breast milk jaundice" disappears within a few days after nursing is interrupted and, curiously, does not recur when breast feedings are reinstituted. During this period, also, certain rare cases of unremitting nonhemolytic jaundice beginning after birth may be diagnosed as Crigler-Najjar syndrome; this diagnosis is made by exclusion or by assay of bilirubin-conjugating activity in liver tissue (which is obtained by percutaneous biopsy). Another extremely rare type of familial jaundice, presumably due to inhibition of conjugation in serum, is known as Lucey-Driscoll syndrome. This condition persists after the first week, but gradually corrects itself.

The diagnosis of hyperbilirubinemia in patients more than two months of age is made in the same way that it is in older children and adults; Ostrow (see Chapter 6) provides an effective method for making the differential diagnosis in this disease.

Most, if not all, conditions associated with unconjugated hyperbilirubinemia in the newborn can be treated successfully, either by direct removal of the toxic pigment by exchange transfusion or by photodegradation of the pigment.

Conjugated Hyperbilirubinemia

All liver diseases and biliary malformations in infancy are associated with conjugated hyperbilirubinemia.[4] Therefore, such terms as obstructive jaundice, surgical jaundice, and cholestatic syndrome are misleading when applied to neonatal conjugated jaundice and should be abandoned.

The first task in a neonatal diagnostic workup is to eliminate rapidly progressive yet eminently treatable conditions. Congenital syphilis and bacterial infections can be controlled with antibiotics, whereas galactosemia and tyrosinosis can be improved with appropriate exclusion diets.

Thereafter, the main diagnostic problem is to distinguish intrahepatic from extrahepatic causes of conjugated jaundice. Unfortunately, the standard liver function tests are not helpful for this purpose in early infancy, with the exception of the occurrence of rapidly rising serum alkaline phosphatase and cholesterol concentrations. This occurrence strongly suggests involvement of the intrahepatic terminal bile ducts in a destructive process, which leads to intrahepatic biliary hypoplasia or paucity of interlobular bile ducts. A further diagnostic aid in detection of intrahepatic biliary hypoplasia is that an unknown but substantial proportion of infants with this condition possess characteristic facies, congenital heart defects (usually pulmonic stenosis), and vertebral malformations, which help to identify this recently described syndrome.[5]

In contrast to older patients, infants normally have lightly and homogeneously colored stools; these may show the presence of bile, thereby ruling out complete extrahepatic biliary obstruction. It should be realized, however, that the absence of bile from stools is not conclusive evidence for extrahepatic obstruction, as it does not exclude the possibility of severe biliary excretory deficiency due to intrahepatic disease. In such cases, a more sensitive measure of bile flow to the intestine is the quantitation of the amount of radioactivity excreted in stools collected for 72 hours following an injection of radioactively labeled rose bengal dye. This test, and a percutaneous liver biopsy specimen analyzed by an experienced pathologist, will allow differentiation of extrahepatic biliary obstruction from other causes of conjugated hyperbilirubinemia in a large majority of cases.[6, 7] Percutaneous liver biopsies should also be performed in infants with idiopathic hepatocellular disease described as "neonatal," the rare instances of familial progressive cirrhosis (Byler disease), and in those suspected of having intrahepatic biliary abnormalities (ie, hypoplasia or atresia of the interlobular bile ducts) or congenital hepatic fibrosis.

Infants in whom percutaneous biopsy specimen shows the characteristic findings of extrahepatic biliary obstruction (proliferation of interlobular bile ducts and periportal fibrosis) should undergo operative cholangiography. Surgical exploration of the porta hepatis for the presence of bile-filled remnants of the biliary tree is indicated when visualization of the extrahepatic bile ducts is not achieved by cholangiography.

References

1. Schmid R: Hyperbilirubinemia, in Stanbury JB, Wyngaarden JB, Frederickson DS (eds): *The Metabolic Basis of Inherited Disease*, ed 3. New York, McGraw-Hill Book Co Inc, 1972, p 1141–1178.
2. Thaler MM: Neonatal hyperbilirubinemia. *Semin Hematol* 1972;9:107.
3. Thaler MM: Cryptogenic liver disease in young infants, in Popper H, Schaffner F (eds): *Progress in Liver Disease*. New York, Grune & Stratton Inc, vol 5, 1976, pp 476–493.
4. Sass-Kortsak A: Management of young infants presenting with direct-reacting hyperbilirubinemia. *Pediatr Clin North Am* 1974;21:777–790.
5. Alagille D, Odievre M, Guatier M, et al: Hepatic ductular hypoplasia associated with characteristic facies, vertebral malformations, retarded physical, mental, and sexual development, and cardiac murmur. *J Pediatr* 1975;86:63–72.
6. Thaler MM, Gellis SS: Studies in neonatal hepatitis and biliary atresia: Part IV. Diagnosis. *Am J Dis Child* 1968;116:280–284.
7. Brough AJ, Bernstein J: Conjugated hyperbilirubinemia in early infancy: A reassessment of liver biopsy. *Hum Pathol* 1974;5:507–516.

Chapter 6

Jaundice in Older Children and Adults

J. Donald Ostrow, MD

Jaundice is the yellow discoloration of the skin and eyes that is caused by retention of bilirubin, the major catabolic product of heme. A few other pigments, such as carotene and lycopene, may also cause yellowing of the skin, but characteristically do not cause discoloration of the sclerae.

The algorithm (Figure 6–1) is intended to apply only to older children and adults; it is not applicable to the differential diagnosis of jaundice in the neonate or very young child. A brief overview of the approach to the differential diagnosis of jaundice is given in an earlier communication,[1] and an audiovisual program that summarizes much of the information to follow is available from the American Gastroenterological Association and the General Services Administration of the US government.[2-4] More detailed overviews of bilirubin metabolism have been given by Schmid[5] and Fleischner and Arias.[6]

The following numbered passages refer to the circled numbers in the algorithms.

1. The initial step in the differential diagnosis of jaundice involves a determination of whether or not there is bilirubin in the urine. If patients state that they have dark urine, this must be confirmed by your own observation. Since other pigments may similarly discolor the urine, the fact that the pigment is indeed bilirubin must be confirmed chemically with commercially prepared tablets (Ictotest), or the older Harrison spot test. A positive urine test for bilirubin indicates retention of conjugated bilirubin in the serum. The tests are positive in about 70% of patients who have a direct-reacting serum bilirubin level of 1 to 2 mg/dL (17.1 to 34.2 μmol/L), and in almost all patients with a direct-reacting bilirubin concentration greater than 2 mg/dL (34.2 μmol/L)[7] (also, written communication, Robert Regan, Ames Co, Elkhart, Indiana). The test is negative in

From: Jaundice in Older Children and Adults. Algorithms for Diagnosis. *JAMA* 1975;234:522–526.

41

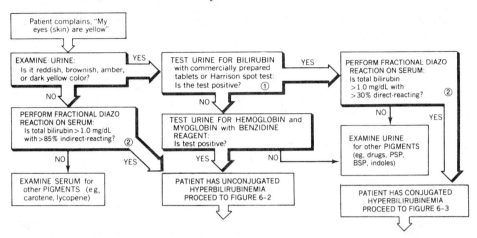

Figure 6–1. Classification of jaundice. PSP = phenolsulfonphthalein; BSP = sulfobromophthalein.

patients with unconjugated hyperbilirubinemia. Pyridium and other highly colored compounds may mask positive reactions, and the instability of bilirubin requires that urine be tested within two hours after passage. Phenothiazines may react with the reagent in the prepared test tablets, and salicylates may react with the Harrison test reagent to yield false-positive reactions.

2. If confirmation of the type of jaundice is desired, the fractional diazo reaction of serum can be performed, although this is usually not necessary. The upper limit of normal for total bilirubin level is 1.0 mg/dL (17.1 μmol/L), with a direct-reacting bilirubin level of less than 0.2 mg/dL (3.42 μmol/L). In pure unconjugated hyperbilirubinemia, at least 85% of the total bilirubin should be indirect-reacting. In conjugated hyperbilirubinemia, there is at least 30%, and usually at least 50%, direct-reacting bilirubin. Obstructive jaundice and acute hepatocellular disease tend to give values greater than 50% direct-reacting, whereas chronic liver disease (cirrhosis) tends to give values in the 30% to 50% range. Patients with 15% to 30% direct-reacting bilirubin usually have hepatocellular or cholestatic jaundice complicated by hemolysis.

3. The separation of unconjugated hyperbilirubinemia into two classes (Figure 6–2), according to whether the indirect-reacting bilirubin value is greater or less than 6.0 mg/dL (102.6 μmol/L) is not exact. Some patients with Gilbert syndrome will occasionally have values as high as 8 mg/dL (136.8 μmol/L), and patients with Arias type II syndrome may occasionally exhibit values as low as 3 mg/dL (51.3 μmol/L).[8]

4. Gilbert syndrome actually consists of multiple entities that cause unconjugated hyperbilirubinemia in excess of levels expected for the rate of bilirubin formation, as estimated from the red blood cell (RBC) lifespan.[9–10] Obviously, many hematologic tests will generally have been performed before the ^{51}Cr-RBC survival study, so that the presence of hemolysis may have been already determined. However, the comparison of serum bilirubin level with RBC lifespan per-

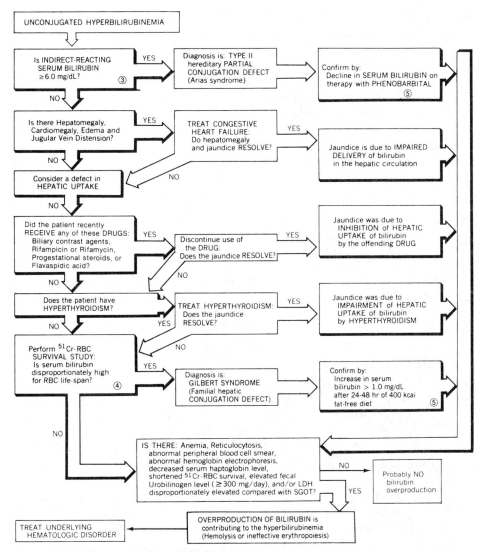

Figure 6–2. Unconjugated hyperbilirubinemia.

mits detection of Gilbert syndrome even in the presence of hemolysis, a very common combination.

5. In both Gilbert syndrome and Arias type II conjugation defect, there is impaired conjugation of bilirubin with glucuronic acid, as measured on liver biopsy specimens by the method of Black et al.[11] However, it is seldom necessary to subject a patient to the risk of liver biopsy in order to confirm these diagnoses biochemically because the clinical indexes in the algorithm usually suffice. Note that the type I complete conjugation defect (Crigler-Najjar) is not listed, since jaundice first develops in such patients during the neonatal period. Even in this

instance, liver biopsy is not indicated, since the diagnosis can be made by show-ing the absence of δ-glucuronide azopigments on chromatography of the ethylan-thranilate azopigments prepared from duodenal bile.[12]

6. For differentiation of cholestatic from hepatocellular jaundice (Figure 6–3), the selection of a serum alkaline phosphatase level of threefold the normal value is somewhat arbitrary.[13] Actually, 90% of the patients with cholestasis will have alkaline phosphatase levels of more than three times normal, and 90% of those with hepatocellular jaundice will have values less than three times normal. Patients with cholestasis from therapy with estrogens, oral contraceptive agents, and anabolic steroids tend to have alkaline phosphatase values in the range of one to three times normal.

7. The findings listed as favoring intrahepatic or extrahepatic cholestasis are not necessarily the usual findings in those syndromes, but, if present, strongly point the way toward one or the other category. Thus, a liver span greater than 15 cm and a decreased serum cholesterol value are unusual in intrahepatic cholestasis, but, when present, strongly suggest that the cholestasis is due to alcoholic hepatitis. Note that extrahepatic obstruction causes some liver enlarge-ment but rarely to greater than 15 cm overall span. A good discussion of the differential diagnoses of cholestasis is found in the report by Leevy et al[14] and Berk et al.[15]

8. Tests for antimitochondrial antibodies are usually positive in primary biliary cirrhosis, and almost always negative in extrahepatic obstruction. The level of α-fetoprotein is characteristically highly elevated in patients with primary hepatocellular carcinoma. Both these tests can be performed in clinical laborato-ries at community hospitals, but it is probably simpler to mail samples to central laboratories or referral centers for analysis.

9. Although the diagnosis of the Dubin-Johnson syndrome can be con-firmed by a liver biopsy specimen that demonstrates the characteristic finding of brown to black centrolobular granular pigment, this is seldom necessary. Sulfo-bromophthalein (BSP) kinetic studies[16] will clearly identify the characteristically minuscule transfer maximum (T_m) for BSP into bile, or analysis of the isomers of coproporphyrins in the urine will show the characteristic increases in the total quantity of the isomer 1 and in the ratio of isomer 1 to isomer 3.[17] These tests as well are more easily done in referral centers.

10. The most difficult problem in the diagnosis of jaundice is the differ-entiation of intrahepatic from extrahepatic cholestasis. On clinical evidence alone, the differentiation can usually be made in 90% to 95% of patients with cholestasis. Of particular importance is an epidemiologic history of exposure to drugs, viruses, or alcohol (which can cause intrahepatic cholestasis). If extrahe-patic obstruction is strongly suspected, transduodenal retrograde or transhepatic cholangiography can be performed, followed by exploratory laparotomy if extra-hepatic obstruction is confirmed or still suspected. The transduodenal cholangio-gram requires great expertise with a special fiberoptic duodenoscope, and should

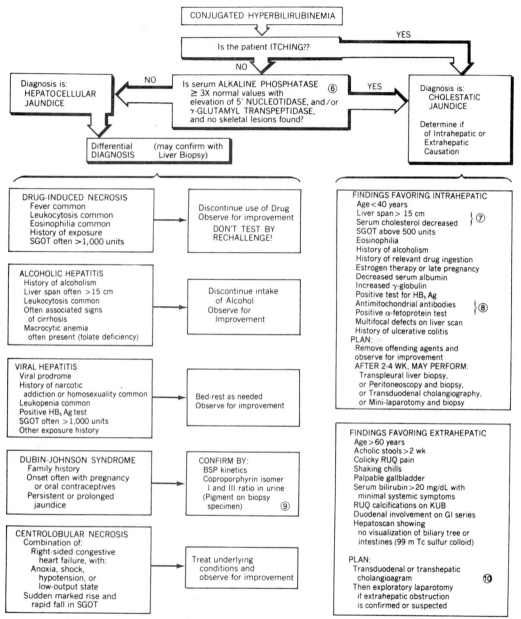

Figure 6–3. Conjugated hyperbilirubinemia. RUQ = right upper quadrant; KUB = plain x-ray film of abdomen; GI = gastrointestinal; BSP = sulfobromophthalein.

45

be performed only at referral centers. The transhepatic cholangiogram can be accomplished at any hospital, but the risks and difficulties in interpretation again indicate that it is best done at referral centers.

In the community hospital, the first invasive study should probably be an exploratory laparotomy, under local anesthesia, through a small right upper quadrant incision. This so-called mini-laparotomy will usually demonstrate quickly whether the cause of the jaundice is intrahepatic or extrahepatic. If it is intrahepatic, the patient has not been subjected to the risks of general anesthesia, a liver biopsy can be performed, and the wound closed. If biliary duct obstruction is discovered, then cholangiography can be performed through the gallbladder, cystic duct, or common duct, and general anesthesia then induced for bypass or removal of the obstruction.

This work was supported by a Medical Investigatorship from the US Veterans Administration.

Rudi Schmid, MD, Irwin M. Arias, MD, Lawrence M. Gartner, MD, and Hyman J. Zimmerman, MD, gave many suggestions that have been incorporated into the final version of the algorithms.

References

1. Ostrow JD: Recent advances in bilirubin metabolism, in *Viewpoints on Digestive Diseases*. Chapel Hill, NC, American Gastroenterologic Association, September 1971.
2. Ostrow JD: *Mechanisms and Differential Diagnosis of Jaundice*, an Audio-Visual Lecture of the National Medical Audiovisual Center. Atlanta, American Gastroenterologic Association, 1974.
3. Ostrow JD: *Unconjugated Hyperbilirubinemia*, an Audio-Visual Lecture of the National Medical Audiovisual Center. Atlanta, American Gastroenterologic Association, 1974.
4. Javitt NB: *The Cholestatic Syndromes*, an Audio-Visual Lecture of the National Medical Audiovisual Center. Atlanta, American Gastroenterologic Association, 1974.
5. Schmid R: Bilirubin metabolism in man. *N Engl J Med* 1972;287:703–709.
6. Fleischner G, Arias IM: Recent advances in bilirubin metabolism. *Am J Med* 1970;49:576–589.
7. Klatskin G, Bungards L: An improved test for bilirubin in urine. *N Engl J Med* 1953;248:712–717.
8. Arias IM, Gartner LM, Cohen M, et al: Chronic non-hemolytic unconjugated hyperbilirubinemia with glucuronyl transferase deficiency: Clinical, biochemical, pharmacologic and genetic evidence for heterogeneity. *Am J Med* 1969;47:395–409.
9. Berk PD, Blaschke TF: Detection of Gilbert's syndrome in patients with hemolysis: A method using radioactive chromium. *Ann Intern Med* 1972;77:527–531.
10. Berk PD, Martin JF, Blaschke TF, et al: Unconjugated hyperbilirubinemia: Physiologic evaluation and experimental approaches to therapy. *Ann Intern Med* 1975;82:552–570.
11. Black M, Billing BH, Heirwegh KPM: Determination of bilirubin UDP-glucuronyl

transferase in needle-biopsy specimens of human liver. *Clin Chim Acta* 1970; 29:27–35.

12. Fevery J, Blanckaert N, Heirwegh KPM: Unconjugated bilirubin and increased proportion of bilirubin monoconjugates in the bile of patients with Gilbert's syndrome and Crigler-Najjar disease. *J Clin Invest* 1977;60:970–979.

13. Zimmerman HJ, West M: Serum enzyme levels in the diagnosis of hepatic disease. *Am J Gastroenterol* 1963;40:387–404.

14. Leevy CM, Chen T, Zaki FG: Differential diagnosis of cholestasis. *Adv Intern Med* 1971;17:323–342.

15. Berk PD, Javitt NB: Hyperbilirubinemia and cholestasis. *Am J Med* 1978;64: 311–326.

16. Quarfordt SH, Hilderman HL, Valle D, et al: Compartmental analysis of sulfobromophthalein transport in normal patients and patients with hepatic dysfunction. *Gastroenterology* 1971;60:246–255.

17. Ben-Ezzer J, Rimington C, Shani M, et al: Abnormal excretion of the isomers of urinary coproporphyrin by patients with Dubin-Johnson syndrome in Israel. *Clin Sci* 1971;40:17–30.

Chapter 7

Cholestatic Jaundice in Adults

Murry G. Fischer, MD
Alvin M. Gelb, MD
Leonard A. Weingarten, MD

In the two prior chapters, algorithms were presented that primarily dealt with the diagnosis of jaundice in the newborn and with medical causes of jaundice in older children and adults. In the latter chapter, the author concluded that "the most difficult problem in the diagnosis of jaundice is the differentiation of intrahepatic from extrahepatic cholestasis." Our algorithms pursue this problem by branching logic using current diagnostic modalities that have become available during the past few years (Figure 7–1).

When conjugated hyperbilirubinemia exists with increasing total bilirubin levels of more than 3 mg/dL (51.3 μmol/L), visualization of the biliary tree by conventional oral or intravenous cholecystography (IVC) is unlikely and should not be attempted.

The following numbered passages refer to the boxed numbers in the algorithms.

1. The initial step is to determine if there has been recent biliary tract surgery. When a T-tube is still in situ, T-tube cholangiography is the simplest way to opacify the biliary tree and clarify the problem. If there is no T-tube entry and bile duct injury is known or suspected, percutaneous transhepatic cholangiography (PTC) should be performed and all other diagnostic modes bypassed.

2. If an enlarged nodular liver is felt on physical examination, and metastatic hepatic disease is suspected, radionuclide liver scan and liver biopsy should be the first diagnostic modalities used for confirmation. When nonconfirmatory, and a high index of suspicion still exists, computed axial tomography (CT) scanning should be performed.

3. For the majority of patients with neither recent biliary tract surgery nor a hard nodular liver, the first major branch point, sonography, has been almost always successful in identifying patients with ductal dilation.[1] If dilation cannot

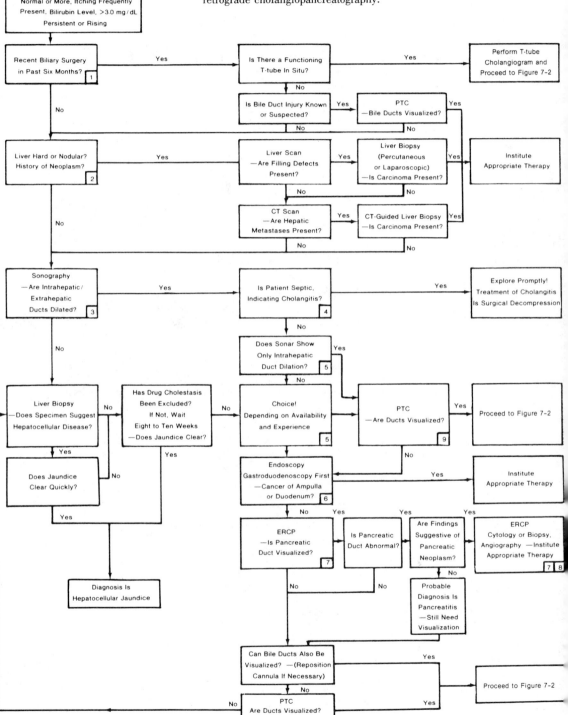

Figure 7–1. Cholestatic jaundice.
PTC = percutaneous transhepatic cholangiography;
CT = computed axial tomography; ERCP = endoscopic
retrograde cholangiopancreatography.

50

be demonstrated by an experienced sonographer, a diagnosis of hepatocellular jaundice is likely and should be confirmed by liver biopsy.

4. If sonography demonstrates ductal dilation in a septic jaundiced patient, further diagnostic testing is unwise, since delay may have tragic consequences. A septic patient is one with high spiking fever, shaking chills, and impending or actual septic shock. These patients should be explored promptly and drained surgically. Direct decompression of the major bile ducts is preferred, since no antibiotic will reach therapeutically effective levels in the severely obstructed biliary system.[2, 3] Patients with mild cholangitis may be treated with antibiotics. If they respond, their diagnostic studies may be continued according to the algorithm.

5. The further workup of the nonseptic patient with sonographically identified dilated biliary ducts depends to some extent on modalities available at any given institution. If sonography shows only intrahepatic duct dilation indicating a probable block at the porta hepatis, the best approach is to perform PTC, since opacification is almost always successful under these circumstances.

6. When a skilled endoscopist is readily available, a more thorough search is possible by first performing gastroduodenoscopy. This will help to identify cases of carcinoma of the ampulla of Vater or duodenum, which have a much more favorable prognosis with radical surgical excision than carcinoma of the pancreas. When such lesions are found, biopsy should be performed. A normal biopsy result, however, does not exclude carcinoma, since the lesion may be submucosal. An abnormal enlargement or protrusion of the ampulla, whether ulcerated or not, should be considered carcinoma until proved otherwise, despite a normal endoscopic biopsy result. Thus, if a lesion of the duodenum or ampulla is visualized endoscopically, one should proceed directly to surgery.

7. If no lesion is seen on duodenoscopy, endoscopic retrograde cholangiopancreatography (ERCP) should be tried and an attempt made to opacify both the biliary tree and the pancreatic ducts. Should pancreatography suggest a pancreatic neoplasm, brush biopsy of the ducts[4] or cell cytology,[5, 6] or transduodenal needle aspiration biopsy[7] can be done to try to confirm the diagnosis preoperatively.

8. When carcinoma of the pancreas is strongly suspected or proved, selective angiography should be performed in patients otherwise suitable for pancreatectomy. Angiography will not only demonstrate the vascular supply and possible abnormalities for the operating surgeon, but may also identify noncurable patients in whom vessel encasement by tumor precludes radical resection.

9. In institutions where endoscopic facilities are not available or when attempts at ERCP visualization have failed, PTC will usually identify the site of obstruction and often suggests the etiology. The technique of PTC is easily learned and is available in most modern radiology departments. The introduction of the Chiba skinny needle has done much to promote its popularity.[8, 9] Many believe that PTC done with the skinny needle has a lower complication rate from bleeding

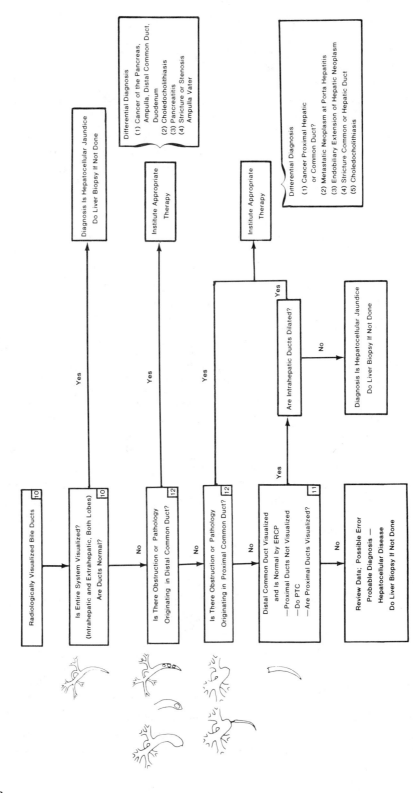

Figure 7–2. Radiologically visualized ducts.

and bile leakage than when a 19-gauge flexible sheath-covered (Teflon) needle is used. While possibly true for patients with hepatocellular disease, this is not borne out in those with obstructed ductal systems.[10, 11] Percutaneous transhepatic cholangiography using the skinny needle is, however, more successful in opacifying nondilated ducts.[8, 9] If a notably dilated biliary tree is demonstrated by PTC, the ducts should be decompressed by a PTC-placed drainage catheter,[12] or the patient should promptly undergo exploratory surgery. Prophylactic antibiotics should be given to patients with suspected or known ductal dilation undergoing PTC.

10. Once the biliary tree is opacified radiologically, the key to diagnosis and therapy has been acquired. If the entire biliary tract is normal, the diagnosis is hepatocellular jaundice and a liver biopsy specimen should be confirmatory. When abnormalities exist, each cause has a characteristic x-ray film configuration. The various diagnostic possibilities are listed in Figure 7–2.

11. Occasionally a normal distal duct will be seen on ERCP but the contrast material will not enter the intrahepatic ducts. Although this may indicate failure to inject sufficient contrast substance, it cannot be so assumed. The possibility exists that a proximal obstructing lesion is present. Opacification of the proximal intrahepatic branches of both hepatic lobes must be obtained by either PTC or repeated ERCP.[13]

12. When an obstructing lesion in the biliary tract is demonstrated by ERCP, and contrast material from above the obstruction does not empty within several hours, a potentially dangerous situation has been created that requires urgent surgical intervention. Bacteria have been introduced by the cannula into the obstructed portion of the biliary tree. Bile, an excellent culture medium, permits rapid bacterial growth under these circumstances, and a fulminant cholangitis may be precipitated.[14] Prophylactic antibiotics should be given to patients with suspected ductal dilation. The addition of antibiotics to the contrast material may also prevent or decrease the incidence of this problem.

Despite attempts to close all loops and consider all options, unusual cases will occasionally present that do not fit into any of the patterns described. Most diagnoses will have been considered by the use of the algorithms, and the remaining possibilities in these unusual cases will be limited. We have found algorithms to function not only as diagnostic road maps, but also as excellent teaching vehicles for all educational levels.

References

1. Goldstein LI, Sample WF, Kadell BM, et al: Gray-scale ultrasonography and thin-needle cholangiography: Evaluation in the jaundiced patient. *JAMA* 1977;238:1041–1044.
2. Ram MD, Watanatittan S: Cephalothin levels in human bile. *Arch Surg* 1974;108:187–189.

3. Keighley MRB, Drysdale RB, Quoraishi AH, et al: Antibiotic treatment of biliary sepsis. *Surg Clin North Am* 1975;55:1379–1390.

4. Osnes M, Serck-Hanssen A, Myren J: Endoscopic retrograde brush cytology of the biliary and pancreatic ducts. *Scand J Gastroenterol* 1975;10:829–831.

5. Blackstone MO, Cockerham L, Kirsner JB, et al: Intraductal aspiration for cytodiagnosis in pancreatic malignancy. *Gastrointest Endosc* 1977;23:145–147.

6. Roberts-Thomson IC, Hobbs JB: Cytodiagnosis of pancreatic and biliary cancer by endoscopic duct aspiration. *Med J Aust* 1979;1:370–372.

7. Tsuchiya R, Henmi T, Kondo N, et al: Endoscopic aspiration biopsy of the pancreas. *Gastroenterology* 1977;73:1050–1052.

8. Redeker AG, Karvountzis GG, Richman RH, et al.: Percutaneous transhepatic cholangiography: An improved technique. *JAMA* 1975;231:386–387.

9. Ferrucci JT, Wittenberg J, Sarno RA, et al: Fine needle transhepatic cholangiography—a new approach to obstructive jaundice. *AJR* 1976;127:403–407.

10. Juler GL, Conroy RM, Fuelleman RW: Bile leakage following percutaneous transhepatic cholangiography with the Chiba needle *Arch Surg* 1977;112:954–958.

11. Kreek MJ, Balint J: Special report: Risks of the skinny needle procedure. Read before the Annual Meeting of the AASLD, Chicago, Nov 7, 1978.

12. Kaude JV, Weidenmier CH, Agee OF: Decompression of bile ducts with the percutaneous transhepatic technique. *Radiology* 1969;93:69–71.

13. Fischer MG, Wolff WI, Geffen A, et al: Combined use of percutaneous transhepatic cholangiography and endoscopic ampullary cholangiography in the diagnosis of 'difficult' jaundice cases. *Am J Gastroenterol* 1975;63:369–380.

14. Davis JL, Milligan FD, Cameron JL: Septic complications following endoscopic retrograde cholangiopancreatography. *Surg Gynecol Obstet* 1975;140:365–367.

Chapter 8

Acute Diarrhea

Terry K. Satterwhite, MD
Herbert L. DuPont, MD

Diarrheal illness is one of the most common disorders of man. In most instances, enteric infection is self-limiting, but in some cases, appropriate specific therapy can shorten the illness, and in a smaller number, similar treatment may be life-saving. This algorithm (Figure 8–1) is one current approach to the management of acute diarrhea.

Hospitalization vs Outpatient Management

Whether the patient should be hospitalized or treated as an outpatient depends on a number of factors, including the nature of the underlying disease and the age of the patient as well as the degree of systemic toxicity, fever, and state of hydration. The following criteria usually should be followed in selecting those patients who should be admitted to the hospital: (1) the very young or elderly with severe diarrhea, or (2) patients of any age with diarrhea and pronounced systemic toxemia, hyperpyrexia, or dehydration. While hospitalized, the patient's condition can be closely monitored and any metabolic disturbances treated while the cause of the diarrhea is being sought. The outpatient's condition can be managed with an oral electrolyte solution while the workup is in progress, and the patient can be admitted if clinical deterioration occurs. The workup is the same for the outpatient or inpatient.

Drug-Induced Diarrhea

Drugs such as antimicrobial agents (especially clindamycin, lincomycin hydrochloride monohydrate, ampicillin, and cephalosporins) as well as warfarin

From: The Patient with Acute Diarrhea. An Algorithm for Diagnosis. *JAMA* 1976;236:2662–2664. Copyright 1976 by the American Medical Association.

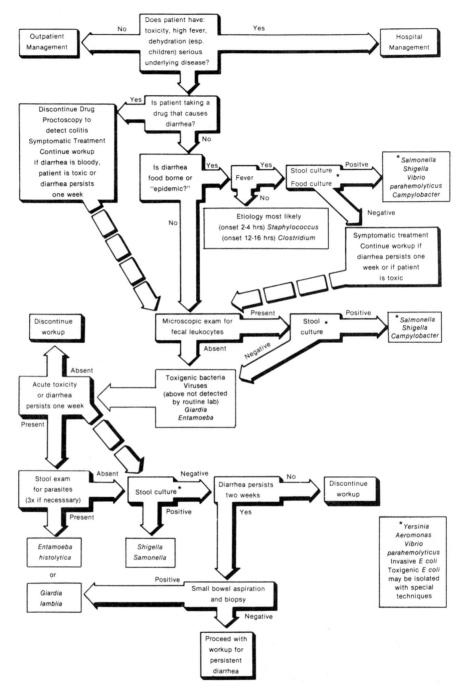

Figure 8–1. The patient with acute diarrhea.

sodium, thyroid replacement, and antimetabolites may cause diarrhea. Antibiotic-induced diarrhea may vary from mild, nonspecific, and watery to severe colitis with pseudomembrane formation. The diarrhea may begin after the drug course has been completed.[1] When drug-associated diarrhea is suspected, the drug therapy should be discontinued and proctoscopy performed to see if a pseudomembrane is present. If there is blood in the stool or if the diarrhea persists one week after treatment with the suspected therapeutic agent has been discontinued, the workup should be continued in quest of an etiologic agent.

Common Source Diarrhea

Important in the patient's history is the finding of other persons with a similar illness following a common exposure (such as a particular food). If there is a logical source (eg, picnic food or warmed-over turkey after Thanksgiving), then the physician must consider the illnesses that are characteristically food-borne. When food-borne enteric disease occurs and none of those involved has fever, a toxin-mediated illness is suspected. If vomiting is out of proportion to diarrhea and if the incubation period is two to four hours, staphylococcal food poisoning is the probable diagnosis. If the onset is 12 to 16 hours after ingestion, *Clostridium perfringens* or possibly other toxigenic bacteria are more likely causative agents. *Bacillius cerceus* produces two toxins, one of which is associated with illness similar to the staphylococcus and another that mimics the illness produced by *C perfringens*.[2]

If fever is present, stool cultures and food cultures should be performed and may show the usual causes of diarrhea in this setting, ie, *Salmonella* or *Shigella*. *Vibrio parahemolyticus* should be suspected during summer months when the patient has eaten a seafood meal that has not been properly cooked or has been recontaminated after cooking. Special salt-containing media (such as thiosulfate-citrate-bile salt-sucrose agar) must be used to isolate *V parahemolyticus*. *Campylobacter jejunis* has become a widely recognized cause of food-borne and water-borne enteritis. A presumptive diagnosis can sometimes be made by examining a recently passed stool with phase contrast or darkfield microscopy. The organisms are cultured on selective media such as Skirrows and grow best at 42°C in 5% to 10% oxygen and 3% to 10% carbon dioxide.[3]

In the case of food-borne diarrheal disease, if the stool and food cultures are negative and the diarrhea persists longer than a week or if toxicity persists despite symptomatic therapy, the diagnostic workup should continue.

Exudative and Nonexudative Diarrhea

In addition to a careful history, the presence or absence of fecal polymorphonuclear or mononuclear leukocytes is a focal point in the subsequent evaluation of patients with diarrhea. The test is easily performed in the physician's office or emergency room. A small fleck of mucus (or if mucus is not present, a drop of liquid stool) is placed on a glass microscope slide with a wooden applicator stick and is thoroughly, yet carefully, mixed with an approximately equal volume of Loffler methylene blue (found in labs where reticulocyte staining is done). A coverslip is placed on the mixture, and after two or three minutes, leukocytes generally are identified under the "high dry" objective of a light microscope in patients with colitis.[4] The fecal specimen can be allowed to dry before heat fixing and staining with methylene blue. Fecal leukocytes are produced by bacteria that invade the colonic mucosa, ie, infection caused by *Salmonella, Shigella, Campylobacter, Yersinia,* and invasive *Escherichia coli.* Other disorders associated with colonic mucosal inflammation and destruction will be positive for fecal leukocytes, eg, ulcerative colitis,[2] and we have observed leukocytes in stools of patients with antibiotic-associated colitis. Fecal leukocytes are usually not present in the stools of those with diarrhea secondary to viruses, toxigenic bacteria, and parasites.[4-9] Special laboratory techniques must be used to identify *Yersinia* and invasive strains of *E coli.*[10, 11]

Presence of Fecal Leukocytes

Those with positive fecal leukocytes should have their stools cultured for *Shigella, Salmonella,* and *Campylobacter,* and blood cultures should be obtained in those with high fever. The usual bacterial causes of fecal leukocytes are *Shigella, Salmonella,* and *Campylobacter.* All microbiology laboratories can culture stools for *Salmonella* and *Shigella* and most also can successfully grow and identify *Campylobacter.* Idiopathic ulcerative colitis also is associated with an exudative stool, yet in such cases, the history of chronicity or intermittency should be sought. Since parasites that cause diarrhea do not usually produce fecal leukocytes, it is not necessary to do stool studies for ova and parasites in the leukocyte-positive cases unless there is an historical clue that would lead one to suspect parasitic infestation or the stool culture is repeatedly negative.

Absence of Fecal Leukocytes

Other agents may produce diarrhea by toxin production *(Staphylococcus, E coli, C perfringens,* and *Vibrio cholerae)* or by inducing a lesion in small-bowel mucosa *(Giardia,* viruses) and thereby cause watery diarrhea without white blood cells in stools. Amebic dysentery usually is not associated with fecal leukocytes.[7-9] Food, travel, and epidemiological history may be helpful and, coupled with food cultures, may lead to the diagnosis. Evidence is accumulating to suggest that toxigenic *E coli* are the most important causes of diarrhea of travelers.[12] Specialized laboratory facilities are necessary to identify toxigenic bacteria, invasive *E coli,* or viruses, but at this time, such facilities are not available to the practitioner. With the purification of bacterial and viral antigens, serologic studies will be forthcoming that will aid the practitioner in detecting these agents. Stools should be examined for protozoa, especially if illness has lasted longer than one week. The common parasitic offenders are *Giardia lamblia* and *Entamoeba histolytica*, but occasionally *Dientamoeba fragilis* and other parasites may cause diarrhea. A total of three freshly obtained, warm stool samples may be necessary for examination for *Amoeba*. *Giardia* are found in stools in approximately 50% of infected patients. If stools are negative for parasites, we would advise that the physician culture the stool for enteric bacterial pathogens (*Shigella* and *Salmonella*), even though this is unlikely to be positive without fecal leukocytes. If the patient has a toxic reaction, the stool culture should be done concurrently with the search for parasites.

Should the diarrhea not abate within two weeks, small-bowel intubation with aspiration and biopsy may show *G lamblia*. If *Giardia* is found, or in an occasional case where intubation is not performed or is unrewarding, therapy for giardiasis may be administered. In the patient with negative workup whose diarrhea persists two weeks, a workup for persistent diarrhea should be instituted.

References

1. Tedesco FJ, Barton RW, Alpers DH: Clindamycin-associated colitis: A prospective study. *Ann Intern Med* 1974;81:429–433.
2. Terranova W, Blake PA: *Bacillus cereus* food poisoning. *N Engl J Med* 1978; 298:143–146.
3. Blaser MJ, Reller LB: *Campylobacter enteritis*. *N Engl J Med* 1981;305:1444–1451.
4. Harris JC, Dupont HL, Hornick RB: Fecal leukocytes in diarrheal illness. *Ann Intern Med* 1972;76:697–703.
5. Ryder RW, Sack DA, Kapikian AZ, et al.: Enterotoxigenic *Escherichia coli* and reovirus-like agent in rural Bangladesh. *Lancet* 1976;1:659–662.
6. Pierce JE, DuPont HL, Lewis KR: Acute diarrhea in a residential institution for the retarded. *Am J Dis Child* 1974;128:772–775.
7. Willmore JG, Shearman CH: On the differential diagnosis of the dysenteries: The diagnostic value of the cell-exudate in the stools of acute amoebic and bacillary dysentery. *Lancet* 1918;2:200–206.
8. Graham D: Some points in the diagnosis and treatment of dysentery occuring in the British Salonika Force. *Lancet* 1918;1:51–55.
9. Anderson J: A study of dysentery in the field: With special references to the cytology of bacillary dysentery and its bearing on early and accurate diagnosis. *Lancet* 1921;2:998–1002.
10. Nilehn B: Studies on Y. enterocolitica: Growth of various solid media at 37°C and 25°C. *Acta Pathol Microbiol Scand* 1969;77:685–697.
11. Du Pont HL, Formal SB, Hornick RB, et al: Pathogenesis of *Escherichia coli* diarrhea. *N Engl J Med* 1971;285:1–9.
12. Gorbach SL, Kean BH, Evans DJ, et al: Travelers' diarrhea and toxigenic *Escherichia coli*. *N Engl J Med* 1975;292:933–936.

Chapter 9

Urinary Tract Infections

Calvin M. Kunin, MD

The diagnosis and management of urinary tract infection rests on two major concepts. The first, *significant bacteriuria*, provides the basis for definitive diagnosis, efficacy of therapy, and follow-up. Until recently, it was relatively expensive to test for significant bacteriuria. Also, results were often available only after the physician had to make a therapeutic commitment. Significant bacteriuria can now be detected by excellent, inexpensive office methods, including microscopic examination of the urine and quantitative culture. In addition, there now are commercially available chemical tests, which when properly used should be helpful for both screening and follow-up.

The second major concept is a *therapeutic concept* that divides urinary tract infection into the so-called *complicated* (or surgical) and *uncomplicated* (or medical) categories of infection. It is relatively easy to treat infection uncomplicated by structural or neurologic lesions. Numerous effective antimicrobial agents are useful both for treatment and prophylaxis. Furthermore, antimicrobial sensitivity tests (which can be performed reliably enough in the office setting) are highly predictive of therapeutic efficacy. Complicated infections (in which there may be a foreign body, neurogenic bladder, or obstructive lesion), on the other hand, are more difficult to manage. In such situations, one achieves transient elimination of infection only to experience recurrence once the antimicrobial agent is no longer given, or when a resistant organism emerges. This situation demands an entirely different therapeutic strategy.

This report contains three strategies for detection and management of urinary tract infection. These include (1) screening programs, (2) examination procedures for the symptomatic patient seen in the office practice, and (3) routine monitoring of patients with indwelling urinary catheters in the hospital. The ra-

From: Urinary Tract Infections. Flow Charts (Algorithms) for Detection and Treatment. *JAMA* 1975;233:458–462. Copyright 1975 by the American Medical Association.

tionale for these concepts was clearly defined by Kass[1] more than 20 years ago and has been refined and amplified by a great number of excellent studies in more recent years.[2, 3]

Significant bacteriuria in the asymptomatic or symptomatic patient is used as the point of entry in each of the flow charts (Figures 9–1 through 9–3). The therapeutic approaches to uncomplicated or complicated infection are interwoven within the framework. Detailed definitions, laboratory methods, and antimicrobial dosage schedules are those published in a manual I have written.[4] Other books and several authoritative monographs are also available for reference.[5–8]

It is my hope that these diagrams will be useful in helping physicians, nurses, and allied health workers to deal more effectively with the detection and management of urinary infections.

Screening Programs

The ultimate place of mass screening programs for detection of bacteriuria remains to be determined. We can, however, define certain high-risk groups and set priorities for detection in office practice (Figure 9–1). The most important element of any program is to provide assurance that high standards of care and follow-up will be available for any patient found to have infection.

The flow chart offers three approaches to screening tests. Two of them (the nitrite test and detection of subnormal levels of glucose in the urine on first morning specimens) are just beginning to be exploited on a mass basis. These chemical methods have the advantage of permitting the patient (or parent) to do the testing at home without obtaining a clean voided specimen. Self-detection of infection has proven feasible with dipslide cultures in a large-scale study conducted among schoolgirls in Oxford, England.[9] The self-administered nitrite test (when used on three different morning specimens) detected 90% of cases in a study that our department recently conducted among women in Madison, Wisconsin.

The diagram indicates that final confirmation should be by quantitative urine culture, preferably in a central laboratory that can also provide the physician with information on identification of organism and antimicrobial sensitivity tests. Large-scale self-screening not only has the potential of greatly reducing the cost of detecting a case, but also permits a much larger group of individuals to be screened. It is my hope that these methods can be adapted to the routine of office practice as well as for community-wide programs.

Symptomatic Patients in Office Practice

The flow chart (Figure 9–2) illustrates the sequence of events that might be followed for a patient who is first seen with signs and symptoms suggestive of

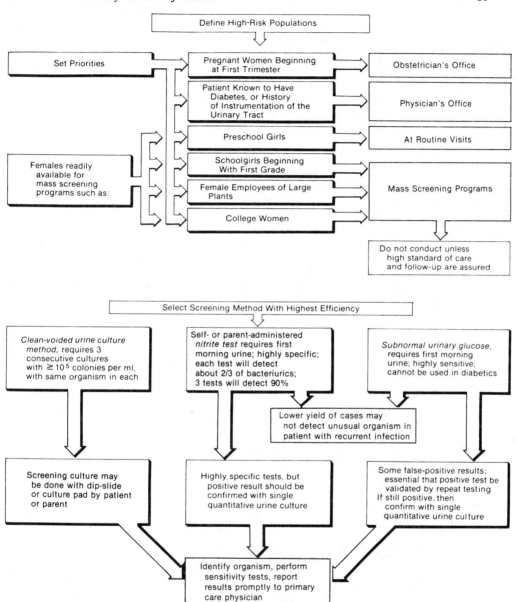

Figure 9—1. Algorithm for screening high-risk groups for significant bacteriuria.

urinary infection in office practice. The quantitative urine culture is used as the point of departure for diagnosis. The criteria for "significant bacteriuria" depend largely on the mode of collection. A single urine specimen may be all that can be obtained prior to making a therapeutic commitment.

For that reason, special emphasis is placed on the use of the Gram's stain

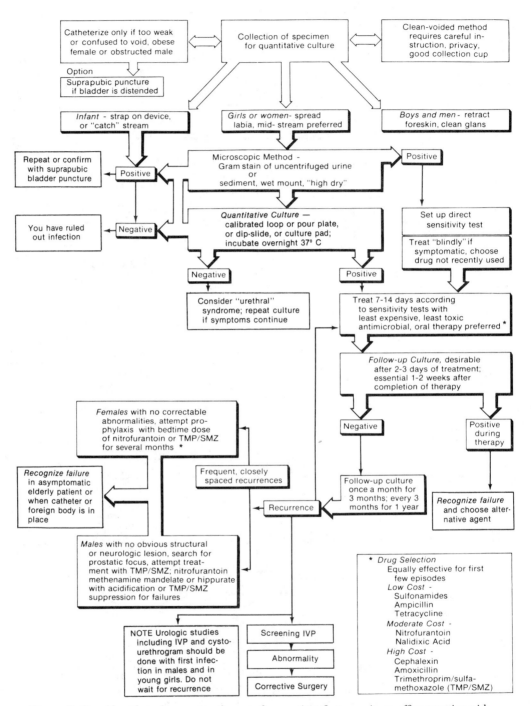

Figure 9–2. Algorithm of sequence of events for a patient first seen in an office practice with signs and symptoms suggestive of urinary infection. IVP = intravenous pyelogram.

of uncentrifuged urine, or wet-mount examination of the sediment for bacteria. Significant bacteriuria requires a bacterial count of ten or more colonies per milliliter of urine when the clean-voided method is used. Lower counts may at times occur when the patient has taken excess fluid, but this is unusual. It is important to emphasize, however, that when a suprapubic aspiration is performed, counts as low as 1,000 colonies per milliliter are indicative of infection.

The chart assumes that there is no antecedent knowledge as to whether the patient has important underlying structural or neurologic disease or a history of recurrent infection. It does point out, however, the indications for at least a screening pyelographic study and emphasizes the importance of urologic evaluation particularly in the young male.

A guide to choice of drugs is given, emphasizing selection according to lowest cost and side-effects. Generally, excellent correlation is found between in vitro sensitivity tests and therapeutic efficacy. Virtually all the commonly used agents are highly effective for the first few episodes of treatment. Thereafter, sensitivity tests are extremely valuable as a guide to choice of drug. It is important to recognize failure if bacteriuria persists during therapy (it usually should be gone after the first day of treatment).

Every writer on the subject of therapy of urinary infection emphasizes the importance of follow-up. This is usually done by periodic urine cultures. In the future, self-administered chemical tests may make follow-up more economical and effective.

Recurrent infection is very common in females and is usually due to reinfection. Recurrent infection in males usually is due to persistence of an infected focus that may require surgical correction. The frequency and pattern of recurrences determine the form of therapy to be used. Generally, it is best to treat isolated instances of recurrence with a 7- to 14-day course of an effective agent. Prophylaxis or suppressive therapy may be necessary when recurrent episodes are frequent and closely spaced.

Monitoring With Indwelling Catheters

Catheter-induced bacterial colonization of the urine is the most common nosocomial infection and the most frequent cause of Gram-negative rod bacteremia. Much of the morbidity and mortality from these infections can be prevented by avoiding unnecessary instrumentation of the urinary tract and by strict aseptic management of the urinary drainage system. In view of the frequency and importance of these infections, it seems reasonable to develop a system to monitor the urine of catheterized patients routinely for evidence of infection and to have the results of bacteriologic identification and antimicrobial sensitivity tests readily available. This may be accomplished by the routine procedure described in Figure 9–3. Procedures for aspirating urine from the catheter and posting data on the bulletin board are presented in detail elsewhere.[1]

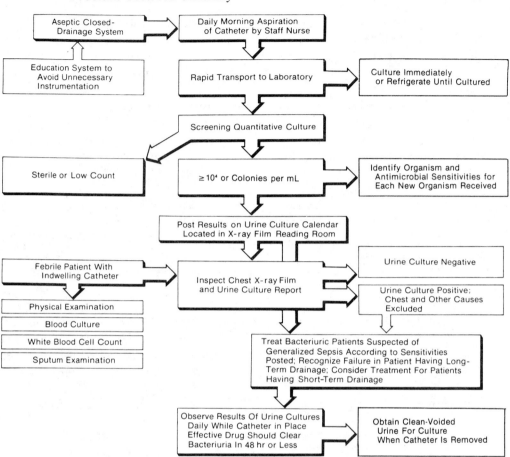

Figure 9–3. Algorithm for routine monitoring of hospitalized patients with indwelling catheters.

There are several benefits that can be derived from routine monitoring of bacteriuria in patients with catheter drainage. These include (1) rapid aid in evaluation of the source of infection in a febrile patient; (2) ability to select immediately the most effective, least toxic, and least expensive antimicrobial agent for patients manifesting sepsis, or infected while short-term catheter drainage is being used; (3) evaluating the efficacy of aseptic technique being used; (4) determination of cross infection on a ward; and (5) recognition that a given drug is effective or ineffective in controlling infection.

It must be emphasized that patients having long-term catheter drainage often do well even though continuously infected and that antimicrobial agents will not clear bacteria from the urine of such patients. For these reasons, therapy is usually reserved for suspected episodes of sepsis arising from the urinary tract. It is important to recognize that persistently positive cultures during treatment with an antimicrobial agent mean that the drug is not effective and treatment with it should be stopped.

Conclusions

The three flow charts, or algorithms, on detection and treatment of urinary tract infections are presented in the hope that they will serve as useful guides for the practicing physician. They represent the current views of many workers in the field. The concept of significant bacteriuria provides the basis for each of the flow charts. It is the most reliable guide to the presence of infection and response to therapy, and is essential for close follow-up of patients. Persistence of significant bacteriuria during therapy means that the drug has failed. Early recognition of failure should allow the physician to reevaluate his or her selection of drugs and seriously consider the cost-benefit ratio of continued treatment.

References

1. Kass EH: Chemotherapeutic and antibiotic drugs in management of infections of the urinary tract. *Am J Med* 1955;18:764–781.
2. Kincaid-Smith P, Fairley KF: *Renal Infection and Renal Scarring*. Melbourne, Australia, Mercedes Publishing Services, 1971.
3. O'Grady F, Brumfitt W (eds): *Urinary Tract Infection*. New York, Oxford University Press, 1968.
4. Kunin CM: *Detection, Prevention and Treatment of Urinary Tract Infections*, ed 2. Philadelphia, Lea & Febiger, 1974.
5. Brumfitt W, Asscher AW: *Urinary Tract Infection*. New York, Oxford University Press, 1973.
6. Kaye D: *Urinary Tract Infection and Its Management*. St. Louis, CV Mosby Co, 1972.
7. Stamey TA: *Urinary Infections*. Baltimore, Williams & Wilkins Co, 1972.
8. Freedman LA: Pyelonephritis and urinary tract infection, in Strauss MB, Welt LG (eds): *Diseases of the Kidney*, ed. 2. Boston, Little, Brown & Co, 1971.
9. Asscher AW, Harrison S, Jones RV, et al: Screening for asymptomatic urinary-tract infection in schoolgirls. *Lancet* 1973;2:1–4.

Chapter 10

Fever of Unknown Origin

Donald M. Vickery, MD
Robert K. Quinnell, MD

Fever of unknown origin (FUO) has been regarded as a supreme diagnostic puzzle. This reputation may be undeserved, since there is a tendency to group many specific syndromes that include fever as one of their symptoms under this heading. The term "FUO" should be reserved for a syndrome in which the fever is prolonged and there are no other specific signs or symptoms that would define a separate syndrome. The first criterion is recognized generally, but neglect of the second has resulted in the implication that fevers associated with polyarthritis, abdominal pain, or rash are all FUOs and may be approached similarly. A third criterion, that the fever is undiagnosed after routine diagnostic tests, is sometimes applied but is too vague to be satisfactory.

The algorithms presented here provide a logical, step-by-step approach to the FUO syndrome. The essential features of this approach are (1) limitation of associated symptoms to malaise, fatigue, weight loss, and chills; (2) fever for at least two weeks before beginning any laboratory investigation; and (3) performance of a limited number of widely available laboratory tests in patients with fever for more than two but less than four weeks. Thus, the algorithm is compatible with the criteria of Petersdorf and Beeson[1]: (1) illness of more than three weeks' duration, (2) fever higher than 38.3°C on several occasions, and (3) diagnosis uncertain after one week of study in the hospital.

Few other syndromes give rise to such a wide variety of possible diagnoses and, therefore, offer as much potential for ineffective use of the laboratory. To avoid inappropriate use of the laboratory while giving optimal care, the physician must appreciate the following: (1) the fundamental importance of the history and physical examination, (2) the use of time as a diagnostic tool, and (3) the anxiety of both the physician and the patient because the diagnosis is not known.

From: Fever of Unknown Origin. An Algorithmic Approach. *JAMA* 1977;238:2183–2188. Copyright 1977 by the American Medical Association.

Normal findings from history and physical examinations are extraordinarily useful. The majority of persons with FUO and no other signs or symptoms will eventually defervesce without the establishment of a definitive diagnosis and without any apparent sequelae. Careful observation is the rational approach with patients who are relatively well and who have no other specific signs or symptoms.

Even when a definitive diagnosis is established, time is often more helpful than the use of sophisticated diagnostic procedures. Most diagnoses are made because new signs or symptoms develop or because a relatively simple laboratory procedure becomes positive. Prognosis is seldom adversely affected by the delay of an appropriate observation period. Prematurely embarking on extensive laboratory investigation is expensive and may be counterproductive. Furthermore, many diagnostic procedures carry a substantial risk to the patient. It is doubly tragic when serious adverse effects result from an unnecessary procedure.

Still, it is exceedingly difficult to tell any patient that the diagnosis is uncertain, but that further testing is not indicated. The patient has come to the physician to find an answer and to put an end to uncertainty. The physician must deal with the anxiety of not knowing what might happen to his or her reputation (and malpractice insurance) if the patient eventually experiences a bad outcome. The importance of "catching it early" is overrated, both by society and the medical profession. Resisting the temptation to "do some tests" requires that the physician have confidence in himself or herself and tests the physician's ability to communicate with the patient.

This is not to deny the value of early detection of a treatable disease. An FUO may involve substantial morbidity: the cost of lost workdays as well as the cost of medical services, and the chance of increased disability due to delayed treatment. But the desirability of early detection of treatable disease must not be confused with the ability to make such diagnoses. It is decision-making rather than diagnosis that matters most. The yield, risk, and cost of each procedure must be weighed against the morbidity, risk, and cost of the illness. Algorithms such as those presented here (Figures 10–1 through 10–4) may be of some help in making these difficult decisions by delineating a logical, step-by-step approach to the problem.[2, 3]

The Algorithms

The algorithms assume that a history has been taken and a physical examination has been performed. Blocks 1 through 3 (Figure 10–1) establish entrance criteria. An oral temperature of 38.1°C has been selected as the minimum temperature that marks a fever. This criterion is arbitrary, but many normal persons may experience temperatures in excess of 37.0°C, especially at the peak of the diurnal variation. Also to be considered is the syndrome of habitual hyperthermia, in which a young woman may experience temperatures of 37.2°C to 38.0°C during the second half of the menstrual cycle. These patients may also

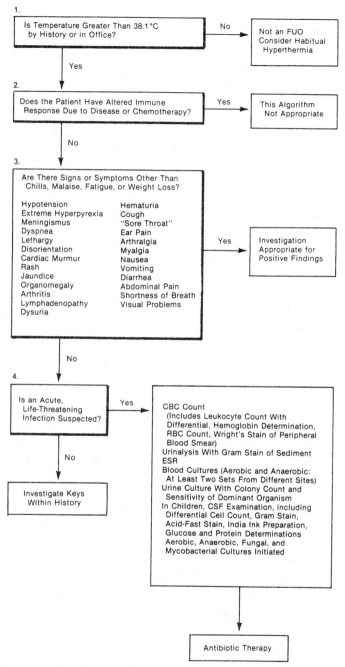

Figure 10–1. Approach to fever of unknown origin (FUO). CBC = complete blood cell; CSF = cerebrospinal fluid; ESR = erythrocyte sedimentation rate.

complain of a number of other symptoms such as insomnia, vague aches and pains, headache, and bowel problems, but this syndrome does not fall into any other recognized disease category.

The patient who has altered immune responses associated with disease (eg, Hodgkin's disease, multiple myeloma) or chemotherapy may have a febrile illness that progresses at an unusual pace and is caused by an organism unlikely to be found in an immunologically competent patient. The approach in these instances must take into account the nature of the underlying disease and the chemotherapy employed; its complexity prevents its inclusion in these algorithms.

Block 3 indicates the need to exclude syndromes that are marked by symptoms other than chills, fever, malaise, fatigue, or weight loss. Some signs and symptoms that often help to define syndromes other than FUO are listed.

The physician should determine at the outset the degree of disability and pace of the illness. If the patient has delayed the first visit for several days or weeks or if the onset of the fever has been slow, the chance of a sudden catastrophe occurring is low. A few patients will have such severe disability that it may be reasonable to shorten some of the indicated time intervals.

Rarely, a patient with sepsis or acute bacterial endocarditis will seek medical care before localizing signs or signs of shock are present. During this early and transient stage, decision-making cannot rely on the laboratory. Only the severeity of the nonspecific symptoms and acute onset in an appropriate setting (eg, in a debilitated patient or in a patient who has had urinary tract instrumentation) can lead the physician to proceed on the hypothesis that a life-threatening infection exists. The leukocyte differential count, erythrocyte sedimentation rate, and urinalysis with Gram stain of the sediment may add weight to this hypothesis but can neither absolutely confirm nor deny it. The same is true of the tetrazolium test and limulus lysate assay when these are employed. It is extremely important to obtain at least two specimens for blood culture (aerobic and anaerobic) from separate sites before antimicrobial therapy is begun.

In children, meningitis from *Hemophilus influenzae* or *Neisseria meningitidis* may be rapidly progressive and, therefore, examination of the cerebrospinal fluid should be made. The simple fact remains that if no localizing signs or signs of shock have developed, there is no certain way to distinguish these cases from the multitude of cases of acute viral illness. All patients with fever cannot and should not be treated as though they have a life-threatening infection. Appropriate use of this hypothesis at such an early stage is a rare and fortuitous event.

Keys Within History

In blocks 5 through 9 (Figure 10–2), specific elements of the history that are important in the investigation of FUO are considered. If possible, all drug regimens should be discontinued, not only because they may cause a fever but also because they may interfere with subsequent laboratory investigations.

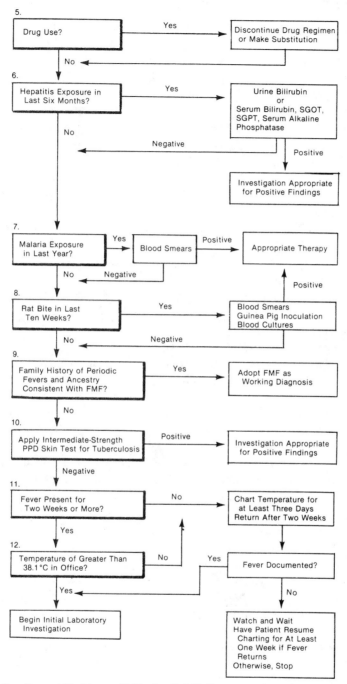

Figure 10–2. Keys within history. FMF = familial Mediterranean fever; PPD = purified protein derivative.

Fever is usually not severe in cases of hepatitis, but this may be the only symptom other than fatigue in the prodrome of this disease. A test of the urine for bilirubin is safe, quick, and inexpensive. Blood tests are less desirable first alternatives, but they do have the advantage of providing more specific information and are necessary should the test for urine bilirubin prove to be positive.

Malaria exposure again has become rare for Americans, but if exposure is reported, then thin smears treated with Wright's or Giemsa stains should be examined. Thick preparations should be made only by those persons familiar with the technique and its interpretation, since artifacts are common.

Rat-bite fever may be caused by two agents. *Spirillum minus* may be identified in blood smears from the patient or through the technique of inoculation into the abdominal cavity of guinea pigs or mice. *Streptobacillus moniliformis* may be cultured from the blood with special media; however, the organism grows slowly and may take from two to seven days to appear.

Fever without accompanying serositis is relatively rare in familial Mediterranean fever, but this diagnosis should be considered in patients with an appropriate family history or ancestry. It has been most commonly reported among peoples of the Mediterranean basin (Sephardic Jews, Armenians, Arabs, and Italians). However, the disease has been reported in many other groups, particularly Ashkenazic Jews and the Irish. The diagnosis can only be made on the basis of the characteristic syndrome of periodic fevers accompanied by peritonitis or pleuritis or both; therefore, the patient should be observed for the appearance of the other characteristics of the syndrome.

Tuberculosis remains the most frequent ultimate diagnosis in FUO. While this diagnosis now is most common in the elderly, it should be considered in all age groups and especially in young, dark-skinned persons. In this latter group, a majority will have extrapulmonary disease only, thus adding to the difficulty of making the diagnosis. The skin test for this disease is quick, safe, and inexpensive. While a positive test does not assure the diagnosis, a negative test makes tuberculosis unlikely. (Anergy in severe tuberculosis is associated with symptoms other than those of the FUO syndrome and, therefore, is unlikely to be a source of error in the algorithm.)

If the fever has not been present for two weeks or if the patient is afebrile when examined, then a period of observation and charting of the temperature is appropriate. Fevers of less than two weeks' duration disappear so frequently without any intervention that even the most modest set of laboratory examinations cannot be recommended.

A great deal has been made of various patterns of fevers. However, the fever pattern in general cannot be relied on to indicate an appropriate line of investigation. Perhaps only the fever of malaria presents so striking a pattern as to suggest a diagnosis. The algorithm calls for several examinations of the blood smear as part of the complete blood cell count if the fever is persistent, even if the patient does not give a history of exposure to malaria and there is no fever pattern.

Initial Laboratory Investigations

When a patient has had a fever for more than two weeks, a few procedures, easily done and with little accompanying risk, should be performed (Figure 10–3). These tests are primarily aimed at giving the greatest possibility of constructing a pattern of laboratory findings and clinical factors that will define a syndrome other than FUO. These tests are more sensitive than specific and should show some abnormality in the most common causes of prolonged fever. If the fever cannot be documented, then a strategy of watchful waiting should be adopted.

If the set of laboratory examinations from block 13 fails to define a syndrome other than FUO, then a further period of observation and charting of temperature is warranted. During this one-week period, an effort should be made to have at least some of the temperatures taken by an independent observer, with the simultaneous recording of pulse. As the number of negative laboratory examinations increases, so does the probability of factitious fever, and this possibility must be given increasing weight. Clues to factitious fever include failure of temperatures to follow the usual diurnal pattern, failure of pulse to correlate with temperature, rapid defervescence without sweating, and high temperatures without accompanying prostration. At the end of this period, if the fever continues and is verified, then a more elaborate set of laboratory examinations is indicated.

After the examinations in block 16 are completed, the majority of patients will have either defervesced spontaneously or will have a syndrome that is distinguishable from FUO. The few remaining patients may be observed for one more week; during this time, it is imperative that as many temperature measurements as possible be taken by an independent observer and that these are correlated with pulse. Only in a small number of patients will it be necessary to consider hospitalization.

Hospitalization

The primary reasons for hospitalization are to (1) objectively document fever during 48 hours in a situation in which the possibility of factitious fever can be minimized, and (2) perform certain procedures that may be difficult or impossible to do on an outpatient basis (Figure 10–4). In general, the best chance is that a syndrome will be defined either through the repeating of laboratory examinations previously done or with the addition of a few more indicated tests. However, bone marrow biopsy and culture and proctosigmoidoscopy have value and may be recommended. Liver biopsy may be especially helpful, primarily because of the propensity of systemic diseases to involve this organ. This is especially true in cases of tuberculosis. The bone marrow may show evidence of malignant disease or infection, and cultures of the aspirate should be performed.

After the results are received from the investigation conducted in the hospital, only the rarest of patients will remain within the category of FUO. In this

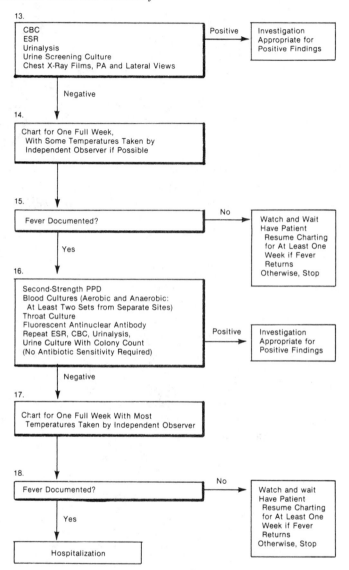

Figure 10–3. Initial laboratory investigations. CBC = complete blood cell; PPD = purified protein derivative; PA = posteroanterior; ESR = erythrocyte sedimentation rate.

situation, the recent literature suggests that the gallium scan has the ability to localize either abscess or tumor at relatively low risk.[4, 5] However, our own experience does not support this, and the recommendation must remain tentative until further information on the utility of the gallium scan is available. Under these circumstances, the probability of any other procedure yielding the answer is low. However, if the patient is incapacitated or is losing weight, then even these low-yield procedures should be considered, although they involve some haz-

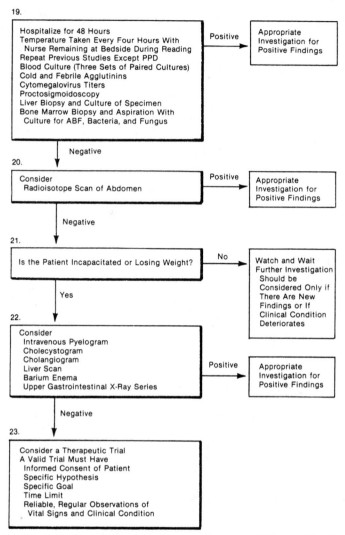

Figure 10—4. Hospitalization. PPD = purified protein derivative; AFB = acid-fast bacilli.

ard to the patient and are expensive. If some of the suggested procedures can be eliminated in the individual case, it will be to the patient's advantage. Fortunately, the probability of having to embark on such a prolonged, extensive investigation is minimal, as the algorithm has defined a patient with more than a month of verified fever, in which all other reasonable laboratory studies have failed to define a syndrome, and in whom there is evidence of disease progress.

A therapeutic trial must be considered in patients who have substantial disability and in whom the diagnosis remains uncertain despite extensive investigation. A valid trial may prevent the needless repetition of expensive laboratory procedures and overcome the difficulty of dealing with equivocal or falsely negative laboratory data as well as cure the illness. One runs the risk of causing drug toxicity and superinfection with this action. To be worthwhile, the trial must be a valid test of a hypothesis. Shotgun antimicrobial therapy is inappropriate in such a trial. There are usually only four classes of therapy to be considered: (1) antituberculous agents, isoniazid with or without a second drug; (2) antibiotics, for endocarditis or sepsis; (3) chloroquine hydrochloride, for amebiasis or malaria; and (4) steroids, for polymyalgia rheumatica only.

The first will be the most frequently used in trials. The last is difficult to use because of nonspecific antipyretic effects. Block 23 outlines the guidelines for a therapeutic trial.

These algorithms do not include laparotomy. Laparotomy cannot be advised at any time without some indication of disease in the abdomen.[6]

James F. Fries, MD, assisted in the preparation of this manuscript.

References

1. Petersdorf RG, Beeson PB: Fever of unexplained origin: Report of 100 cases. *Medicine* 1961;40:1–30.
2. Feinstein AR: An analysis of diagnostic reasoning: III. The construction of clinical algorithms. *Yale J Biol Med* 1974;46:5–32.
3. Lundberg GD: The modern clinical laboratory: Justification, scope, and directions. *JAMA* 1975;232:528–529.
4. Habibian MR, Staab EV, Matthews HA: Gallium citrate GA 67 scans in febrile patients. *JAMA* 1975;233:1073–1076.
5. Kumar B, Coleman RE, Alderson PO: Gallium citrate GA 67 imaging in patients with suspected inflammatory processes. *Arch Surg* 1975;110:1237–1242.
6. Baker RR, Tumulty PA: The value of exploratory laparotomy in fever of unexplained etiology. *Johns Hopkins Med J* 1969;125:159–165.

Chapter 11

Joint Pain or Arthritis

James F. Fries, MD
Donald M. Mitchell, MD

One of six patient visits to a primary care physician is for a musculoskeletal complaint. Usually, the complaint is pain near joints or is attributed to "arthritis." In the terminology of many patients, "arthritis" is a synonym for musculoskeletal pain, rather than the medically understood synovial inflammation. We will attempt to provide guidelines for investigation of these complaints and for clinical formulation and decisions.

The American Rheumatism Association recognizes more than 100 musculoskeletal and articular conditions.[1] Many of these conditions closely resemble others, and precise diagnosis is, at times, extremely difficult.[2] We will deal only with the most common problems. The guidelines presented will be useful in the majority of cases and will provide a logical framework within which to categorize the problems.

We have considered three questions, each developed with a flow sheet, or algorithm: (1) Is laboratory evaluation required? (2) If required, which investigations are indicated? (3) After evaluation, how can the results of the investigations be used?

Laboratory Evaluation

Is laboratory evaluation required? In general, no. Of patients with musculoskeletal complaints in the primary care setting, the majority will not have "arthritis" or other joint disease by the definition of a physician. Most will have localized traumatic conditions or nonspecific myalgic syndromes. Only a small percentage will have significant rheumatic disease. Moreover, even when disease is considered likely, in most cases no therapeutic opportunity will have been missed by a delay of weeks or even months.

From: Joint Pain or Arthritis. *JAMA* 1976;235:199–204. Copyright 1976 by the American Medical Association.

Table 11–1.
Laboratory Investigations.

Procedure	Location		
	Physician's Office Laboratory	Community Hospital Laboratory	Referral Hospital Laboratory
Serum chemistry			
Uric acid		●	
Triiodothronine (T$_4$)		●	
Creatine phosphokinase		●	
Aldolase		●	
Hematology			
Complete blood cell count (hematocrit; hemoglobin; white blood cell, differential cell counts; platelets on smear)	●		
Erythrocyte sedimentation rate	●		
Serologic tests			
Latex fixation (rheumatoid factor) titer		●	
Fluorescent antinuclear antibody		●	
Antistreptolysin O		●	
Anti-DNA antibody			●
Serum complement			●
X-ray films			
Affected area		●	
Sacroiliac joints		●	
Barium swallow		●	
Small-bowel series		●	
Barium enema		●	
Cultures			
Blood		●	
Cervix		●	
Joint fluid		●	
Synovial fluid			
Joint fluid crystals		●	
Biopsy			
Muscle (proximal)		●	
Temporal artery		●	
Electromyogram			●
Sigmoidoscopy	●		
Genotype			
HLA-W27			●

Excessively aggressive laboratory investigations may be detrimental in several ways. The total charge for the laboratory procedures listed in Table 11–1 exceeds $800 in most facilities. While serious harmful effects from these tests are rare, inconvenience and discomfort may occur with several. False-positive laboratory results leading to further tests, excessive concern, patient dependency,

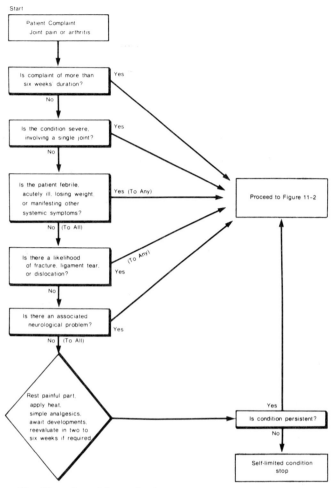

Figure 11—1. Algorithm of need for evaluation.

erroneous diagnostic labeling, and unnecessary and hazardous drug administration are common in this disease area.

Therefore, usually, no laboratory investigation is indicated when a patient is first seen in the primary care setting. Ordinarily, rest, heat, and mild analgesic treatment provide a reasonable initial therapeutic approach. Observation, patience, and periodic reevaluation are appropriate. If the condition is persistent for more than two to six weeks, more complete investigation is indicated.

Important exceptions to the general approach of symptomatic treatment, observation, and reevaluation are indicated in Figure 11—1. On occasion, the severity of the condition or associated objective clinical signs mandate immediate thorough investigation. These include single joint involvement, where septic arthritis, acute gouty or "microcrystalline" arthritis, and significant trauma with a possibility of fracture, ligament injury, or dislocation may require immediate attention. When systemic symptoms such as fever, weight loss, skin rash, or other evidence of multisystem disease are present, thorough evaluation should proceed unless an obvious self-limited condition is present. Such patients may have systemic lupus erythematosus, underlying malignancies, subacute bacterial endocarditis, or other major and treatable illnesses. Associated neurological problems such as pain in a sciatic nerve distribution, the carpal tunnel syndrome, and cervical nerve root compression syndromes are benefited by immediate attention. When this algorithm is applied, the large majority of patients with initial complaints of "joint pain" or "arthritis" will be found *not* to have serious conditions requiring immediate evaluation.

Indicated Investigations

Table 11–1 lists nine types of laboratory investigation, each of which is sometimes required in evaluation of joint pain or arthritis. On some occasions, additional investigations may be necessary. For most patients, only a few tests are required. If a test has been recently performed or the clinical situation is obvious, even these tests need not be invariably ordered. Most listed are widely available. Some are not, but are included because of their importance in categorization of the patient with rheumatic disease. Without all tests, the algorithms in Figures 11–2 and 11–3 are less complete but are still useful. For example, anti-DNA antibody and serum complement are of particular use in identification and stratification of patients with systemic lupus erythematosus. Identification of the white blood cell histocompatibility antigen, HLA-W27, is assuming increasing importance in diagnosis. In certain of the previously termed "rheumatoid variants" such as ankylosing spondylitis and Reiter syndrome, this antigen is nearly always present.

Many laboratory investigations in rheumatic disease often yield false-positive or false-negative results. This is exemplified by rheumatoid arthritis and rheumatoid factor tests, gouty arthritis and serum uric acid elevation, and inflammatory diseases and the erythrocyte sedimentation rate (ESR). A few tests are relatively specific: demonstration of urate or calcium pyrophosphate crystals in joint fluid, culture of a specific organism, identification of myositis or temporal arteritis by biopsy, and perhaps the identification of HLA-W27. Occasionally, even these tests may give a normal result even when there is disease. The fluorescent antinuclear antibody test and the ESR are useful particularly because of their sensitivity. However, their specificity is low, with relatively frequent false-positive results.

Figure 11–2 presents a framework for choosing particular tests in individual clinical situations. It begins with the assumption that the first algorithm (Figure 11–1) has indicated a need for further investigation by the presence of arthritis or joint pain and a severe, systemic, persistent, or monoarticular problem.

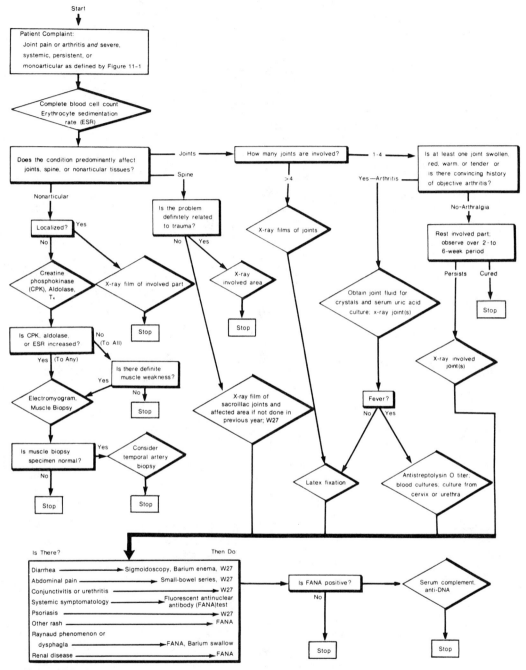

Figure 11–2. Algorithm of indicated investigations. Proceed through algorithm until a "stop" box is reached, then go to Figure 11–3.

Usually, a complete blood cell count and ESR are obtained. This provides a base line against which future disease progression or drug toxicity can be compared, a screening for serious diseases not discussed in these algorithms, and an aid to differentiation of organic and functional disease. Further choice of tests depends on the particular clinical manifestations. The initial branch requires identification of the condition as *predominantly* affecting the joints, the spine, or the nonarticular tissues; when the condition predominantly affects the joints, determine the number of joints involved and whether *objective* arthritis is present. Joint fluid examination should be carried out when objective arthritis involves only a few joints. In such cases, it is essential to search for crystals and to culture for organisms. On occasion, synovial white blood cell count and mucin clot test may be of use in distinguishing inflammatory from noninflammatory processes. With polyarticular conditions, determination of the latex fixation titer is frequently more important. Accompanying complaints may suggest involvement of other organ systems; these require additional investigation as indicated in the large box. "Fever" refers to an oral temperature above 37.5°C (99.6°F). When appropriate, studies to verify preceding streptococcal disease, concurrent sepsis, or venereal infection should be performed at this stage. In patients with polyarthritis, x-ray examination usually does not require a complete survey of all joints. Posteroanterior views of the hands and the most severely involved joints will frequently suffice. The usual clinical error is to order an unnecessarily wide "skeletal survey." In general, changes on x-ray film occur slowly and require considerable disease duration before detectable change.

When the condition predominantly affects the spine or sacroiliac joints, determination of its relationship to trauma is important. If a traumatic cause is not obvious, consideration of possible associated conditions is indicated.

Nonarticular conditions are frequently the most perplexing to categorize satisfactorily. Usually, such problems are less severe and more likely to be self-limited. The localized nonarticular problem usually requires little evaluation beyond appropriate x-ray films; these may not even be required in all patients. The generalized problem requires investigation for the possible presence of an active myositis or polymyalgia rheumatica; most patients will have less well-defined musculoskeletal syndromes. When a biopsy of muscle tissue is indicated, a symptomatic, proximal muscle such as the deltoid is preferred.

Clinical Interpretation

Figures 11–1 and 11–2 have used a limited clinical and laboratory database. Obviously, such a database is not adequate for rigorous diagnosis in every case. However, the data are suitable for accurate clinical categorization, and in most cases will provide sufficient information to allow differentiation between the entities of the particular category. Moreover, categorization of rheumatic conditions under the eight proposed headings provides a useful guide to clinical thinking, and has therapeutic implications.

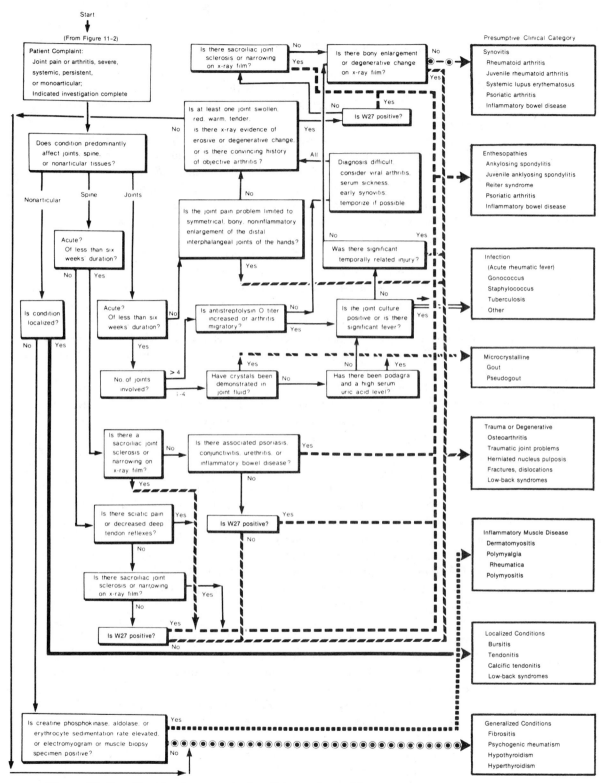

Figure 11–3. Algorithm for categorization of rheumatic conditions.

Figure 11–3 may be applied after completion of the preceding two algorithms. Here, consideration is given to patients in whom the indicated investigations are complete. Use of this algorithm will result in assigning a particular patient to a clinical category.

The first category is that of synovitis, in which the pathologic process consists primarily of an inflammatory reaction in the synovial tissue. Rheumatoid arthritis is the classic example; this process is also seen in juvenile rheumatoid arthritis, systemic lupus erythematosus, psoriatic arthritis, and other conditions.

We have used the term "enthesopathy" for the second category.[3] This suggests that the primary site of inflammation is the enthesis, which is the narrow region where tendon and ligament attach to and become, in transition, bone. This group of diseases was previously termed the rheumatoid variants. There is a strong predilection for involvement of the spine and sacroiliac joints, for serologic abnormalities such as rheumatoid factor to be extremely uncommon, and for the pathologic process to be characterized by periostitis and new bone formation.[4] Primary involvement appears to be outside of the synovial space. More recently, entities in this category have been linked by the common presence of the genotype, HLA-W27. The W27 antigen is found in only 5% of the normal population. Ankylosing spondylitis is the prototype disease, and W27 is present in virtually every patient.[5] Some traditional diagnostic entities, such as psoriatic arthritis and arthropathies accompanying inflammatory bowel disease, sometimes fall in the synovitis category, and sometimes within the group of enthesopathies.

Third is infection. The prototype condition here is direct infection of the synovial space, but we have included in this category acute rheumatic fever, which is not an infection in the usual sense but follows streptococcal disease. An electrocardiogram may be of additional help in this setting.

The fourth category is that of microcrystalline synovitis, in which the pathologic process is characterized by crystal formation within the synovial space and an accompanying strong inflammatory reaction. Gout is the prototype condition, but crystals other than uric acid can provoke similar syndromes.

Fifth are the syndromes associated with trauma or degenerative change. The largest single entity in this category is osteoarthritis, and indeed, this condition is the most common rheumatic disease problem.

Sixth is muscle disease in which the primary pathologic condition consists of inflammation predominantly involving the skeletal muscle. Polymyositis and dermatomyositis are the best known of these entities. Polymyalgia rheumatica is probably more common. In this recently emphasized entity, myalgia is prominent but inflammation in the muscles has not been conclusively demonstrated.

In the seventh category we have included a variety of localized conditions. Many of these are not diseases in the usual sense but are local inflammatory or traumatic problems.

Finally, we have noted the group of generalized conditions, which also are not clearly defined disease entities. In some circumstances, a condition defined as "fibrositis" implies organic pathologic causes although objective evidence is lacking. In other cases, psychogenic factors appear clearly the most important. These conditions are nonprogressive but often recalcitrant.

In the rheumatic diseases, use of clinical information requires integration of clinical observations with laboratory tests. In following Figure 11–3, both clinical findings and laboratory results are used. Some tests obtained in response to Figure 11–2 are not used in Figure 11–3, but remain important in distinguishing entities within a clinical category, in staging severity of condition, as a baseline for following future progression, and for prognosis.

Management programs are associated with particular clinical categories. The rational therapeutic approach to synovitis is an attempt to reduce inflammation in the synovial membrane. Therapeutic doses of salicylates, gold salts, hydroxychloroquine sulfate, synovectomy, and other therapeutic modalities may be required. Antibiotics or pure analgesics without anti-inflammatory actions are much less appropriate. In the enthesopathies, anti-inflammatory agents are again indicated; however, aspirin treatment is frequently disappointing. Phenylbutazone and indomethacin are particularly effective in these disorders. Inflammation induced by microcrystals again responds somewhat differently to therapy. In this instance, colchicine, phenylbutazone, and indomethacin are generally the most useful agents. Infection in the joint space is, of course, best managed by appropriate systemic antibiotic therapy, sometimes in conjunction with drainage procedures.

The traumatic and degenerative arthritides are managed with mild analgesics, weight reduction, physical methods, and sometimes with surgery. Major anti-inflammatory approaches are of little benefit in most cases. Inflammation in the muscles usually requires corticosteroids for control. Localized conditions, on the other hand, usually require only localized therapeutic approaches. Resting the involved part, heat, and local infiltration of procaine or corticosteroids are frequently successful. Finally, the generalized conditions are managed conservatively and with appropriate attention to the psychological factors operating. Thus, significant differences exist in the treatment of patients in different clinical categories.

Comment

Clinical judgment in utilizing these guidelines is required.[6] On occasion, a test may be redundant or obviously unnecessary. On other occasions, repeat evaluation of dubious laboratory values or elaboration by further tests not discussed is indicated. Any complicated problem mandates a complete history and physical examination. Some rheumatic diseases are not discussed here. Conditions omitted are either sufficiently rare that they would not be expected to be encountered in 1,000 consecutive patients seen in the primary care setting, or are quite unlikely to manifest as "joint pain."

If these algorithms are applied widely, the implications are profound but conjectural. The number of patients with these problems is large; hence, any major change in investigative or therapeutic strategy would be expected to have a large effect. However, there are no data presently available from which to calculate the direction of this effect. If fewer tests are currently being performed than are advocated in these algorithms, the cost of diagnosis could rise by their consistent application. If tests are currently used less selectively, or with less diagnostic usefulness, the cost of care might go down. In either case, the effect on the quality of care is uncertain. As teaching aids, use of algorithms has obvious advantages. They provide information with brevity and clarity. Knowledge is represented in the context of logic, resulting in explicit notation of decision processes. Clearly, alternative formulations to those presented here are possible, and could also possess the virtues of clarity, brevity, and explicit definition of logic. There is presently no way to compare alternative constructions against objective data and in terms of clinical outcome.[7] Thus, the placing of undue reliance on these algorithms either by individual physicians or by health care planners might prove unwise. The technology for collecting and analyzing large bodies of actual clinical data for these purposes is in place.[8, 9] The questions raised by clinical constructs such as the foregoing raise the critical issue of accumulating data for verification, optimization, and validation.

This study was supported by a Clinical Scholar award and Clinical Center grant from the Arthritis Foundation, Clinical Immunology Center grant AI 11313 from the National Institutes of Health, and a grant from the Canadian Arthritis and Rheumatism Society.

References

1. *Primer on Rheumatic Diseases*. The Arthritis Foundation, 1972.
2. Hollander JL, McCarty DJ: *Arthritis and Allied Conditions: A Textbook of Rheumatology*. Philadelphia, Lea & Febiger, 1972.
3. Ball J: Enthesopathy of rheumatoid and ankylosing spondylitis. *Ann Rheum Dis* 1971;30:213–223.
4. Moll JMH, Haslock I, Macras IF, et al: Associations between ankylosing spondylitis, psoriatic arthritis, Reiter's disease, the intestinal arthropathies, and Behcet's syndrome. *Medicine* 1974;53:343–364.
5. Brewerton DA, Caffrey M, Nicholls A, et al: The histocompatibility antigen (HL-A 27) and its relation to disease. *J Rheumatol* 1974;1:249–253.
6. Fries JF: Experience counting in sequential computer diagnosis. *Arch Intern Med* 1970;126:647–651.
7. Fries JF, Hess EV, Klinenberg J: A standard database for rheumatic disease. *Arthritis Rheum* 1974;17:327–335.
8. Fries JF: Time-oriented patient records and a computer databank. *JAMA* 1972; 222:1536–1542.
9. Fries JF, Weyl S, Holman HR: Estimating prognosis in systemic lupus erythematosus. *Am J Med* 1974;57:561–565.

Chapter 12

Infertility in the Male

Ronald S. Swerdloff, MD
Stephen P. Boyers, MD

The first and most important rule in the evaluation of infertility is to consider the problem from the standpoint of both members of the couple. Too often a woman is extensively investigated only to discover later that her husband is azoospermic, and, likewise, a man undergoes lengthy treatment for oligospermia while his wife has undiagnosed tubal obstruction or has anovulatory cycles. The evaluation of both the man and woman should proceed in parallel until a significant problem is uncovered. Ideal management is attained in a clinical setting where the couple is seen by a team of physicians. In the usual case, where the man is under the care of either an endocrinologist or a urologist and the woman is under the care of a gynecologist, communication between physicians must be ongoing.

The male partner should undergo a complete history and physical examination with special emphasis on the reproductive system. The history should include questions regarding prescribed medications; alcohol, other drug, and marijuana abuse; systemic illnesses; and exposure to industrial and environmental toxins. Potency, sexual techniques, and frequency of intercourse must be queried. Evidence of underandrogenization includes decreased beard, mustache, and chest hair, eunuchoid proportions, and gynecomastia. Hypospadias may represent a mechanical cause of impaired sperm delivery or indicate underandrogenization during early fetal development. Scrotal examination will detect abnormal testes, spermatocele, varicoceles, and absent vas deferens. Small testes (<4.0 cm in longest diameter or <15 cc by orchidometer) indicate impaired germinal tissue mass, either due to primary testicular failure or hypothalamic-pituitary insufficiency. Scrotal examination of a standing patient performing the Valsalva maneuver will assist in the diagnosis of smaller varicoceles.

The semen analysis is the cornerstone of the evaluation of the potentially infertile man.[1] Semen samples should be collected by masturbation (after one to

---

From: Evaluation of the Male Partner of an Infertile Couple. An Algorithmic Approach. *JAMA* 1982;247:2418–2422. Copyright 1982 by the American Medical Association.

two days' abstinence) in a clean, dry, widemouthed container provided by the physician. The specimen should be obtained either in the physician's office or at home, but in the latter case, the specimen should be kept warm and be transported to the physician's office within one hour of collection. If the patient objects to masturbation for personal or religious reasons, coitus interruptus or collection in a special plastic condom can be used. Strict Roman Catholics may require perforation of the condom before collection. The time of collection should be noted on all specimens. Sperm count, motility, and morphology must be assessed. Since there is considerable variability in sperm number in semen samples from individual fertile patients, a minimum of three semen samples must be obtained before a patient can be identified as being azoospermic (no sperm) or oligospermic (low sperm concentrations). While the lower limit for a normal sperm concentration is somewhat controversial, we have defined oligospermia as less than 20 million sperm per milliliter. Once the patient is determined to be either azoospermic or consistently oligospermic, hormonal testing should be done. Because of the sporadic nature of hormone secretion, we routinely obtain three blood samples at least 20 minutes apart and pool the serum before measurement of luteinizing hormone (LH), follicle-stimulating hormone (FSH), and testosterone levels.[2-4] The results of these tests are essential for the characterization of the patient's problem and determination of the therapeutic approach.

Azoospermia

In the azoospermic patient, four hormonal patterns may be seen.

Low Serum Testosterone, Elevated LH, Elevated FSH (Figure 12–1). Such patients have primary testicular failure involving both the Leydig cells (testosterone secretion) and germinal elements (sperm production). The elevated serum gonadotropin levels distinguish primary testicular insufficiency from hypothalamic-pituitary disease. Patients with pantesticular insufficiency do not respond to any known therapy, and artificial insemination-donor (AID) or adoption should be discussed.

Normal Testosterone, Normal LH, Elevated FSH (Figure 12–1). These results may be seen in azoospermic or severely oligospermic patients with primary germinal tubular failure without associated Leydig cell damage. The reason for the increase in the FSH level is unclear, but many believe that these patients have a deficiency of a selective FSH inhibitor (inhibin) that is normally produced in the spermatogenic tubules (Sertoli cells).[5] From a therapeutic standpoint, these patients are similar to the primary panhypogonadal patients described previously, and AID or adoption should be discussed.

Low Testosterone, Low LH, Low FSH (Figure 12–2). Such patients have hypogonadotropic hypogonadism on either a congenital or acquired basis. Anosmia is often found in patients with congenital LH and FSH deficiency. All patients with hypogonadotropic hypogonadism should be tested for deficiencies of other pituitary hormones (thyroid-stimulating hormone [TSH], adrenocorticotropic hor-

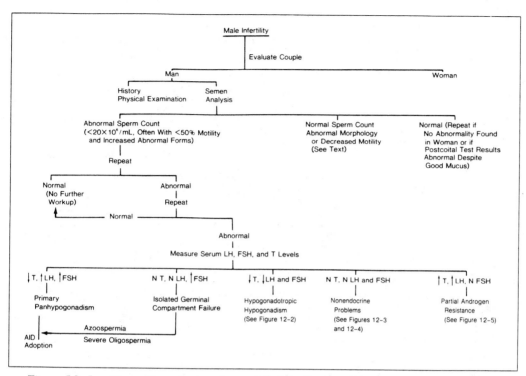

Figure 12–1. Diagnostic evaluation of potentially infertile man. LH = luteinizing hormone; FSH = follicle-stimulating hormone; T = testosterone; N = normal; AID = artificial insemination-donor.

Figure 12–2. Evaluation and treatment of patient with hypogonadotropic hypogonadism. T = testosterone; LH = luteinizing hormone; FSH = follicle-stimulating hormone; ACTH = adrenocorticotropic hormone; TSH = thyroid-stimulating hormone; GH = growth hormone; PRL = prolactin; hCG = human chorionic gonadotropin; hMG = menotropins (human menopausal gonadotropin); LHRH = gonadotropin-releasing hormone (leuteinizing hormone-releasing hormone).

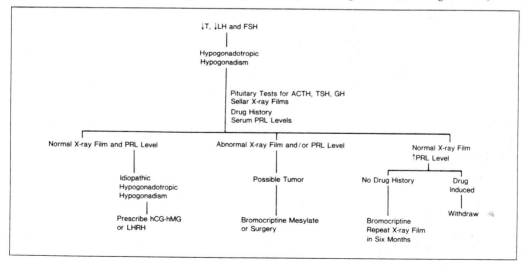

mone [ACTH], and possibly growth hormone [GH]). Serum prolactin level should be measured, as it is elevated in many patients with pituitary tumors.[4] A careful neurologic examination, including visual field testing and appropriate sellar films, which may include sellar polytomograms, should be performed. Anorexia nervosa and severe malnutrition will be suggested by physical examination. Abnormal sellar x-ray films with or without an elevated serum prolactin level suggest a pituitary adenoma. Such patients may require further endocrinologic evaluation. Some patients may have hyperprolactinemia without a detectable sellar abnormality. The list of pathogenic mechanisms is extensive, but these most commonly occur with antidopaminergic drugs and small pituitary microadenomas.

Patients with hypogonadotropic hypogonadism can be treated for infertility with replacement gonadotropins. Human chorionic gonadotropin (hCG) and menotropins (human menopausal gonadotropin, hMG [Pergonal]) are used for this purpose. Experimental treatment with a regimen of frequent small pulse doses of the hypothalamic hormone, gonadotropin releasing hormone (luteinizing hormone-releasing hormone [LHRH]), has been successful in inducing fertility.[6] Treatment of patients with pituitary tumors is beyond the scope of this chapter on the evaluation of the infertile patient. However, patient management may include either surgery, radiotherapy, or bromocriptine mesylate.

Normal Testosterone, LH, and FSH (Figure 12–3). Azoospermic patients with this hormonal pattern have either retrograde ejaculation or an obstruction of the ejaculatory system. Azoospermia due to impaired spermatogenesis without obstruction is usually associated with an elevated level of serum FSH.[7] The distinction between these disorders is important, since many obstructive problems can be approached surgically.

Figure 12–3. Diagnostic evaluation of azoospermic man. N = normal; T = testosterone; LH = luteinizing hormone; FSH = follicle-stimulating hormone.

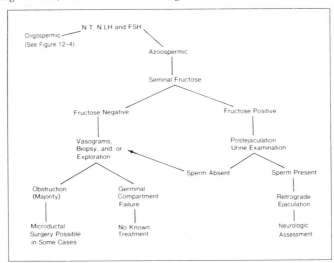

Fructose is normally produced by the seminal vesicles and transported into the vas deferens by the ejaculatory ducts. Absent seminal fructose usually indicates congenital absence or obstruction of the seminal vesicles and vas deferens. Such patients may have the absence of the cauda epididymis and vas deferens noted on the physical examination of the scrotal contents.

In most patients, an obstruction of the seminal excretory pathway occurs proximal to the excretory ducts of the seminal vesicles with resultant normal semen fructose concentrations and normal testicular mass on examination. In such patients, exploration, vasograms, and testicular biopsy may be required to define the nature of the obstructive defect.

Retrograde ejaculation is suspected by the presence of autonomic neuropathy and is most frequently seen in patients with diabetes mellitus. The presence of large numbers of sperm in postejaculation urine specimens confirms the diagnosis.

Oligospermia

Low Testosterone, Elevated LH, Elevated FSH (Figure 12–1). These patients have primary gonadal insufficiency and are treated in general as in the first azoospermic group. If the oligospermia is moderate (10 to 20 $\times$ 10^6 sperm per milliliter), insemination with the first portion of a split ejaculate may be worthwhile.

Normal Testosterone, Normal LH, Elevated FSH (Figure 12–1). These patients usually have severe oligospermia secondary to damage of the germinal elements. They are treated as the second azoospermic group.

Low Testosterone, Low/Normal LH and FSH (Figure 12–2). These oligospermic patients usually have partial deficiencies of gonadotropin secretion, most likely on the basis of acquired hypothalamic or pituitary disease. A serum prolactin level should be measured in these patients. An elevated serum prolactin level may indicate a pituitary tumor. Treatment must be determined by the nature of the pathologic findings, but lowering of the serum prolactin level frequently returns gonadal function to normal.[8] Patients with a hypothalamic-pituitary cause for oligospermia are treated as described for the third azoospermic group.

The majority of very obese men and an occasional lean patient may have normal serum LH and FSH levels and a low total testosterone level. The latter finding occurs as a result of decreased sex hormone binding protein.[9] Such patients are not actually hypogonadal as confirmed by a normal serum free-testosterone level.

Normal Testosterone, LH, and FSH (Figure 12–4). This hormonal pattern is seen in the majority of oligospermic patients. Patients with varicoceles should be treated by ligation of their internal spermatic vein. The remainder of these patients are now categorized as having idiopathic oligospermia, and several forms of therapy have been proposed. These include insemination with the first

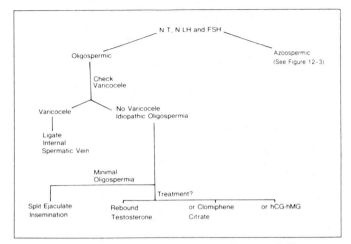

Figure 12—4. Diagnostic evaluation of oligospermic man. N = normal; T = testosterone; LH = luteinizing hormone; FSH = follicle-stimulating hormone; hCG = human chorionic gonadotropin; hMG = menotropins (human menopausal gonadotropin).

portion of a split ejaculate, rebound treatment with testosterone, or treatment with clomiphene citrate or with hCG-hMG.[1] None of these treatments has been shown to be unequivocally beneficial in carefully controlled studies. If one of these therapies is instituted, a time limit should be invoked, after which the options of AID or adoption should be discussed. When the man has oligospermia, the woman should be evaluated to ensure that subfertility does not exist in both members of the couple.

High-Normal-to-Elevated Testosterone and LH, With Low-Normal-to-Low FSH (Figure 12–5). These patients have partial androgen resistance (a deficient cellular response to testosterone) resulting in a secondary increase in serum LH level. Because the testes are continually stimulated by LH, the secretion rate of testosterone and estradiol is increased. Since a small percentage of testosterone is normally converted to estradiol by aromatization, serum estradiol levels are usually elevated. Serum estradiol measurement will support this diagnosis. The increased estradiol/testosterone ratio often produces gynecomastia. Many patients have evidence of impaired androgen response during fetal genital development, resulting in pseudohermaphroditism, which in its mild form may present as hypospadias. Germinal failure presumably occurs as a result of decreased testosterone effect at the germinal cell level. Diagnosis is likely on the basis of the above hormonal pattern, but absolute confirmation requires the measurement of tissue androgen receptors in specialized laboratories. No known therapy is available for the oligospermia seen in such patients.

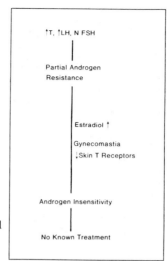

Figure 12–5. Diagnostic evaluation of patient with partial androgen resistance. T = testosterone; LH = luteinizing hormone; FSH = follicle-stimulating hormone; N = normal.

Normal Sperm Counts but Abnormal Morphology or Motility

Necrospermia. Dead sperm can be identified with supravital stains. While no treatment is available for necrospermia, recent discovery of abnormal sperm metabolism in several such patients may presage a period of specific therapies.[1]

Abnormal Sperm Motility or Morphology. This is usually seen in oligospermic specimens but can occur in men with normal counts. Abnormal sperm forms indicate impaired spermatogenesis. Decreased motility may occur with structural or metabolic defects of sperm or may represent a hostile semen environment. The presence of inflammatory cells suggests genital tract infection, indicating the need for appropriate culture and antibiotic treatment.

Agglutination may indicate the presence of antisperm antibodies. Serum sperm agglutination antibodies (usually IgG) can be measured with positive titers found in the sera of 2% to 13% of subfertile men and up to 2% of fertile men.[10–12] These autoantibodies rarely get into the seminal plasma, but their presence in serum may serve as a marker for local production of IgA antisperm antibodies in the genital tract. A causal relationship between serum sperm agglutinating antibodies and male infertility has not been unequivocably established.

Conclusion

This algorithmic approach to the evaluation of the male partner of an infertile couple uses the combination of careful history and physical examination, careful semen analysis, and specific hormonal testing procedures to aid the physician in the diagnostic assessment of the patient's problem. We believe this approach is helpful in planning therapy. Unfortunately, we are hampered in the evaluation of the infertile man by insufficient understanding of the pathogenesis of many causes of impaired spermatogenesis, inadequate means of assessing the true fertility potential of patients with oligospermia, and insufficient data evaluating therapeutic approaches to the latter problems.

References

1. Sherins RJ, Howards SS: Male infertility, in Harrison JH, Gittes RF, Perlmutter PD, et al (eds): *Campbell's Urology*, ed 4. Philadelphia, WB Saunders Co, 1979, pp 715–776.

2. Swerdloff RS, Glass AR: Male reproductive abnormalities, in Hershman JM (ed): *Endocrine Pathophysiology: A Patient Oriented Approach*. Philadelphia, Lea & Febiger, 1977, p 177.

3. Swerdloff RS: Physiology of male reproduction—hypothalamic-pituitary function: The hypothalamic-pituitary-gonadal axis, in Harrison JH, Gittes RF, Perlmutter PD, et al (eds): *Campbell's Urology*, ed 4. Philadelphia, WB Saunders Co, 1979, pp 125–133.

4. Odell WD, Swerdloff RS: Abnormalities of gonadal function in man. *Clin Endocrinol* 1978;8:149–180.

5. Baker HWG, Bremner WJ, Burger HG, et al: Testicular control of FSH secretion. *Recent Prog Horm Res* 1976;37:1429–1465.

6. Keogh EJ, Bertolini J: Treatment of Kallmann's syndrome by pulsatile administration of GnRH, in Abstracts of the Serono Symposium: Endocrinology of Human Infertility. Oxford, England, September 1980.

7. DeKretser DM: The endocrinology of male infertility. *Br Med Bull* 1979;35:187–192.

8. Franks S, Jacobs HS, Martin N, et al: Hyperprolactinemia and impotence. *Clin Endocrinol* 1978;8:277–287.

9. Glass AR, Swerdloff RS, Bray GA, et al: Low serum testosterone and sex-hormone-binding-globulin in massively obese men. *J Clin Endocrinol Metab* 1977;45:1211–1219.

10. Hendry WF, Morgan H, Stedronska J: The clinical significance of antisperm antibodies in male subfertility. *Br J Urol* 1977;49:757–762.

11. Halun A, Antonia D: Autoantibodies to spermatozoa in relation to male infertility and vasectomy. *Br J Urol* 1973;45:559–562.

12. Marmar JL: Functional role of spermagglutinating antibodies in men. *Fertil Steril* 1980;34:365.

Chapter 13

Splenomegaly

Edward R. Eichner, MD
Charles L. Whitfield, MD

Splenomegaly may be a presenting or dominant feature of certain diseases. Since the spleen enlarges in many conditions, a systematic approach may facilitate timely and cost-effective diagnosis of the cause of splenomegaly. The algorithms herein attempt to present a rational, step-by-step diagnostic approach. They consider the causes of splenomegaly in the rough order of their frequency, and they stress clues from the history, physical examination, and routine laboratory test results.

Normal Functions of the Spleen

In many instances, the spleen enlarges as it performs its normal functions. The four most important normal functions of the spleen are (1) clearance of microorganisms and particulate antigens from the bloodstream; (2) synthesis of immunoglobulin and properdin factors; (3) destruction of effete or abnormal red blood cells; and (4) embryonic hematopoiesis, which can reactivate as extramedullary hematopoiesis in certain diseases.

Mechanisms of Splenomegaly

There are six basic pathophysiologic mechanisms of splenomegaly: (1) immune response "work hypertrophy," as in subacute bacterial endocarditis, infectious mononucleosis, or Felty's syndrome; (2) red blood cell destruction "work hypertrophy," as in hereditary spherocytosis or thalassemia major; (3) congestive, as in cirrhosis or splenic vein thrombosis; (4) myeloproliferative, as in chronic myelocytic leukemia or myeloid metaplasia; (5) infiltrative, as in sarcoidosis,

From: Splenomegaly. An Algorithmic Approach to Diagnosis. *JAMA* 1981;246:2858–2861. Copyright 1981 by the American Medical Association.

amyloidosis, or Gaucher's disease; and (6) neoplastic, as in chronic lymphocytic leukemia, the lymphomas, and, rarely, in metastatic cancer. Miscellaneous causes of splenomegaly include trauma, cysts, and hemangiomas. The algorithms (Figures 13–1 and 13–2) include all of these conditions.

Detection and Significance of Splenomegaly

The following algorithms assume that splenomegaly has been documented. It might be noted that spleen size is not a reliable guide to spleen function, because palpable spleens are not always abnormal, and abnormal spleens are not always palpable. Patients with low diaphragms have palpable but normal-sized spleens, as do 3% of healthy college freshmen and almost 5% of hospital patients.[1] In contrast, clinical splenomegaly is rare in idiopathic (autoimmune) thrombocytopenic purpura, despite avid splenic destruction of antibody-coated platelets.

A careful physical examination for splenomegaly should include palpation with the patient supine and also in the right lateral decubitus position, with the knees up. Only light fingertip pressure should be applied, and the patient should inspire slowly. Some believe that splenic percussion can identify borderline enlargement; in the presence of splenomegaly, the percussion note in the lowest intercostal space in the left anterior axillary line changes from resonant to dull with full inspiration. It is clear, however, that mild splenomegaly may not be detectable on even the most careful physical examination. Roentgenographic examination of the abdomen can give a better evaluation of spleen size, but is of no help when the splenic outlines are not seen. A spleen length of more than 15 cm on roentgenogram will usually correlate with splenomegaly, but a normal spleen length on roentgenogram does not exclude moderate splenomegaly. Sometimes gastrointestinal barium studies can help outline an enlarged spleen.

The radioisotopic spleen scan with technetium Tc 99m sulfur colloid and gamma scintillation camera technique gives an excellent index of spleen size, provided that careful measurements are made in both the lateral and posterior projections. When the largest spleen area from these two projections is calculated, even mild splenomegaly can be distinguished from a normal spleen.[2] With splenic enlargement, the lateral area increases more than the posterior area. If only length is measured, or if splenic size is only approximated visually, the radioisotopic spleen scan can fail to identify mild splenomegaly. Although the computed tomographic (CT) scan has not yet been systematically applied to spleen sizing, the authors have seen a few instances in which the CT scan showed splenomegaly (increased horizontal dimension especially) where the radioisotopic spleen scan had been interpreted as normal. With careful measurements as described earlier, however, the radioisotopic scan is at least as good as the CT scan for spleen size, and is preferred because it also gives a picture of splenic reticuloendothelial function. For example, an enlarged spleen may show major areas of decreased radioisotope uptake in children with sickle cell anemia and in patients with extensive splenic infiltration with sarcoidosis or amyloidosis.[1] The CT scan, however, is probably more sensitive than the radioisotope scan in detecting small splenic lacerations, and should thus be considered when splenic trauma is suspected.[3]

Scope and Limitations of the Algorithms

The following algorithms are for adolescent and adult patients, not for children, and emphasize diseases found in the United States. They do not include therapy. The division into one algorithm for acute or subacute illness and another for chronic illness and for asymptomatic splenomegaly is arbitrary, but conforms to the authors' experience. The listing of disorders in rough order of their frequency is the authors' best estimate from personal experience and from review of the literature.[4-8] It is understood that an algorithm does not supplant a careful history and physical examination. Indeed, a careful history and physical examination may point to the obvious diagnosis and supplant the need for an algorithm.

Splenomegaly With Acute or Subacute Illness

Acute left upper quadrant pain with an enlarged, tender spleen suggests subcapsular hematoma or frank rupture of the spleen (Figure 13–1). By far the most common setting will be after trauma, as the algorithm indicates. Pathologic or spontaneous rupture of the spleen, however, is a well-known complication of acute infectious diseases, notably malaria, typhoid fever, and infectious mononucleosis, and also occurs in the acute and chronic leukemias, and, rarely, in the lymphomas.[9] Symptoms, physical findings, and routine roentgenograms can be helpful but sometimes misleading. The spleen scan is the mainstay for diagnosing subcapsular hematoma or rupture but sometimes produces false-negative results. The CT scan is increasingly valuable in diagnosing splenic laceration and is generally more readily available than selective splenic angiogram. Splenic angiogram is probably the most specific test for diagnosing splenic infarction, but a careful spleen scan often suffices here. Splenic abscesses, seen most often in subacute bacterial endocarditis, after seeding from peritonitis or abdominal surgery, or with disease in a contiguous organ, are usually, but not always, detected by spleen scan. In theory, the gallium citrate Ga 67 scan should complement the routine spleen scan in detecting splenic abscess, but such gallium scans are often difficult to interpret and are not yet recommended routinely.[10]

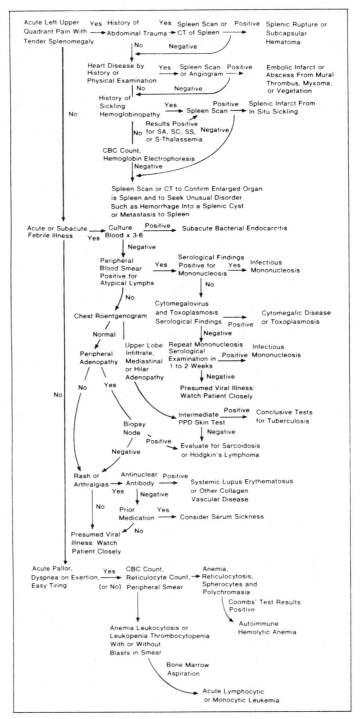

Figure 13–1. Algorithm for diagnostic assessment of splenomegaly with acute or subacute illness. CBC count = complete blood cell count; CT = computed tomography.

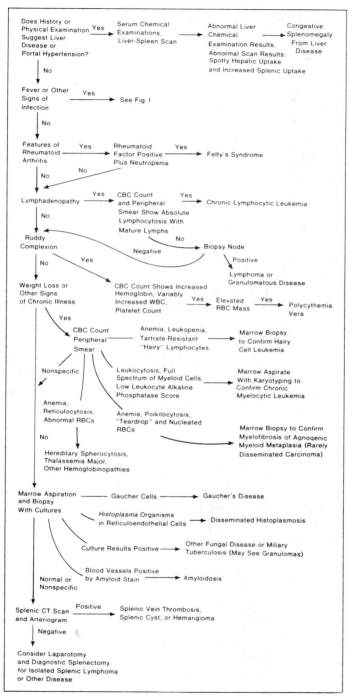

Figure 13—2. Algorithm for diagnostic assessment of splenomegaly with chronic illness or asymptomatic splenomegaly. CBC count = complete blood cell count; CT = computed tomography.

Splenomegaly With Chronic Illness or Asymptomatic Splenomegaly

Liver disease with portal hypertension is probably the most common cause of splenomegaly in this setting (Figure 13–2). Usually the liver disease is obvious by history, physical examination, or routine laboratory test results, such as the serum multichannel chemistry analysis. The liver-spleen scan usually shows decreased and patchy hepatic uptake along with increased splenic uptake ("reversed ratio"). Sometimes, however, the liver disease is occult and perhaps "burned out" so that the chemical test results for liver function are normal. Rarely, even the liver scan is normal. In these cases, liver biopsy may be necessary.

Patients with congestive splenomegaly from liver disease or from splenic vein thrombosis can be asymptomatic. Other common causes of asymptomatic splenomegaly are agnogenic myeloid metaplasia, Gaucher's disease, splenic cysts,[6] and, in the authors' experience, sarcoidosis, amyloidosis, and mild hereditary spherocytosis. While patients in the early stages of polycythemia vera or chronic myelocytic leukemia may be asymptomatic, the complete blood count and peripheral blood smear immediately suggest the diagnosis. The algorithm in Figure 13–2 shows the sequential diagnostic approach to all of these conditions.

In the United States, the following are among the relatively few diseases that now cause giant splenomegaly (defined as ten times or more the usual upper limit of normal weight of about 200 g) as a presenting or early feature: (1) agnogenic myeloid metaplasia, (2) chronic myelocytic leukemia, (3) hairy cell leukemia, (4) isolated splenic lymphoma, (5) Gaucher's disease, and (6) sarcoidosis. The algorithm also includes these diseases.

The decision to do diagnostic laparotomy to exclude isolated splenic lymphoma is sometimes difficult. While this decision will vary from patient to patient, the consensus seems to hold that when complete diagnostic studies fail to disclose the cause of splenomegaly, when the operative risk is not prohibitive, and especially when the patient has other signs of illness, splenomegaly of undetermined cause is an indication for splenectomy.[5]

References

1. Eichner ER: Splenic function: Normal, too much and too little. *Am J Med* 1979;66:311–320.
2. Westin J, Lanner L-O, Larsson A, et al: Spleen size in polycythemia: A clinical and scintigraphic study. *Acta Med Scand* 1972;191:263–271.
3. Mall JC, Kaiser JA: CT diagnosis of splenic laceration, *AJR* 1980;134:265–269.
4. Dameshek W: Splenomegaly—a problem in differential diagnosis. *Med Clin North Am*, 1957, pp 1257–1267.
5. Hermann RE, DeHaven KE, Hawk WA: Splenectomy for the diagnosis of splenomegaly. *Ann Surg* 1968;168:896–900.

6. Silverstein MN, Maldonado JE: Asymptomatic splenomegaly. *Postgrad Med* 1970; 45:80–85.

7. Goldstone J: Splenectomy for massive splenomegaly. *Am J Surg* 1978;135:385–388.

8. Traetow WD, Farti PJ, Carey LC: Changing indications for splenectomy. *Arch Surg* 1980; 115:447–451.

9. Andrews DF, Hernandez R, Grafton W, et al: Pathologic rupture of the spleen in non-Hodgkin's lymphoma. *Arch Intern Med* 1980; 140:119–120.

10. Chun CH, Raff MJ, Contreras L, et al: Splenic abscess. *Medicine* 1980;59:50–65.

Chapter 14

Evaluation of Obesity

George A. Bray, MD
Henry A. Jordan, MD
Ethan A. H. Sims, MD

Obesity ranks as one of the most common medical disorders in this country. Its importance lies in its association with many common diseases that may enhance morbidity and mortality. Yet, until recently, it has been one of the least-accurately characterized. When gross endocrine or other disease can be excluded, it is often the practice to categorize patients as having "exogenous obesity." Since all obesity is exogenous with respect to energy balance, this term contributes little to the understanding of the problem and ought to be discarded. Indeed, the term exogenous obesity has acquired a connotation of blaming the patient for allowing such a condition to develop. This term implies that obesity is a simple consequence of overeating and is in turn ascribed to human frailty or to emotional instability.[1] This is perhaps in part a consequence of our frustration in treating a difficult clinical problem.

Rapidly expanding knowledge has brought out important physiologic deviations from the norm in many types of obesity.[2] These and many other aspects of this problem are summarized in the report of the recent Fogarty International Conference on Obesity.[3] Many of the concepts presented here are derived from this Conference. The assessment of a patient with obesity extends beyond the mere attempt to identify specific metabolic disorders or disease states. Even if no disease entity or clinical syndrome can be pinpointed, there are many factors contributing to the obesity that can be identified and often modified. Evaluation of modes of optimal treatment depends both on proper identification of the type of obesity involved and on the various secondary factors working to perpetuate the disorder. Our purpose is to suggest a framework by which such an identification may be facilitated.

From: Evaluation of the Obese Patient. 1. An Algorithm. *JAMA* 1976;235:1487–1491. Copyright 1976 by the American Medical Association.

Assessment of the obese patient requires both clinical and laboratory techniques. These procedures are used to sharpen our diagnostic acumen and to aid in understanding natural history, prognosis, and approaches to therapy, which may be indicated. Table 14–1 provides a broad outline of one approach toward classifying obese patients, which is described in greater detail else-where.[3–5] It includes both an anatomic and etiologic diagnosis. Table 14–2 lists those contributory factors that may not be diagnostic entities, but must be taken into consideration in caring for patients and aiding them in changing their eating behavior.

Anatomic Diagnosis

The number of adipose cells normally increases until adolescence and thereafter remains relatively fixed.[6] In one major category of obesity, we now know that there is hypercellularity of the adipose tissue, which at times may be increased as much as three to five times above normal (Table 14–1). These individuals also show varying degrees of enlargement of fat cells. The onset of this type of obesity is usually in early or late childhood.[7] The distribution of fat tends to be generalized and to be associated with less metabolic disorder than the type of obesity of later onset, which involves mainly hypertrophy.[8] Diagnosis of the hypercellular type of obesity can be made with certainty only by techniques not yet generally available. These involve measurement of the lipid content of the adipocytes together with an estimate of total body fat. A presumptive diagnosis may, however, be made on clinical grounds when the onset is in childhood and the distribution of the fat is universal.

On the other hand, when the onset of the obesity is during adult years or during pregnancy, it involves mainly enlargement of adipose tissue cells with lipid and tends to be more central in distribution. These forms of obesity are often associated with metabolic disorders such as non-insulin-dependent diabetes mellitus, hyperlipemia, or hypertension. Sustained reduction in weight to a point where the adipose cells have a normal content of lipid should at least theoretically be more feasible in this category of patients than in those with severe cellular hyperplasia. In the latter group, weight reduction to the normal range must result in less than the normal range of lipid per cell, since cell number is relatively fixed. We do not yet know whether long-term maintenance of a reduced body weight can bring about a reduction in the number of fat cells.

Etiologic Diagnosis

A distinct etiologic classification other than "obesity of unknown origin" can be made for only a small number of patients (Table 14–1). It is important, however, to consider the possibility of *endocrine* abnormalities in every patient,

---
Table 14–1.
Classification of Obesity.

Anatomic

   Hypercellular

      With increase in no. of adipocytes and variable degrees of enlargement; onset usually early or late childhood

   Normocellular

      With increase in size but not in no. of adipocytes; onset usually in adult years or during pregnancy

Etiologic

   Endocrine

      Excess of insulin or of adrenocortical hormones

      Associated with other endocrine disorder

         Diabetes mellitus, non-insulin-dependent

         Ovarian dysfunction

         Thyroid dysfunction

         Cushing disease

   Hypothalamic

   Genetic

      Unusual syndromes associated with obesity

      Familial obesity (reserve for obesity with strong familial incidence)

   Obesity of undetermined origin

since many of these diseases can be treated definitively. *Genetic* diagnoses include such rare conditions as Prader-Labhart-Willi syndrome, hyperostosis frontalis interna, and others. Much more uncertainty surrounds a diagnosis of familial obesity, since in humans the effects of environment are difficult to separate from those of heredity. Studies of twins with obesity[9] and particularly of children adopted at an early age, who tend to resemble their true rather than their foster parents,[10] give support to the concept of a strong familial tendency of obesity in humans. With knowledge of a patient's familial background of obesity and other disorders, it may be possible to ease his or her unwarranted feelings of guilt. Finally, the category of obesity of undetermined origin will in the present state of our knowledge remain the largest category, but in the individual patient, attention to the clinical course and progression of laboratory findings may lead to more specific diagnosis.

Contributory Factors

The fact that so many patients fall into the category of obesity of undetermined origin makes it all the more important that we identify the constellation of factors that contribute to and perpetuate the obesity in a given patient. Table 14–2 provides an abbreviated checklist of such factors. These, again, are described in more detail elsewhere.[3] Information regarding the circumstances surrounding abnormal eating patterns and decreased physical activity may form a basis for effective treatment through behavior modification.

An approach to planning tests for obese patients is outlined in Figure 14–1. This algorithm is a flow chart by which most of the common known etiologic factors can be identified. Because the techniques for determining the total numbers of adipocytes are not now readily available, we have omitted the procedure from the algorithm, but would recommend that it be performed where possible, particularly in the forms of obesity with juvenile onset. Many of the measurements in Figure 14–1 should be performed on obese and also on nonobese individuals who enter the health-care system for treatment. In particular, measurement of blood pressure, of serum triglyceride and cholesterol concentrations, and some assessment of glucose metabolism provide important information with respect to potential avenues of treatment. In addition, through these tests, the patients themselves may gain insight into their burden of correctable complicating disorders, such as pulmonary insufficiency (in its extreme form, Pickwickian syndrome), hyperlipemia, or abnormal glucose tolerance and may thus become better motivated to lose weight.

Consideration of various special modes of therapy is beyond the scope or mission of this discussion. It should be emphasized, however, that the risks associated with modest degrees of overweight (body mass index <27; 30% overweight) are often minimal, and thus the potential therapies to be used should have the lowest possible risk (Table 14–3). For detailed consideration of current modes of therapy, the reader is again referred to the report of the Fogarty Conference[3] and to other sources.[4, 5]

This study was supported in part by grants RR 425 (GAB), AM 15165 (GAB), and AM 10254 (EAHS) from the National Institutes of Health.

Table 14–2.

Factors Contributory to Obesity.

Information Relevant to Obesity

Family history

Obesity

Diabetes mellitus

Hyperlipemia

Accelerated arteriosclerosis

Profile of patient's obesity

Rate of progression at various stages of life

Current rate of weight gain or loss

Contributing Factors

Factors influencing eating behavior, such as circumstances of eating, social factors, psychiatric disorders such as depression

Frequency and pattern of eating; nibbling or gorging pattern; night feeding, compulsive eating

Factors affecting amount eaten, such as occupation of cook, composition of diet, perceived satiety

Physical activity; previous experience with exercise programs; current physical fitness, daily routine; living conditions; opportunities for extra exertion and exercise

Pharmacologic and endocrine factors

Use of oral contraceptives

Insulin excess from ill-advised use of insulin or substitutes

Glucocorticoid administration

Phenothiazine drugs or other tranquilizers

Addiction

Alcohol (type and amount drunk)

Tobacco smoking or recent cessation of smoking

Marijuana smoking

1. Overweight is defined as weight/height^2 >27 (see Table 14–3).[11]

2. Obesity may be defined in three ways (criteria for children are presented elsewhere[12]):
   Triceps + subscapular fatfold = 36 mm[11]
   Triceps >18 mm (males); >25 mm (females)[13]
   Body fat >30% (females); >25% (males)[14, 15]

3. Blood pressure[16]:

	Normal	Borderline	Hypertensive
Systolic	<140	141–160	>160
Diastolic	<90	91–95	>95

   (*Note:* When upper arm is large, accurate measurement can only be obtained by intra-arterial manometry.[17])

4. Cortisol suppression:
   Plasma cortisol, 5 μg/dL at 8 AM, 9 h after 1 mg of dexamethasone orally

5. To assess hypothyroidism, measurement of serum thyroxine (competitive binding or radioimmunoassay) is the preferred test, coupled with a triiodothyronine resin uptake (T_3RU) if alterations in thyroxine-binding globulin are suspected.

   Serum thyroxine, μg/dL

Normal	>5.5
Borderline	4.0–5.5
Abnormal	<4.0

   (*Note:* The lower limits of normal may vary from laboratory to laboratory and with the specific method used.)
   If thyroxine level is borderline or if independent confirmation of a low value is desired, a serum thyrotropin determination would be the additional tests of choice.

   Serum thyrotropin, μU/mL

Normal	<7
Borderline	7–10
Abnormal	>10

6. Measurement of serum glucose two hours after a standard meal or a standard load of glucose is desirable for any obese patient, particularly of the adult-onset type. This test is of more value than a fasting glucose value in excluding diabetes mellitus. It may need repetition from time to time in patients who are at high risk of diabetes mellitus (ie, those with a family history of it or women who have given birth to unusually large infants).

   Serum glucose, mg/dL

	Fasting	2 h after standard meal or glucose load
Normal	<110	<140
Borderline	110–125	140–175
Abnormal	>125	>175

   More reliance may be placed on a series of glucose values, but these must be interpreted with care, since they increase with age and may vary from normal to abnormal and back. After a standard glucose load of 75 g or 1.75 g/kg, to a maximum of 75 g for children, measurements of fasting level and the level one and two hours after the glucose load can be added (Σglucose$_{0-2}$) for interpretation.[18]

   Sum of glucose, mg/dL

	Age 20–50 yr	Age 70 yr
Normal	<440	<480
Borderline	440–460	480–540
Abnormal	>460	>540

7. Suggested upper limits for normal[19] (values of children presented elsewhere[20]):

Age, yr	Cholesterol, mg/dL	Triglycerides, mg/dL
0–19	230	140
20–29	240	140
30–39	270	150
40–49	310	160
50–59	330	190

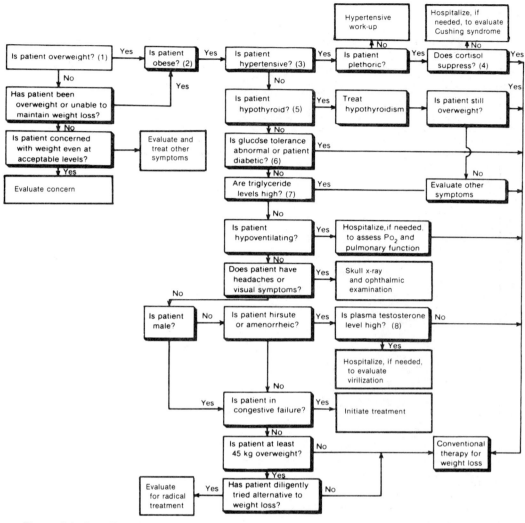

Figure 14—1. Algorithm for evaluating obesity. Numbers in the algorithm refer to listed criteria.

8. Plasma testosterone is high if >300 ng/dL in females.

9. Measurements (unless recently done):
   Complete blood cell count
   Urinalysis
   Chest film (if indicated)
   Electrocardiogram (before beginning a vigorous exercise program or if otherwise indicated)
   Glucose tolerance (or fasting and 2 h postprandial)
   Carbohydrate intake should be 200 g or more for two days before test; loading dose of 40 g/m^2 should be used
   Electrocardiogram (before exercise program or if patient is more than 40 years of age)

Table 14–3.
Body Mass Index.*

Height		Weight, kg (lb)								
Inches	Meters	45.3 (100)	49.90 (110)	54.43 (120)	58.97 (130)	63.50 (140)	68.04 (150)	72.57 (160)	77.11 (170)	81.65 (180)
55	1.397	23.24	25.56	27.89	30.21	32.54	34.86	37.19	39.51	41.84
56	1.422	22.43	24.67	26.92	29.16	31.40	33.65	35.89	38.13	40.37
57	1.448	21.64	23.80	25.96	28.13	30.29	32.46	34.62	36.79	38.95
58	1.473	20.90	22.99	25.08	27.17	29.26	31.35	33.44	35.53	37.62
59	1.498	20.20	22.22	24.24	26.26	28.28	30.29	32.32	34.33	36.35
60	1.524	19.53	21.48	23.43	25.39	27.34	29.29	31.25	33.20	35.15
61	1.549	18.89	20.78	22.67	24.56	26.45	28.34	30.23	32.12	34.01
62	1.575	18.29	20.12	21.95	23.78	25.61	27.44	29.26	31.09	32.92
63	1.600	17.71	19.48	21.26	23.03	24.80	26.57	28.34	30.11	31.88
64	1.626	17.16	18.88	20.60	22.31	24.03	25.75	27.46	29.18	30.90
65	1.651	16.64	18.30	19.97	21.63	23.30	24.96	26.62	28.29	29.95
66	1.676	16.14	17.75	19.37	20.98	22.60	24.21	25.82	27.44	29.05
67	1.702	15.66	17.23	18.79	20.36	21.93	23.49	25.06	26.62	28.19
68	1.727	15.20	16.72	18.24	19.77	21.29	22.81	24.33	25.85	27.37
69	1.753	14.77	16.24	17.72	19.20	20.67	22.15	23.63	25.10	26.58
70	1.778	14.35	15.78	17.22	18.65	20.09	21.52	22.96	24.39	25.83
71	1.803		15.34	16.74	18.13	19.52	20.92	22.32	23.71	25.10
72	1.829		14.92	16.27	17.63	18.99	20.34	21.70	23.05	24.41
73	1.854		14.51	15.83	17.15	18.47	19.79	21.11	22.43	23.75
74	1.879		14.12	15.41	16.69	17.97	19.26	20.54	21.83	23.11
75	1.905			14.99	16.25	17.50	18.75	20.00	21.25	22.50
76	1.930			14.61	15.82	17.04	18.26	19.47	20.69	21.91

*Expressed as weight (kg)/height (meters)^2.

86.18 (190)	90.72 (200)	95.25 (210)	99.79 (220)	104.33 (230)	108.86 (240)	113.40 (250)	117.93 (260)	122.47 (270)	127.01 (280)	131.54 (290)	136.08 (300)
42.62											
41.12	43.28										
39.71	41.80	43.89									
38.37	40.39	42.41	44.43								
37.11	39.06	41.01	42.96	44.92	46.87	48.82	50.78	52.73	54.68	56.64	58.59
35.90	37.79	39.68	41.57	43.46	45.35	47.24	49.13	51.02	52.90	54.79	56.68
34.75	36.58	38.41	40.24	42.07	43.90	45.72	47.55	49.38	51.21	53.04	54.87
33.66	35.43	37.20	38.97	40.74	42.51	44.28	46.06	47.83	49.60	51.37	53.14
32.61	34.33	36.05	37.76	39.48	41.20	42.91	44.63	46.34	48.06	49.78	51.49
31.62	33.28	34.94	36.61	38.27	39.94	41.60	43.26	44.93	46.59	48.26	49.92
30.67	32.28	33.89	35.51	37.12	38.74	40.35	41.96	43.58	45.19	46.81	48.42
29.76	31.32	32.89	34.46	36.02	37.59	39.15	40.72	42.29	43.85	45.42	46.99
28.89	30.41	31.93	33.45	34.97	36.49	38.01	39.53	41.05	42.57	44.09	45.61
28.06	29.53	31.01	32.49	33.96	35.44	36.92	38.39	39.87	41.35	42.82	44.30
27.26	28.70	30.13	31.57	33.00	34.44	35.87	37.30	38.74	40.17	41.61	43.04
26.50	27.89	29.29	30.68	32.08	33.47	34.87	36.26	37.66	39.05	40.45	41.84
25.77	27.12	28.48	29.84	31.19	32.55	33.90	35.26	36.62	37.97	39.33	40.69
25.07	26.39	27.71	29.02	30.34	31.66	32.98	34.30	35.62	36.94	38.26	39.58
24.39	25.68	26.96	28.25	29.53	30.81	32.10	33.38	34.66	35.95	37.23	38.52
23.75	25.00	26.25	27.49	28.75	30.00	31.25	32.50	33.75	35.00	36.25	37.50
23.13	24.34	25.56	26.78	27.99	29.21	30.43	31.65	32.86	34.08	35.30	36.52

References

1. Astwood EB: The heritage of corpulence. *Endocrinology* 1962;71:337–341.
2. Sims EAH, Danforth E Jr, Horton ES, et al: Endocrine and metabolic effects of experimental obesity in man. *Recent Prog Horm Res* 1973;29:457–487.
3. Bray GA (ed): *Obesity in Perspective,* Fogarty International Center Series on Preventive Medicine. Government Printing Office, 1976, vol 2, pt 1 and 2.
4. Bray GA: The varieties of obesity, in Bray GA, Bethune JE (eds): *Treatment and Management of Obesity*. Hagerstown, Md, Harper and Row, 1974, chap 5, pp 61–76.
5. Bray GA: The overweight patient, in *Advances in Internal Medicine*. Chicago, Year Book Medical Publishers, 1976, vol 21, pp 267–308.
6. Hirsch J, Knittle JL: Cellularity of obese and nonobese human adipose tissue. *Fed Proc* 1970;29:1516–1521.
7. Salans LB, Cushman SW, Weismann RE: Studies of human adipose cell size and number in nonobese and obese patients. J Clin Invest 1973;52:929–941.
8. Bjorntorp P: Effects of age, sex and clinical conditions on adipose tissue cellularity in man. *Metabolism* 1974; 23:1091–1102.
9. Newman HN, Freeman FN, Holzinger KJ: Twins: A study of heredity and environment. Chicago, University of Chicago Press, 1937, pp 72–75, 325–363.
10. Withers RF: Problems in the genetics of human obesity. *Eugen Rev* 1964; 56:81–90.
11. Keys A, Aravanis C, Blackburn H, et al: Coronary heart disease: Overweight and obesity as risk factors. *Ann Intern Med* 1972;77:15–27.
12. Seltzer CC, Mayer J: A simple criterion of obesity. *Postgrad Med* 1965;38:101–107.
13. *Ten-State Nutrition Survey, 1968–70*. Government publication CHSM 72–8131.
14. Durnin JVGA, Womersley J: Body fat assessed from total body density and its estimation from skinfold thickness: Measurements on 481 men and women aged from 16 to 72 years. *Br J Nutr* 1974;32:77–97.
15. Steinkamp RC, Cohen NL, Siri WE, et al: Measures of body fat and related factors in normal adults, I. *J Chronic Dis* 1965;18:1279–1289.
16. Chiang BN, Perlman LV, Epstein FH: Overweight and hypertension: A review. *Circulation* 1969;39:403–421.
17. Kvols LK, Rohling BM, Alexander JK: A comparison of intra-arterial and cuff blood pressure measurements in very obese subjects. *Cardiovasc Res Center Bull* 1969; 7:118–123.
18. Prout TE: Use of screening and diagnostic procedures: Oral glucose tolerance test in diabetes mellitus, in Sussman K, Metz RJS (eds): *Diagnosis and Treatment*, ed 4. New York, American Diabees Association, 1975.

19. Levy RI, Frederickson DS, Shulman R, et at: Dietary and drug treatment of primary hyperlipoproteinemia. *Ann Intern Med* 1972;77:267–294.
20. Friedmann G, Goldberg SJ: Normal serum cholesterol values: Percentile ranking in a middle-class pediatric population. *JAMA* 1973;225:610–612.

Chapter 15

Clinical Findings in Obesity

George A. Bray, MD
William T. Dahms, MD
Frank L. Greenway, MD
Molly Marriott Solares, RN
Mark Molitch, MD
Richard L. Atkinson, MD

In the previous chapter, we provided an algorithm for use in evaluating the cases of obese patients. To determine the frequency of abnormalities among the various measurements in this algorithm, we have evaluated a large group of obese patients, and the results are reported in this chapter.

Measures and Methods

Obese patients telephoning the Harbor General Hospital in response to an article in the daily newspaper were offered the opportunity to obtain a free medical evaluation in our Obesity Clinic. Each patient was seen once, on one of three separate weekends (Table 15–1). They were requested not to eat for 12 hours before the clinic appointments. Upon arrival, they filled out questionnaires concerning their present and past history of obesity. A blood sample was obtained on each patient, and those attending the third clinic received 40 g/m^2 of a dextrose solution. A second blood sample was drawn two hours later. Patients were weighed and their height recorded. They were then interviewed by a physician who measured skinfold thickness in the triceps and subscapular regions. Blood pressure was determined using an automatic blood pressure recorder. The initial blood samples on all patients were submitted for measurement of glucose, triglyceride, and cholesterol levels.

On the patients seen in the third clinic, samples were also analyzed for blood urea nitrogen (BUN), uric acid, albumin, alkaline phosphatase, total protein, serum glutamic oxaloacetic transaminase, lactic dehydrogenase, and bilirubin levels. Determination of thyroxine level by radioimmunoassay was performed on the 57 samples containing sufficient serum and on those patients who were not taking birth control pills.

From: Evaluation of the Obese Patient. 2. Clinical Findings. *JAMA* 1976;235:2008–2010. Copyright 1976 by the American Medical Association.

Results

Distribution of the 261 patients in this study by age and sex for each of the three clinics is shown in Table 15–1. There were very few patients under 18 or over 60 years of age. The highest frequency was observed in the third, fourth, and fifth decades. The distribution of body weights by 20-kg and 20-pound intervals for the 234 women in this study is plotted in Figure 15–1. This figure also contains the frequency distribution and cumulative percentile of body weights for women aged 35 to 44 years, as obtained from the National Center for Health Statistics Survey of 1960 to 1962.[1] More than one third of our patients were above the 99th percentile of weights for women aged 35 to 44 years. The peak frequency of weight among our patients was in the interval between 95 and 104 kg.

Using the body mass index (weight/height^2) as suggested in the previous chapter, we found that 95% of the patients were overweight. (See Figure 14–1 on p 111.) The body mass index was between 27 and 30 in 21 and was above 30 in all the rest. Percent overweight was calculated from the midpoint of the weight range for men or women with medium frames[2] using the Metropolitan Life Insurance Tables. All patients were more than 10% overweight, and 91% were more than 20% overweight. The median degree of overweight was 62%. Using a triceps skinfold greater than 18 mm for males and greater than 25 mm for females as a criterion for obesity,[3] we found that 98% of our patients were obese. Thus nine patients who are obese by skinfold measurements were not overweight using a body mass index greater than 27.

The prevalence of hypertension is calculated using the criteria from the previous chapter. Of the 249 patients for whom data are available, 39 (16%) had

Table 15–1.

Age and Sex Distribution of Patients Seen in Obesity Clinic.*

| | *Clinic Weekend* | | | | | |
| | *1* | | *2* | | *3* | |
Age, yr	F	M	F	M	F	M
<18	0	0	2	0	2	0
18–30	13	4	21	2	28	3
31–40	15	1	33	2	23	3
41–50	3	3	30	3	22	3
51–60	2	0	16	1	14	0
>60	0	0	5	1	5	1
Total	33	8	107	9	94	10

*261 patients were seen on only one weekend.

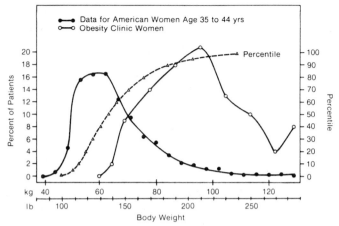

Figure 15–1. Distribution of body weight. Frequency distribution for women aged 35 to 44 years is shown by closed circles and cumulative percentage as triangles (from *National Health Survey, 1960 to 1962*[1]). Distribution of weights among our 234 female patients is shown by open circles.

a diastolic blood pressure above 95 mm Hg and 84% were normotensive. Only five (2%) had diastolic blood pressures of more than 100 mm Hg, but nearly 10% had blood pressures that were in the borderline range (90 to 95 mm Hg). The systolic blood pressure likewise showed a substantial frequency of elevation. Systolic blood pressures above 160 mm Hg were present in 7% of the patients. None of the hypertensive patients was plethoric. Serum thyroxine concentrations were reported for 57 patients who were not taking oral contraceptives. All of the 57 patients were normal except two; one had a value of 2.8 μg/dL (36.1 nmol/L) and the other had a value greater than 14 μg/dL (180.6 nmol/L). Thus, two out of 57 (4%) showed abnormalities in serum thyroxine concentrations. The prevalence of abnormal glucose values was determined in the third clinic. Fasting serum glucose values were higher than 110 mg/dL (6.1 mmol/L) in three of 104 patients, between 90 mg/dL (5.0 mmol/L) and 110 mg/dL in 33, and lower than 90 mg/dL in 68. The levels of serum glucose two hours after an oral load of 40 g/m^2 were above 140 mg/dL (7.8 mmol/L) in 25 of the patients, between 120 mg/dL (6.7 mmol/L) and 140 mg/dL in 24, and below 120 mg/dL in 54. All of the patients with abnormally high fasting blood glucose levels knew that they had diabetes mellitus.

Two patients had serum triglyceride concentrations in excess of 500 mg/dL (5.6 mmol/L). If we use the criteria published by the National Institutes of Health (NIH)[4] (see also chapter 14), 63 patients (25%) had abnormally elevated values. Fourteen patients had serum cholesterol levels above 300 mg/dL (7.8 mmol/L), and 48 others had values between 251 mg/dL (6.5 mmol/L) and 300 mg/dL. According to the upper limits of normal values for cholesterol provided by the NIH,[4] 27 of 237 patients (11%) had elevated levels of cholesterol. Thus, in this group of obese patients, both hypertriglyceridemia and hypercholesterolemia were serious abnormalities. However, we could find no statistically significant correlation between body weight and either serum cholesterol or triglyceride values.

Pulmonary hypoventilation and congestive heart failure were not detected in this group of patients. Medical data were adequate for assessing menstrual history in 167 patients. Of this group, two were amenorrheic, 23 had irregular periods, 16 had undergone surgical hysterectomy, and four were postmenopausal. Thus, menstrual abnormalities were present in 27% (45 of 167). One woman had secondary amenorrhea and a history of headaches. She had been evaluated previously for these symptoms and had been told she had a pituitary tumor. We admitted her to the hospital for reevaluation and treatment with external radiation.

The results from serum analyzed by a multichannel automated system of chemical analysis are presented in Table 15–2. Several abnormalities were ob-

——— **Table 15–2.** ———
Data From Multichannel Analyzer.

Test	Normal Range	Obese Mean ± 2 SD	Range	No. of Abnormally High Values
Creatinine, mg/dL	0.5–1.2	0.72 ± 0.24	0.48–0.96	0
Total protein, g/dL	6.0–8.0	7.4 ± 0.90	6.6–8.4	8
Albumin, g/dL	3.0–6.0	4.1 ± 0.66	3.40–4.72	0
Calcium, mg/dL	8.5–11.0	9.2 ± 0.82	8.4–10.0	0
Phosphorus, mg/dL	2.5–4.5	3.39 ± 0.98	2.41–4.37	1
Uric acid, mg/dL	2.5–8.0	5.87 ± 3.22	2.6–9.1	7
Alkaline phosphatase, international units	36.0–92.0	59.6 ± 32.8	26.8–92.4	7
Bilirubin, mg/dL	0.1–1.2	0.44 ± 0.34	0.1–0.8	0
Blood urea nitrogen, mg/dL	10.0–20.0	13.8 ± 6.24	7.6–20	3
Cholesterol, mg/dL	150–300	202 ± 75	127–277	1

served in this group of tests. Total protein levels were high in eight of the patients due to an increase in globulin. Uric acid and alkaline phosphatase levels were elevated in seven patients. Other tests for liver function were normal. The meaning of these abnormalities is uncertain, and additional study is required to clarify it.

Comment

The present study on 27 obese men and 234 obese women showed several abnormalities when the algorithm for laboratory investigation was used. Elevation in blood pressure and serum triglyceride levels and abnormalities in glucose tolerance were commonly observed and justify their inclusion in the algorithm (see Figure 14–1). In addition to elevated triglyceride level, we found that 11% of the patients had elevated levels of cholesterol, and measurement of cholesterol should thus be added to the algorithm. Question 6 should read "Are triglyceride or cholesterol levels high?" Substantial elevations in alkaline phosphatase and uric acid levels were observed in 7% of the obese patients. This may indicate the need to include these tests too, but more data are needed before we could routinely recommend this. In two of 57 patients, thyroxine values were abnormal, one being high and one low. On the basis of these data, it would appear that the measurements of thyroxine are warranted, since thyroid disease is treatable. Use of the algorithm in chapter 14 will thus be expected to uncover a substantial number of abnormalities in the obese patient.

This investigation was supported in part by grants RR 425 and AM 15165. Carol Frey and Irene Holbrook assisted in organizing this project.

References

1. *National Health Survey (National Center for Health Statistics) Weight, Height and Selected Body Dimensions of Adults, United States 1960–1962*. Public Health Service No. 1000, Series 11, No. 8, June 1965.
2. Bray GA (ed): *Obesity in Perspective: Fogarty International Center Series on Preventive Medicine*, part 1. DHEW Publication No. (NIH) 75–708, US Government Printing Office, 1975, p 72.
3. *Ten State Nutrition Survey 1968–1970*. DHEW Publication No. (HSM) 72–8131, 1972.
4. Levy RI, Frederickson DS, Shulman R, et al: Dietary and drug treatment of primary hyperlipoproteinemia. *Ann Intern Med* 1972; 77:267–294.

Chapter 16

Chest Pain

J. Willis Hurst, MD
Spencer B. King III, MD

The algorithm presented here emphasizes the workup of a patient who has chest "pain" whose clinical features might be associated with myocardial ischemia caused by coronary atherosclerosis. Note that the arrows in the algorithm are numbered and correspond to related numbered paragraphs in the discussion. The discussion highlights some of the information one needs to consider to move from one place in the algorithm to another.

The physician whose goal is to give comprehensive care should define in advance the items in the history, physical examination, and laboratory workup (which includes a chest roentgenogram and ECG) that should be done on every patient. Items done occasionally are not included in the initial data-gathering process. With this approach, the physician should be able to identify the cause of the chest discomfort in the majority of instances without resorting to additional diagnostic studies. While such an approach is often correct, it is not invariably correct. We now know that many diagnostic errors occur and that more data are often needed to determine with certainty if a patient does or does not have atherosclerotic coronary heart disease. An approach to this problem is presented in the algorithm (Figure 16–1).

Algorithm for Evaluation of Chest Pain

1. The physician believes that the patient does not have myocardial ischemia but has another condition. Furthermore, the physician believes that additional workup is not needed. Examples of this situation are anxiety and hyperventilation syndrome (neurocirculatory asthenia) or muscular pain of unknown cause requiring no further workup other than proper follow-up.

From: The Problem of Chest Pain. Emphasis on the Workup of Myocardial Ischemia. *JAMA* 1976;236:2100–2103. Copyright 1976 by the American Medical Association.

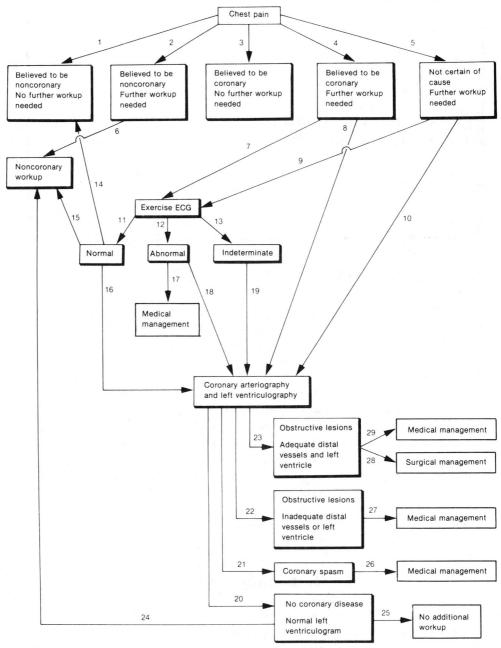

Figure 16—1. Algorithm for the evaluation of chest pain. Numbers correspond to discussion in text.

2. The physician believes that the pain is noncoronary in origin and that further workup is needed to clarify the cause or severity of the problem. An example of this situation is esophageal reflux, in which the symptoms are definite but gastric and esophageal abnormalities must be further delineated by appropriate workup. Noncoronary, cardiac causes of chest pain can often be elucidated by echocardiography. This is discussed under "Comment."

3. The physician believes the pain is coronary in origin. Furthermore, the physician sees no need for additional workup, since other data are sufficient to eliminate the need for exercise ECG or coronary arteriography. An example of this situation is the 75-year-old patient with typical angina pectoris that is produced by effort. The angina is not disabling and has been present for several years.

4. The physician believes that the patient has chest pain caused by coronary atherosclerotic heart disease. The physician also believes that either an exercise ECG, a radionuclide scan, or a coronary arteriogram is needed to make an appropriate decision regarding the management of the patient's condition. Patients with disabling stable angina pectoris, unstable angina pectoris, or recurrent episodes of prolonged pain thought to be caused by myocardial ischemia are in this group. Radionuclide scans are discussed under "Comment."

5. The physician is not certain as to the true nature of the patient's chest pain. In such cases, the physician is unwilling to dismiss the problem as unimportant and believes that further workup is needed to manage the situation: (1) The chest discomfort has a few symptoms suggesting myocardial ischemia, but the real problem is that the physician is unable to get a reliable history related to the chest pain. The physician is shrewd enough to know that further questioning may simply create a false-positive history. (2) The history might be clear enough, but some features suggest symptoms caused by coronary atherosclerosis, and others do not. The physician remembers that classic angina pectoris with effort is misdiagnosed 10% of the time and that more prolonged chest discomfort occurring intermittently over a period of weeks is misdiagnosed 30% of the time. The physician knows that the diagnostic error rate in women is about 50%. Knowing this, the physician turns to more definitive methods of study.

6. The physician, using the available data, has decided that the chest discomfort is not related to coronary atherosclerotic heart disease but is related to some other problem such as an esophageal disorder.

7. The physician believes that the chest discomfort is caused by coronary atherosclerotic heart disease. Furthermore, the physician believes that an exercise ECG will be useful by adding support to the contention or by identifying certain features that indicate the severity of the problem.[1-9] The development of angina pectoris during the test often teaches the patient and physician a great deal. The stage of the exercise test in which the angina pectoris occurs is very important. The development of 2-mm ST segment displacement signifies high-grade obstructive disease in the left main coronary artery or its equivalent (ie,

tight lesions in the proximal left anterior descending and circumflex or severe triple-vessel disease). We believe that this finding is even more meaningful if it occurs in stage 1 or 2 of the Bruce exercise test.

Since the exercise test is dangerous in some patients, it is wise to think through in advance whether the results of the exercise test are going to be useful. For example, ST segment displacement may develop during the stress test in patients with aortic stenosis, aortic regurgitation, hypertension, cardiomyopathy (especially obstructive cardiomyopathy), or the click-murmur syndrome. In some of these, myocardial ischemia may indeed be present, but it may not be directly related to coronary atherosclerosis. The following conditions may invalidate the ECG changes during the stress test: digitalis medication, neurocirculatory asthenia, hypokalemia, Wolff-Parkinson-White syndrome, and left and right bundle-branch block. An exercise test may still be useful in patients with these conditions, since telltale symptoms may be identified during the test.

The physician must be familiar with incidence of false-positive and false-negative responses in various population groups, or errors will be made in the use of the results of the test.

The exercise test is contraindicated immediately after recent myocardial infarction. The test is used in patients with chest pain when the symptoms do not contraindicate the test and when the results will assist the physician in clarifying the problem. The test may be used in patients with stable angina pectoris to assess the amount of work the patient can perform without symptoms or ECG evidence of myocardial ischemia. The test may be performed in certain carefully selected patients who are thought to have unstable angina pectoris or episodes of myocardial ischemia in order to determine if chest discomfort or ST segment displacement occurs with exercise. Considerable clinical judgment and experience is needed to select these patients, and if there is any concern for the safety of the patient, it is proper to obtain a coronary arteriogram rather than require an exercise stress test.

8. The physician recognizes that the chest discomfort has been progressive and for this reason believes that the exercise stress test is dangerous to the patient and elects to obtain a coronary arteriogram as quickly as possible, since coronary bypass surgery may be indicated. Patients with evidence of myocardial necrosis in the ECG or elevated serum enzymes are not usually candidates for coronary arteriography except when emergency surgery is required. Emergency surgery may be considered when the patient continues to have bouts of chest pain caused by myocardial ischemia following a myocardial infarction. This is an interesting subset of patients in which there is evidence of step-by-step severe myocardial ischemia and necrosis. Surgery for fresh infarction is now being studied.

9. The physician is not certain as to the cause of the chest discomfort. The chest pain has certain features that suggest myocardial ischemia and none of the features that contradict the performance of an exercise ECG stress test. The result of the exercise stress test may be of value in such patients, but the clinician

must be familiar with the frequency of false-positive and false-negative responses in the exercise ECG in different population groups. When this information is ignored, the stage is being set for confusion and misinterpretation of the significance of a positive or negative response in the stress ECG. Some physicians would also perform a radionuclide stress test in addition to the ECG stress test. The results of the combination of tests may enable the physician to increase his or her diagnostic accuracy, but the error rate may still be unacceptably high when compared to the accuracy of coronary arteriography.

10. The physician is not certain as to the cause of the patient's discomfort but believes that myocardial ischemia caused by coronary atherosclerotic heart disease is a good possibility. Furthermore, the characteristics (frequency and duration) of the discomfort support the idea that if the discomfort is caused by myocardial ischemia due to coronary atherosclerosis, then an exercise stress test is contraindicated (see discussion in item 7). Therefore, it is necessary to have a coronary arteriogram performed in order to clarify the problem.

11. Results of the exercise stress test are normal. One must keep in mind that false-negative exercise stress test responses occur in 20% or more of certain population groups, or else total reliance may be placed on the result of the test. Accordingly, a coronary arteriogram may be needed in some patients with a normal exercise ECG. The same applies to patients with a negative radionuclide stress test. (See "Comment.")

12. Results of the exercise stress test are abnormal. One must keep in mind that false-positive exercise test responses do occur. In fact, false-positive exercise test responses occur in more than one third of women less than 40 years of age. Accordingly, by the time an exercise test is done for chest discomfort simulating myocardial ischemia, it is often necessary to perform a coronary arteriogram to clarify the clinical picture. When the exercise ECG is abnormal, it is necessary to decide if the patient's condition should be managed medically without a coronary arteriogram or whether to move toward surgical management by obtaining a coronary arteriogram. Patients with chest pain who have an abnormal exercise ECG, stable disabling angina, or unstable angina should have coronary arteriography.

13. Results of the exercise test could not be interpreted. There are many legitimate reasons why this occurs, including inadequate rate response and borderline changes of the ST segments.

14. The physician believes that the normal results of the exercise test assist him or her in excluding coronary atherosclerotic heart disease and that the clinical features exhibited by the patient do not justify any additional workup.

15. The physician believes that the normal results of the exercise test exclude coronary atherosclerotic heart disease, but the clinical features exhibited by the patient require that additional noncoronary workup be done.

16. The physician is still concerned that the clinical features exhibited by the patient may be caused by coronary atherosclerotic heart disease even

though the exercise ECG is normal. Some physicians would perform a radionuclide exercise stress test in such patients. Negative results of such a test are strong evidence against the patient's symptoms being due to coronary disease. We are more inclined to move on to coronary arteriography in such patients.

17. The physician believes the abnormal results of the exercise stress test support the contention that the chest pain is caused by coronary atherosclerotic heart disease but that medical management is the preferred method of treatment at that point in time.

18. A coronary arteriogram is needed to delineate the anatomy of the coronary arteries to determine whether coronary bypass surgery or percutaneous transluminal coronary angioplasty is feasible. Patients with stable disabling angina and unstable angina belong to this group. When 2-mm ST segment displacement occurs in the exercise ECG, there is an increased likelihood of a left main coronary obstruction or its equivalent. We believe this is especially likely if the 2-mm displacement occurs during stage 1 or 2 of the Bruce test. This should stimulate one to move more rapidly to coronary arteriography in certain patients.

19. Results of the stress test cannot be interpreted, and a coronary arteriogram is needed to determine the presence or absence of obstructive coronary disease.

20. The coronary arteriogram shows no obstructive lesions, and the left ventriculogram is normal. Workup for a noncoronary cause of chest pain may not be indicated (see items 24 and 25).

21. The coronary arteriogram shows abnormal coronary artery spasm that is accompanied by chest pain and Prinzmetal ST segment change in the ECG. Further plans are discussed in item 26.

22. The coronary arteriogram shows obstructive lesions, inadequate distal vessels, or inadequate ventricular function. Neither coronary bypass surgery nor percutaneous transluminal coronary angioplasty may be performed.

23. The coronary arteriogram shows obstructive lesions, distal arteries that are bypassable, and adequate left ventricular function. Coronary bypass surgery can be done if conditions justify the procedure. Percutaneous transluminal coronary angioplasty may be performed when the obstruction is located in the proximal portion of a single-vessel coronary artery.

24. No obstructive coronary disease was found, but the physician believes additional noncoronary workup is needed to clarify the cause of the chest pain (see "Comment").

25. The normal coronary arteriogram and normal left ventriculogram eliminate a diagnosis of coronary atherosclerotic heart disease, which was the only real concern the physician had about the patient. The other clinical features are such that no additional workup seems necessary.

26. Medical management is indicated for a patient who has been shown to have coronary artery spasm without obstructive lesions. Coronary bypass surgery has not been proved to be effective in such patients.

27. Medical management is required because coronary artery surgery is not feasible, since the coronary arteries distal to the obstructive lesions do not permit the placement of a graft, or left ventricular function is inadequate for surgical intervention.

28. Coronary bypass surgery or percutaneous transluminal coronary angioplasty is indicated.[10-17] While the indications will change as time passes, our current inclination is to operate (or have angioplasty) on patients with disabling stable angina pectoris, certain patients with one of the numerous subsets of unstable angina pectoris, patients with episodes of prolonged myocardial ischemia, and carefully selected patients with repeated bouts of myocardial ischemia after infarction has occurred. Surgery is indicated in patients with significant obstruction of the following: the left main coronary artery even if the patients have mild angina; proximal obstructions of the left anterior descending coronary artery, right coronary artery, and circumflex coronary artery when there is evidence of myocardial ischemia (angina or positive exercise ECG stress test); and proximal obstruction of the proximal portion of the left anterior descending artery plus obstruction of the right or circumflex coronary artery when there is evidence of myocardial ischemia (angina or positive exercise ECG stress test). Patients with obstruction of the proximal portion of the left anterior descending artery with disabling stable angina or unstable angina and young patients with obstruction of the proximal portion of the left anterior descending artery with mild angina and a positive exercise ECG stress test may be candidates for percutaneous transluminal coronary angioplasty and/or, if this is not possible, coronary bypass surgery. Patients with obstruction of the right coronary artery or circumflex coronary artery who have disabling stable angina or unstable angina may be candidates for percutaneous transluminal coronary angioplasty or, if this is not possible, coronary bypass surgery.

29. Medical management might be appropriate for certain patients with chest pain caused by myocardial ischemia secondary to coronary atherosclerotic heart disease. For example, a patient who has stable angina pectoris provoked by moderate exertion and an obstructive lesion in the right coronary artery would be treated medically.

Comment

The algorithm shown in Figure 16–1 emphasizes the use of coronary arteriography in the identification of obstructive lesions due to atherosclerosis. We believe the results of the coronary arteriogram and left ventriculogram are recognized as the gold standard for the diagnosis of this common and serious disease. We suspect that the reader will wonder when echocardiography and radionuclide studies might be useful in the workup of a patient who is suspected of having atherosclerotic coronary disease, whereas these techniques are mentioned earlier following additional suggestions.[17]

The echocardiogram may be quite valuable in diagnosing idiopathic hypertrophic subaortic stenosis (IHSS). Patients with this condition may have chest pain due to myocardial ischemia that may have the characteristic of angina pectoris, or they may have prolonged myocardial ischemia. The ECG may be abnormal in such patients suggesting infarction or ischemia. If the patient is less than 35 or 40 years of age, has the typical murmur and atrial gallop of idiopathic hypertrophic subaortic stenosis, and has large QRS voltage in the ECG, it may not be necessary to have coronary arteriography and left ventriculography; and one might be satisfied with a positive result indicating IHSS in the echocardiogram (see arrow 2 in Figure 16–1).

Sometimes IHSS may be suspected for the first time upon viewing the left ventriculogram. Such a patient may need an echocardiogram to further delineate the condition.

Physicians must always be aware that two conditions can coexist. Accordingly, in older patients, it is often necessary to have a coronary arteriogram performed in patients with echocardiographic evidence of IHSS since atherosclerotic coronary disease and IHSS may be present in the same patient.

The same problem exists in patients with chest pain who also have evidence of mitral valve prolapse on physical examination. An echocardiogram may give adequate information of mitral valve prolapse in a young patient, and a coronary arteriogram might not be needed (see arrow 2 in Figure 16–1).

Sometimes the echocardiogram is used to clarify a borderline observation in the left ventriculogram when prolapse was not suspected earlier.

Atherosclerotic coronary disease and mitral valve prolapse can coexist, and for this reason, it is often necessary to have a coronary arteriogram performed in patients with echocardiographic-proven mitral valve prolapse who are suffering from chest pain.

Radionuclide tests are quite useful and will become increasingly useful in the future. They do not solve all diagnostic problems, however, and care must be exercised to use them properly. For example, radionuclide tests may be used to clarify the problems shown at arrows 3, 4, and 5. Note we have written in boxes 1 through 4 that the physician *believed* the chest pain was or was not coronary in origin, and in box 5 we have written that the physician was uncertain of the cause of the chest pain. There are times when additional studies are needed to shift the physician's thinking into a more definite position. In other words, if the history is of low predictive value and the stress ECG and stress radionuclide tests are normal, the physician may be willing to state that the patient's chest pain is not due to coronary atherosclerosis. There are times that a negative radionuclide stress test may sway the physician away from a diagnosis of myocardial ischemia due to coronary atherosclerosis even when the ECG stress test is positive if the patient's symptoms are not truly characteristic of myocardial ischemia. In patients who have a high prevalence of coronary disease, such as those with a typical history, a negative radionuclide examination cannot exclude coronary disease. We realize the value of radionuclide studies in nudging the physician to make a choice in diagnosing myocardial ischemia or not diagnosing myocardial ischemia. We do point out that the error rate of such an approach depends upon the expertise of the physician in determining the predictive value of a given history, and when the predictive value of a positive or negative exercise ECG stress test and the predictive value of positive and negative exercise radionuclide stress test are known. Knowing all of that, the physician then has to determine how satisfied he or she is with the error rate that is associated with such a noninvasive approach. There are times we accept this approach, and there are times when we do not.

It is not uncommon for us to use radionuclide exercise stress testing *after* we review the results of the coronary arteriogram. For example, a patient with unstable angina or bouts of prolonged myocardial ischemia is considered to have severe coronary atherosclerosis until proven otherwise by coronary arteriography. If, however, the coronary arteriogram shows mild lesions in the coronary arteries and no evidence of coronary spasm can be elicited, we then perform a radionuclide stress test to determine if the lesions observed are actually causing ischemia. If the radionuclide exercise stress test is normal, we may deduce that the symptoms may not be from the mild lesions we have found and that a noncoronary workup is in order.

We also believe it is important to consider the cost of a workup. If noninvasive workups are performed in every case of chest pain, the cost of a diagnostic workup will be very expensive because a significant number of patients will need coronary arteriography to clarify the problem the noninvasive test did not clarify. So, if one discovers that he or she is ordering noninvasive *and* invasive tests in most patients with chest pain, it may be that money will be saved if another approach is used. It may be wiser and cheaper to select those patients for noninvasive studies when the physician will be satisfied if a given result is produced. In other words, if the result is negative, the physician will be satisfied he or she can live with the diagnostic error rate. On the other hand, if the physician determines in advance that he or she cannot accept the result of the noninvasive test as being acceptably conclusive, then he or she should not perform it and should move directly to coronary arteriography, the results of which are the gold standard of diagnostic work.[17]

References

1. Blackburn H, Taylor HL, Keys A: The electrocardiogram in prediction of five-year coronary heart disease incidence among men aged 40 through 59. *Circulation* 1970;41(suppl 1):154–161.
2. Cohen MV, Cohn PF, Herman MV, et al: Diagnosis and prognosis of main left coronary artery obstruction. *Circulation* 1972;45(suppl 1):57–67.

3. Profant GR, Early RG, Nilson KL, et al: Responses to maximal exercise in healthy middle-aged women. *J Appl Physiol* 1972;33:595–599.

4. Redwood DR, Epstein SE: Uses and limitations of stress testing in the evaluation of ischemic heart disease. *Circulation* 1972;46:1115–1131.

5. Barnard RJ, MacAlpin R, Kattus AA, et al: Ischemic response to sudden strenuous exercise in healthy men. *Circulation* 1973;48:936–942.

6. Cumming GR, Dufresne C, Samm J: False-positive ECGs in women. *Can Med Assoc J* 1973;109:108–111.

7. Cheitlin MD, Davia JE, deCastro CM, et al: Correlation of 'critical' left coronary artery lesions with positive submaximal exercise tests in patients with chest pain. *Am Heart J* 1975;89:305–310.

8. Siegel W, Lim JS, Proudfit WL, et al: The spectrum of exercise test and angiographic correlations in myocardial revascularization surgery. *Circulation* 1975;51(suppl 1):156–162.

9. Froelicher VF, Thompson AJ, Longo MR, et al: Value of exercise testing for screening asymptomatic men for latent coronary artery disease. *Prog Cardiovasc Dis* 1976;18:265–276.

10. Krauss KR, Hutter AM, DeSanctis RW: Acute coronary insufficiency. *Circulation* 1972;45(suppl 1):66–71.

11. Bruschke AVG, Proudfit WL, Sones FM: Progress study of 590 consecutive nonsurgical cases of coronary disease followed five to nine years: I. Arteriographic correlations. *Circulation* 1973;47:1147–1153.

12. Bruschke AVG, Proudfit WL, Sones FM: Progress study of 590 consecutive nonsurgical cases of coronary disease followed five to nine years: II. Ventriculographic and other correlations. *Circulation* 1973;47:1154–1163.

13. Cheanvechai C, Effler DB, Loop FD, et al: Aortocoronary artery graft during early and late phases of acute myocardial infarction. *Ann Thorac Surg* 1973;16:249–260.

14. Spencer FC, Isom OW, Glassman E, et al: The long-term influence of coronary artery bypass grafts on MI and survival. *Ann Surg* 1974;180:439–451.

15. Reul GJ Jr, Cooley DA, Wukasch DC, et al: Long-term survival following coronary artery bypass. *Arch Surg* 1975;110:1419–1424.

16. Sheldon WC, Rincon G, Pichard AD, et al: Surgical treatment of coronary artery disease: Pure graft operations, with a study of 741 patients followed three to seven years. *Prog Cardiovasc Dis* 1975;28:237–252.

17. Hurst JW, King SB III, Walter PF, et al: Atherosclerotic coronary heart disease: angina pectoris, myocardial infarction, and other manifestations of myocardial ischemia, in Hurst JW (ed): *The Heart*, ed 5. New York, McGraw-Hill Book Co, 1982, p 1009.

Chapter 17

Sore Throat

Anthony L. Komaroff, MD

The clinician often regards the problem of a sore throat as intellectually trivial or clinically unimportant. Neither attitude is justified. Many etiologic agents remain to be identified, the differential diagnosis is difficult, determination of a treatment strategy is complicated, and the symptom of a sore throat can be associated with or lead to serious illness. Primarily because of its prevalence, sore throat is also a costly problem. Data from the National Ambulatory Medical Care Survey, coupled with cost studies by our group, suggest that as much as $300 million per year may be spent on laboratory tests and medications ordered for this problem. A recognition of the substantial costs involved makes it imperative that the actions taken by clinicians in the evaluation and treatment of patients with sore throat be carefully scrutinized. I will present an explicit strategy for management, while discussing some important aspects of the diseases in question.

Differential Diagnosis

Streptococcal pharyngitis and viral pharyngitis, including infectious mononucleosis, are the most common known causes of sore throat. However, the cause of almost half of the cases of sore throat is unknown, even when techniques are applied to diagnose many viral and other respiratory pathogens.[1] Other known, treatable pathogens are not often considered, particularly *Neisseria meningitidis*, *Corynebacterium diphtheriae*, *Treponema pallidum*, and *Mycobacterium tuberculosis*. While these potentially serious agents may produce sore throats only rarely, they should not be forgotten.

Two more common, treatable, and usually unrecognized pathogens, the mycoplasmas and *Neisseria gonorrhoeae*, should be considered. Although gener-

From: A Management Strategy for Sore Throat. *JAMA* 1978;239:1429–1432. Copyright 1978 by the American Medical Association.

ally thought of as a bronchopulmonary pathogen, *Mycoplasma pneumoniae* has been isolated in approximately 10% of children aged 12 to 19 years with sore throat,[1] and a sore throat commonly precedes a cough in mycoplasma broncho-pulmonary infections.[2] *N gonorrhoeae* has been cultured from the throat in 10% of patients with genital gonorrhea; patients who engaged in orogenital intercourse, particularly male homosexuals, were at special risk; most patients with gonococcal pharyngitis were asymptomatic.[3] Diagnosis requires a culture of a throat swab on Thayer-Martin media.

Initial Visit Strategy

In presenting this strategy, I will raise the principal management questions that apply to adults and children who can volunteer reliably the symptom of a sore throat. Although the strategy focues on the symptom of a sore throat, patients with this single presenting complaint clearly should have other respiratory symptoms evaluated as well.

Why Bother to Diagnose and Treat Streptococcal Pharyngitis? The answer to this question is less clear than one might think. Treatment may slightly accelerate relief of symptoms if begun within 24 hours of symptom onset, but probably does not alter the clinical course in most cases.[4] Treatment probably further reduces an already low rate of suppurative complications, although we know of only one study that provides direct evidence of this.[5] Treatment does reduce the likelihood of spread to close contacts. Treatment probably does not prevent acute glomerulonephritis.[6]

Treatment does prevent acute rheumatic fever. However, this fact does not of itself imply that the diagnosis and treatment of streptococcal pharyngitis is worthwhile. The benefit of diagnosis and treatment must be weighed against its cost.[7] The incidence of rheumatic fever in the United States has been dropping steadily since 1910. Even among children in low-income urban areas in whom incidence is highest, rheumatic fever attack rates from endemic infection are by now probably no greater than 1%[8] and in most communities may be much lower.[9]

Against this background of progressively diminishing potential benefit, the costs of treatment must be considered: the cost of diagnostic tests and medication; the cost of clinician time, patient time, and transportation; costs in dollars and human suffering of treatment side effects; and certain theoretical costs of suppressing type-specific immunity.

Given available information on costs and benefits, we believe that it is wisest to diagnose and treat this usually self-limited condition (streptococcal pharyngitis) when clinical or epidemiologic data suggest that its presence is reasonably likely or when risk from infection is relatively great.

How Does One Diagnose Streptococcal Pharyngitis? Streptococcal pharyngitis means infection with group A streptococci, the only group clearly associated with acute rheumatic fever. *Infection* is defined as a positive culture *plus* an antibody response to streptococcal antigens; the *carrier state* is a positive culture without an antibody response. The most commonly measured evidence of an antibody response has been a fourfold or greater change in tube dilution level of antistreptolysin O on convalescent serum obtained one to six months later. By this definition, the majority of patients with sore throat and with positive throat cultures will not be infected but, rather, will be carriers.[10, 11]

The antistreptolysin O level in the acute serum specimen is of no value in diagnosing the presence of current infection.[12] Hence, there is currently no practical way for the clinician to distinguish the carrier state from the infected state at the time treatment is being considered. It therefore seems wisest to treat the patient with a culture positive for group A streptococci, though many such patients will be uninfected carriers.

How Should a Throat Culture Be Obtained? For proper isolation of group A streptococci, two cotton or Dacron swabs should be rubbed firmly, under direct vision, over the tonsils and posterior pharyngeal wall. The second swab will yield group A streptococci when the first swab has not in about 10% of patients. Use of a liquid transport medium preserves the specimen for at least 48 hours before culturing. Cultures should be plated on sheep-blood agar, since nongroup A streptococci and other pharyngeal saprophytes can produce β-hemolysis (a clear hemolytic zone) on horse-blood agar. Plates should be kept under relatively anaerobic conditions to enhance β-hemolysis.

Occasionally, group A streptococci will not be β-hemolytic. More important, 5% to 50% of β-hemolytic colonies will not be group A.[13, 14] Inhibition of growth by a 0.01-unit bacitracin disk, and fluorescent antibody techniques, are rapid, simple, and effective means of identifying which β-hemolytic organisms are group A.

Other pharyngeal bacteria that grow on sheep-blood agar rarely cause pharyngitis. Therefore, unless one is ordering a repeated culture in a patient with persistent symptoms, it is unnecessary and wasteful to order a complete throat culture in which all organisms are identified and antibacterial sensitivities reported.

When Should a Throat Culture Be Obtained? If particular clinical findings allowed one to predict confidently the presence or absence of streptococcal pharyngitis without obtaining a throat culture, then the culture might be avoided and treatment might be confidently given or withheld. Unfortunately, as Wannamaker[15] and Kaplan et al[10] have shown, no combination of clinical data is a perfect predictor of a positive throat culture. The question then becomes: Should all patients with a sore throat have cultures taken, or should a particular strategy for limiting cultures be formulated? I will take the latter course, recognizing that any such strategy is arbitrary and involves risks.

Table 17–1 is a decision table that displays management strategies, relating certain findings to particular actions. As indicated in column 1, because the risk of acute rheumatic fever is greatest between the ages of 5 and 25 years, we would take a culture from all such patients regardless of clinical findings. In

Table 17–1.
Strategy for Sore Throat Management Displayed in a Decision Table.*

	1	2	3	4	5	6	7	8	9	10	11	12
History												
Sore throat duration >6 days	…	…	…	…	P	…	…	…	…	…	…	…
Age <25 yr	P	…	…	…	…	…	…	…	…	…	…	…
Streptococcus exposure in past week	P	…	…	…	…	…	…	…	…	…	…	…
Anticipated difficulty with follow-up	…	P	…	…	…	…	…	…	…	…	…	…
History of acute rheumatic fever	P	…	P	…	…	…	…	…	…	…	…	…
Diabetic	P	…	P	…	…	…	…	…	…	…	…	…
Known epidemic of meningococcal meningitis	…	…	…	…	…	…	P	…	…	…	…	…
Diphtheria	…	…	…	…	…	…	P	…	…	…	…	…
Streptococcal pharyngitis	P	…	…	…	…	…	…	…	…	…	…	…
Nephritogenic *Streptococcus*	…	P	…	…	…	…	…	…	…	…	…	…
Mononucleosis symptoms	…	…	…	…	…	P	…	…	…	…	…	…
Physical Examination												
Temperature >37.7°C, by mouth	P	…	…	P	P	…	…	…	…	…	…	…
Epiglottis swollen, red	…	…	…	…	…	…	P	P	…	…	…	…
Unilateral tonsillar swelling	…	…	…	…	…	…	…	…	…	…	P	…
Diphtheritic membrane	…	…	…	…	…	…	P	…	…	…	…	…
Gingivitis	…	…	…	…	…	…	…	…	P	…	…	…
Pharyngeal ulcers	…	…	…	…	…	…	…	…	…	P	…	…
Exudate	P	…	…	P	P	…	…	…	…	…	…	…

continued on next page

*Each column represents a particular strategy. Any one datum when present (P) leads to an action (X) in the same column; multiple data are required for action in columns 4 and 5. Actions usually involve ordering tests or treatments, but can include the collection of clinical data (column 6).

Table 17–1. *Continued.*

	1	2	3	4	5	6	7	8	9	10	11	12
Physical Examination (continued)												
Tender anterior cervical nodes	P	...	...	P	P	...	...	...	...	...	...	...
Posterior cervical nodes	...	...	...	...	...	P	...	...	...	...	...	...
Stiff neck	...	...	...	...	...	...	...	...	...	...	...	P
Scarlatiniform rash	P	P	...	...	...	...	...	...	...	...	...	...
Axillary and inguinal adenopathy	...	...	...	...	...	P	...	...	...	...	...	...
Splenomegaly	...	...	...	...	...	P	...	...	...	...	...	...
Actions												
Culture for group A *Streptococcus*	X	X	...	...	...	...	...	...	...	...	...	...
WBC count/differential cell counts	...	...	...	...	...	X	...	...	...	...	...	...
Mononucleosis spot test	...	...	...	...	...	X	...	...	...	...	...	...
Culture on appropriate media	...	...	...	...	...	...	X	...	...	...	...	...
Syphilis serology	...	...	...	...	...	...	...	...	...	X	...	...
Evaluate for tuberculosis	...	...	...	...	...	...	...	...	...	X	...	...
Consider lumbar puncture	...	...	...	...	...	...	...	...	...	...	...	X
Treatment, penicillin	...	X	X	X	X	...	...	...	X	...	...	...
Treatment, ampicillin sodium or chloramphenicol	...	...	...	...	...	...	...	X	...	...	...	...
Observe for respiratory obstruction	...	...	...	...	...	...	...	X	...	...	...	...
Incision and drainage	...	...	...	...	...	...	...	...	...	...	X	...

patients older than 25 years, cultures might be obtained when certain findings suggest streptococcal pharyngitis: exposure to a living-mate with culture-confirmed streptococcal pharyngitis; oral temperature greater than 37.7°C; tonsillar or pharyngeal exudate; tender anterior cervical adenopathy; or scarlatiniform rash. A past history of acute rheumatic fever is associated with more frequent recurrences of streptococcal pharyngitis and with recurrences of rheumatic fever[16]; the clinician should always inquire about past acute rheumatic fever in a patient with a sore throat. Diabetics combat bacterial infections poorly and thus are at particular risk from streptococcal pharyngitis. For all these reasons, any one of the items shown to be present in column 1 should lead to a throat culture.

When Should Immediate Treatment Be Given—Before Culture Results Are Known? Columns 2 through 5 deal with this question. We assume that all patients with positive cultures would be treated. If difficulty is anticipated in reaching the patient several days later when the culture result returns, immediate treatment can be justified, particularly in persons at higher risk. If there is a known epidemic of nephritogenic streptococci, immediate treatment is justified despite its questionable efficacy. A scarlatiniform rash, although uncommon even in children with streptococcal pharyngitis, nevertheless strongly suggests it when present and should trigger therapy. Infectious mononucleosis and other viral infections can produce a maculopapular exanthem, but this usually would not be confused with a scarlatiniform rash. For the aforementioned reasons, a past history of acute rheumatic fever, particularly with carditis, justifies immediate treatment, as may diabetes (column 3). A patient with a temperature of greater than 37.7°C and exudate and tender anterior cervical nodes (a combination strongly suggestive of streptococcal pharyngitis) might justifiably receive immediate treatment (column 4). Winickoff et al[17] found that such a strategy would lead to unnecessary treatment in only 1% of adults with negative throat cultures. If the patient's sore throat has lasted for more than six days, immediate treatment might be given if any two of three findings were present, since treatment is most effective in preventing acute rheumatic fever if given within the first nine days of symptoms (column 5).

What Should the Treatment Regimen Be? Prevention of rheumatic fever requires treatment that eradicates *Streptococcus;* it is surest when treatment is begun within the first nine days after the onset of symptoms.[18] Efficacy of treatment in preventing the initial attack of acute rheumatic fever has been shown definitively only with parenteral penicillin.[18] However, it is assumed that adequate regimens of oral penicillin, or erythromycin, which demonstrably eradicate the organism, therefore will prevent rheumatic fever. Acceptable treatment regimens in adults are penicillin G benzathine, 1.2 million units intramuscularly; oral penicillin V potassium, 250 mg four times a day for ten days; and erythromycin, 250 mg four times a day or 500 mg twice a day for ten days.

Tetracyclines and sulfonamides are less effective in eradicating *Streptococcus* and have no demonstrated effectiveness in preventing rheumatic fever.[13, 18]

Chloramphenicol has not been shown to prevent rheumatic fever and entails unnecessary risks; it should never be used to treat presumptive streptococcal pharyngitis. Penicillinase-resistant penicillins, even when throat cultures also show staphylococci, offer no advantage over penicillin preparations.[19] Injectable preparations that contain shorter-acting penicillins in addition to penicillin V benzathine are not superior to penicillin V benzathine alone.[20] An excellent recent review of streptococcal diseases discusses many of these issues.[13]

How Does One Diagnose Infectious Mononucleosis? The syndrome of infectious mononucleosis is diagnosed primarily by two characteristic hematologic abnormalities, relative ($>$50% lymphocytes) or absolute ($>$4,500 lymphocytes/mm^3) lymphocytosis, the latter being more accurate when superimposed bacterial infection has provoked a neutrophilic response; and by the presence of ($>$10%) atypical lymphocytes. Taking these hematologic findings to define the infectious mononucleosis syndrome (Figure 17–1), Epstein-Barr virus is the etiologic agent in perhaps 95% of the cases, with cytomegalic virus accounting for a few cases.[21] About 90% of the cases, all of them caused by Epstein-Barr virus, are associated with an abnormal heterophil test result; in the 10% of heterophil-normal patients, each of the two viruses accounts for about half of the cases.[21]

The standard serologic diagnostic test, the Paul-Bunnell heterophil test, has been largely replaced by various differential slide tests (spot tests), which are easier to perform and may be more sensitive—they are virtually never falsely negative when the heterophil test result is abnormal, and may be abnormal in some cases of heterophil-normal infectious mononucleosis. The spot tests are also

Figure 17–1. Spectrum of infectious mononucleosis; 100% of patients have lymphocytosis and atypical lymphocytes. Group is divided into two clinical syndromes, two serologic (heterophil) categories, and two etiologic agents.

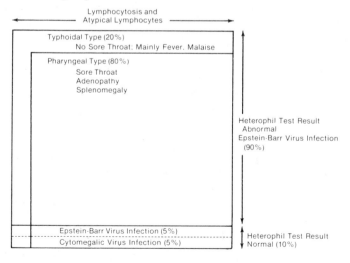

specific but, because they can be falsely positive in 0% to 10% of cases, some physicians recommend performing a confirmatory heterophil test.

When and How Should Patients Be Examined for Infectious Mononucleosis? Column 6 deals with this question. Posterior cervical adenopathy is a sensitive indicator, being absent in less than 10% of patients with infectious mononucleosis.[22] Therefore, we generally would require this finding in a patient with a sore throat before inquiring further about symptoms that tend to be specific for infectious mononucleosis (eg, gradual evolution of symptoms, supraorbital puffiness), before taking the extra time required to examine for axillary or inguinal adenopathy and for splenomegaly, and before ordering diagnostic tests (column 6). Both the characteristic hematologic and serologic abnormalities occur within one week from the onset of symptoms in 80% of patients,[22] but either may be absent in a given patient. Therefore, we recommend ordering total and differential WBC counts and an infectious mononucleosis spot test when posterior cervical adenopathy is found (column 6). Because infectious mononucleosis almost never recurs, some would argue that an investigation of it as the cause of sore throat is unnecessary in patients with serologically verified infectious mononucleosis in the past.

Special Cases. One should culture on appropriate media for meningococci or *C diphtheriae* when known epidemics raise the possibility of these otherwise rare pharyngeal pathogens (column 7). A diphtheritic membrane may be absent in cases of diphtheria,[23] and a pseudomembrane may be seen in infectious mononucleosis and illnesses other than diphtheria. Nevertheless, an apparent membrane, especially when covering the uvula or soft palate as well, should trigger culture for *C diphtheriae* (column 7). A swollen, red epiglottis indicates likely epiglottitis, a condition unusual in children and rare in adults. Furthermore, the patient should be treated immediately for presumed epiglottitis; since *Hemophilus influenzae* is the usual pathogen, ampicillin sodium or chloramphenicol is an appropriate agent. The patient should be watched closely for respiratory obstruction, a life-threatening event (column 8). Notable gingivitis in association with pharyngeal inflammation suggests Vincent's angina, a mixed infection with a spirochete and fusiform Gram-negative bacillus, which responds to penicillin therapy (column 9). A single pharyngeal ulcer, while it most often manifests a *Fusobacterium* infection, can be a primary chancre or a tuberculous granuloma; serologic testing for syphilis and an evaluation for tuberculosis should be undertaken (column 10). Several ulcers, especially in association with a rash, may represent secondary syphilis and should lead to serologic testing. Unilateral tonsillar swelling, if fluctuant, suggests a peritonsillar abscess requiring incision and drainage (column 11); on rare occasions, a hard, nonfluctuant unilateral tonsillar mass can manifest a carcinoma or lymphoma. All patients with sore throat should be examined for stiff neck, especially those patients with a prominent headache; a lumbar puncture should be performed in suspicious cases (column 12).

Follow-up Strategy

In a patient with a positive throat culture for group A *Streptococcus*, a sore throat unresponsive for one week to penicillin suggests several possibilities: poor compliance with the penicillin regimen, infectious mononucleosis, gonococcal pharyngitis, or mycoplasma infection. Cervical adenopathy should remit within one month in streptococcal pharyngitis and within two months in infectious mononucleosis; failure to remit suggests lymphoma, leukemia, granulomatous diseases, or a malignant neoplasm of the head, neck, or chest. Contacts of patients with streptococcal pharyngitis who become symptomatic, or asymptomatic living-mates of those patients who are at high risk from infection (eg, past history of acute rheumatic fever, indigent people living in crowded conditions) should have cultures taken and be treated if the culture is positive.[20]

This report was supported by grant HS 02063-02 with the National Center for Health Services Research, as well as a grant from the Max C. Fleischmann Foundation.

Mark Aronson, MD, Frank Bragg, MD, David Feingold, MD, Gerald Friedland, MD, Charles Rammelkamp, MD, Arnold Smith, MD, Harold Sox, MD, Richard Tompkins, MD, Donald Vickery, MD, and Richard Winickoff, MD, provided background work, editorial advice, or references.

References

1. Glezen WP, Clyde WA, Senior RJ, et al: Group A streptococci, mycoplasmas, and viruses associated with acute pharyngitis. *JAMA* 1967;202:455–460.
2. Alexander ER, Fox HM, Kenny GE, et al: Pneumonia due to mycoplasma pneumoniae. *N Engl J Med* 1966;275:131–136.
3. Bro-Jorgensen A, Jensen T: Gonococcal pharyngeal infections. *Br J Vener Dis* 1973;49:491–499.
4. Brumfitt W, Slater JDH: Treatment of acute sore throat with penicillin. *Lancet* 1957; 1:8–11.
5. Chamovitz R, Rammelkamp CH Jr, Wannamaker LW, et al: The effect of tonsillectomy on the incidence of streptococcal respiratory disease and its complications. *Pediatrics* 1960; 26:355–367.
6. Weinstein L, Le Frock J: Does antimicrobial therapy of streptococcal pharyngitis or pyoderma alter the risk of glomerulonephritis? *J Infect Dis* 1971;124:229–231.
7. Tompkins RK, Burnes DC, Cable WE: An analysis of the cost-effectiveness of pharyngitis management and acute rheumatic fever prevention. *Ann Intern Med* 1977;86:481–492.
8. Siegel AC, Johnson EE, Stollerman EG: Controlled studies of streptococcal pharyngitis in a pediatric population. *N Engl J Med* 1961;265:559–571.
9. Pantell RH: Cost-effectiveness of pharyngitis management and prevention of rheumatic fever. *Ann Intern Med* 1977;86:497–499.
10. Kaplan EL, Top FH, Dudding BA, et al: Diagnosis of streptococcal pharyngitis:

Differentiation of active infection from the carrier state in the symptomatic child. *J Infect Dis* 1971;123:490–501.

11. Role of β-hemolytic streptococci in common respiratory disease, Commission on Acute Respiratory Diseases. *Am J Public Health* 1945;35:675–682.

12. Bisno AL, Stollerman GH: Streptococcal antibodies in the diagnosis of rheumatic fever, in Cohen AS (ed): *Laboratory Diagnostic Procedures in the Rheumatic Diseases*. Boston, Little Brown & Co, 1975, p 223.

13. Peter G, Smith AL: Group A streptococcal infections of the skin and pharynx. *N Engl J Med* 1977;297:311–317, 365–370.

14. Bisno AL, Pearce IA, Stollerman GH: Streptococcal infections that fail to cause recurrences of rheumatic fever. *J Infect Dis* 1977;136:278–285.

15. Wannamaker LW: Perplexity and precision in the diagnosis of streptococcal pharyngitis. *Am J Dis Child* 1972;124:352–358.

16. Spagnuolo M, Pasternack B, Taranta A: Risk of rheumatic fever recurrences after streptococcal infections. *N Engl J Med* 1971;285:641–647.

17. Winickoff RN, Ronis A, Black WL, et al: A protocol for minor respiratory illnesses. *Public Health Rep* 1977;92:473–480.

18. Catanzaro RJ, Stetson CA, Morris AJ, et al: The role of the *Streptococcus* in the pathogenesis of rheumatic fever. *Am J Med* 1954;17:749–756.

19. Rosenstein BJ, Markowitz M, Goldstein E, et al: Factors involved in treatment failure following oral penicillin therapy of streptococcal pharyngitis. *Pediatrics* 1968;73:513–520.

20. Kaplan EL, Bisno A, Derrick W, et al: Prevention of rheumatic fever. *Circulation* 1977;55:51–54.

21. Klemola E, van Essen R, Henle G, et al: Infectious-mononucleosis-like disease with negative heterophil agglutination test. *J Infect Dis* 1970;121:608–614.

22. Hoagland RJ: Infectious mononucleosis. *Am J Med* 1952;13:158–171.

23. Fernbach D, Starling K: Infectious mononucleosis. *Pediatr Clin North Am* 1972;19:957–968.

Chapter 18

Lymphadenopathy

Sheldon Greenfield, MD
M. Colin Jordan, MD

Enlarged lymph nodes occur in many conditions, either as a reaction to a local inflammatory process or associated with a systemic disease whose central focus is not in the lymph system. In some patients, enlarged nodes are the initial or the most prominent manifestation of whatever disease is present and are the starting point for investigation. The algorithms presented here develop guidelines for evaluation of lymph node enlargement of the primary or secondary type.

Scope and Limitations

These algorithms are designed to be applied only to adolescents and adults, because a different array of diseases underlies enlarged lymph nodes in infants and children. They do not include therapy for any of the conditions detected. Following the model of protocols or clinical algorithms for primary care, they do not include diagnostic evaluation of rare diseases. On the other hand, nonspecific findings are included to alert the reader to consider more remote diseases and to avoid premature closure of a line of investigation. The algorithms focus on ambulatory patients, not on the appearance of enlarged nodes in patients in whom serious or chronic disease has been diagnosed. They address only peripheral nodes, confirmed by palpation by the physician, and not those detected by x-ray film, such as hilar nodes.

The algorithms correspond to the principles of decision analysis.[1] The order of the sequential tests in the algorithms implies our estimate of the highest probability of detecting a disease, given information already collected, combined with the importance of its detection, penalty for delay, and the least expense, time, risk, and inconvenience of the test for the patient. The logistics and eco-

From: The Clinical Investigation of Lymphadenopathy in Primary Care Practice. *JAMA* 1978;240:1388–1393. Copyright 1978 by the American Medical Association.

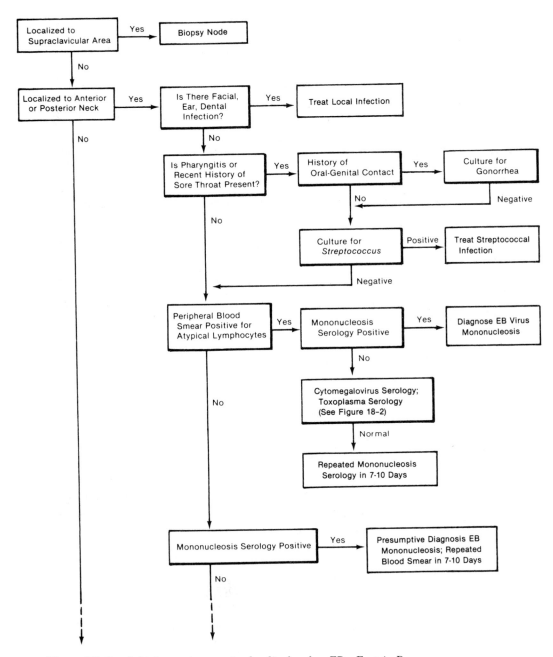

Figure 18–1. Initial steps in assessing localized nodes. EB = Epstein-Barr.

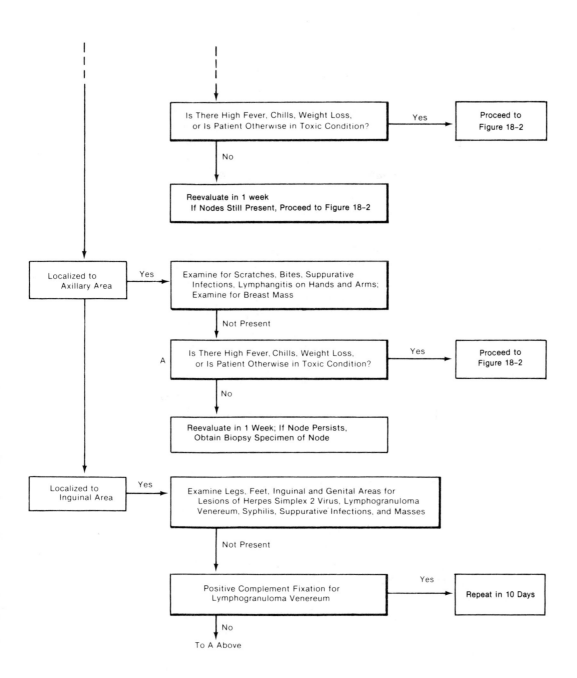

nomics of practice may not permit following the temporal sequence of highest to lowest yield test. For instance, it may be necessary to order a mononucleosis slide test and serological tests for cytomegalovirus and toxoplasma simultaneously rather than await the results of the initial slide test that points to the disease with a considerably higher prevalence.

Substantial enlargement of lymph nodes requiring investigation is defined as one or more nodes estimated to be equal to or greater than 1 cm in diameter, newly recognized, and not known to arise from a previously recognized cause. Multiple small nodes may also indicate investigation. Because of the unreliability of clinical findings in general and the well-recognized difficulty in distinguishing those requiring investigation from shotty nodes, no further refinement of the definition of substantially enlarged nodes will be attempted.

Initial Steps

Investigation is organized according to localization and diffuseness of the enlarged nodes. The attribute of tenderness does not adequately discriminate between enlarged nodes of infectious origin and those produced by other causes, such as Hodgkin's disease. Figure 18–1 presents the initial investigation according to where the nodes occur. Palpable supraclavicular nodes often result from tumors at a distant focus, and a biopsy specimen should be obtained. Enlarged nodes confined to the neck may result from infection that is not obvious. Healing infection of the face, otitis externa without pain, or dental abscess unaccompanied by pain or local swelling at the time of presentation may be the source of the enlarged nodes. Pharyngitis, even mild, or a history of recent sore throat points to throat infection, and culture should be done. Gonococcal pharyngitis should be considered if there has been recent orogenital contact.

In the absence of facial, dental, throat, and ear infection, the possibility of a mononucleosis-like disorder must be considered. Many patients with mononucleosis-like disorders have atypical clinical features, such as localized lymphadenopathy, and often are hospitalized for extensive diagnostic studies that are unnecessary and hazardous.[2] These conditions may be difficult to diagnose since the characteristic laboratory abnormalities are not always present when the patient is seen initially.[3] For example, the onset of relative lymphocytosis with atypical cells may not be present for the first one to three weeks of illness, and the slide or heterophile agglutination tests may become positive only late in the course of the disease.

Further, the occurrence of disorders with clinical and hematologic findings identical to classical heterophile-positive infectious mononucleosis but with negative heterophile reactions has been stressed recently in several publications.[2-5] Therefore, infection with cytomegalovirus or toxoplasmosis should be considered in these instances, as well as Epstein-Barr (EB) virus, and diagnosis must be made by serological investigation. However, in office practice it is easier to start with the peripheral blood smear. If 10% or more atypical lymphocytes are seen and the serological findings for mononucleosis are positive, a definite diagnosis of classic EB virus mononucleosis can be made. If the serological findings for mononucleosis are negative in the presence of atypical lymphocytes, the heterophile-negative mononucleosis syndromes caused by cytomegalovirus and toxoplasma should be considered.

If the blood smear is negative and the serological findings for mononucleosis are positive, a diagnosis of EB virus mononucleosis may be correct. If atypical lymphocytes present on a blood smear that has been repeated after seven to ten days, there is further confirmation of the diagnosis.

If mononucleosis-like syndromes are not detected and if the patient has a toxic reaction, a more extensive investigation, as shown in Figure 18–2, should

Figure 18–2. Investigation of persistent enlarged nodes. EB = Epstein-Barr; PPD = purified protein derivative.

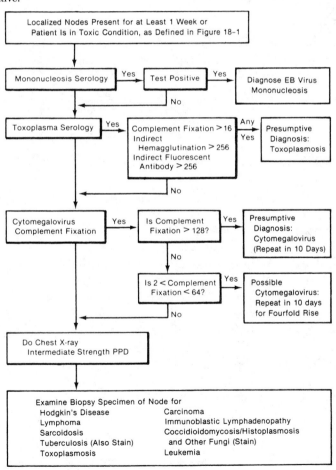

be undertaken. If the patient does not have a toxic reaction, observation and reevaluation in seven to ten days will suffice. If the nodes still persist at that point, further workup as shown in Figure 18–2 should proceed.

Localization of lymph node enlargement to the axilla presents a different spectrum of possible local conditions. Here, cat-scratch fever, sporotrichosis, tularemia, staphylococcal and streptococcal infection, and Hodgkin's disease or lymphoma should be considered. Tumors of the extremity or, more commonly, breast may be covert and heralded by enlargement of an axillary node. Toxoplasmosis and cytomegalovirus infection are less frequently associated with axillary nodes and need not be sought unless the patient has signs of active systemic disease. For these reasons, if the node persists without obvious local cause, a biopsy specimen should be obtained.

With regard to enlarged nodes localized to the inguinal area, local infections not noticed by the patient may be detected by careful examination of the feet, legs, and inguinal and genital areas. Syphilis, lymphogranuloma venereum, genital herpes, malignant melanoma, and other tumors may manifest themselves by an accidental discovery by the patient or the physician of an enlarged node. Because a genital lesion may not be evident at the same time as an enlarged node resulting from lymphogranuloma infection, a complement fixation test for lymphogranuloma-venereum antibodies can be performed. A fourfold rise in titer is necessary for a definite diagnosis and usually requires serum samples obtained ten to 14 days apart. As with axillary nodes, a biopsy specimen should be obtained if the node persists without definitive diagnosis.

Persistent Enlarged Lymph Nodes

Figure 18–2 suggests the approach to take for patients whose enlarged nodes have persisted for at least one week or who are manifesting high fever, chills, or weight loss. A repeated mononucleosis serology test may be positive, although the initial test was negative, because of the delayed heterophile antibody response. At this point, other causes of adenopathy should be pursued more aggressively. Toxoplasmosis antibodies may be measured in several ways. While a fourfold titer rise or fall is usually diagnostic, levels in excess of certain values for each test (as detailed in Figure 18–2) are highly suggestive of acute toxoplasma infection.[4] Recently, cytomegalovirus infection has been noted to be associated with a spontaneous mononucleosis-like syndrome.[5] This illness may be characterized by pharyngitis, splenomegaly, fever, rash, and either localized or diffuse adenopathy, but in any given patient the lymphadenopathy may be the most prominent sign. A fourfold rise in antibody titer is strongly suggestive of this condition and is the most practical diagnostic test if facilities for virus isolation (urine or saliva) are not available.

At this point, after local lesions or infections, toxoplasmosis, cytomegalovirus and EB virus mononucleosis have been effectively excluded, other systemic conditions must be pursued by biopsy of the enlarged node. Pathological examination of the biopsy specimen should include search for Hodgkin's disease, leukemia, lymphoma, sarcoidosis, tuberculosis, toxoplasmosis, carcinoma, coccidioidomycosis, histoplasmosis, and other fungal infections. In recent years the syndrome of immunoblastic lymphadenopathy has been recognized as a cause of protracted fever and lymph-node enlargement.[6] Cultures and stains for tuberculosis and fungi should be done routinely. Chest roentgenogram and tuberculin skin test aid in interpretation of the biopsy specimen. Nonspecific inflammation and hyperplasia do not exclude any of these diseases, and if the patient remains symptomatic or if the nodes persist or enlarge, another node biopsy or biopsy of other involved tissue may be necessary.

Generalized Adenopathy

Generalized adenopathy is often caused by systemic infections, but a drug reaction should also be considered, as indicated in Figure 18–3. In addition to the infectious diseases investigated in Figure 18–2, bacterial endocarditis,

Figure 18–3.   Generalized adenopathy. PPD = purified protein derivative.

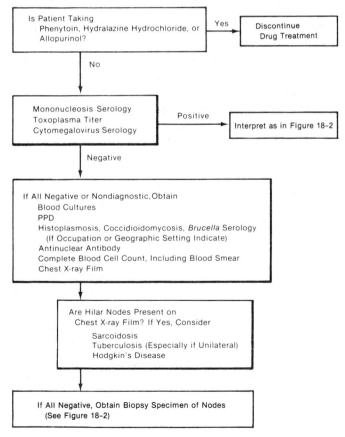

brucellosis, and other less common infections might be implicated. Clues in the history and physical examination may provide some direction: A new murmur or history of intravenous drug administration suggests endocarditis, and blood cultures should be pursued more vigorously. Similarly, a history of having contact with sheep, working in a slaughterhouse, or drinking unpasteurized milk indicates possible brucellosis. Coccidioidomycosis and histoplasmosis are often suspected from the geographic setting and particular exposure histories. Rash, arthritis, and proteinuria are nonspecific but turn attention to lupus erythematosus. A history of contact with someone with tuberculosis should provide added impetus to the investigation of tuberculosis.

Comprehensive detail of pertinent history and physical examination for these diseases is too extensive to be considered here. Further, these clues are too often nonspecific in patients whose primary symptom is adenopathy; thus, laboratory examinations must proceed. Whether they are performed together or sequentially after determining results of prior tests depends on the setting and particular economic situation. If the diagnosis cannot be made securely with the aid of any of these laboratory tests, biopsy specimens should be obtained to look for the conditions mentioned earlier.

Precautions in Applications of Algorithms

While these simple algorithms may serve as a guideline for rapid and cost-efficient diagnosis, much of the clinical information contained is not validated and awaits further testing. Whether following these algorithms will save money and be more efficient than other general approaches is unknown. Further, substituting one sequence of test ordering for another within the general guidelines of the algorithm may improve diagnostic accuracy, decrease inconvenience, and reduce costs. Clinical studies have shown that nurses and physician assistants, guided by protocols or clinical algorithms, are at least as effective and efficient as physicians in the diagnosis and management of certain complaints.[7-12] Until testing has been performed, caution must be exercised in interpreting and following the algorithms presented here.

Our own experience and interpretation of the literature indicate that the approaches we have outlined will be useful in encouraging physicians to think carefully about each sequential step of the diagnostic investigation, with attention at each point to the choice of further tests or procedures. The use of logic, parsimony, and uncluttered approaches may seem best; however, the circumstances of today may not permit a sequential approach to diagnostic reasoning. It may be less expensive to order multiple tests that might provide a clue to the enlarged nodes rather than have the patient return for more office visits or await the results of tests while in the hospital. The cost of the delay in terms of revisits, inconveniences, hospital days, or individual tests vs packages may offset the putative savings of a logical and intellectually satisfying approach to diagnosis. No studies to data have directly addressed this question, and individuals should, according to their own judgment, consider all dimensions of an evaluation, including cost, rapidity, accuracy, and feasibility, as they affect each patient.

References

1. McNeil BJ, Keeler E, Adelstein SJ: Primer on certain elements of medical decision making. *N Engl J Med* 1975;293:211–215.
2. Jordan MC: Nomenclature for mononucleosis syndromes. *JAMA* 1975;234:45–46.
3. Horowitz CA, Henle W, Henle G, et al: Clinical and laboratory evaluation of elderly patients with heterophil-antibody positive infectious mononucleosis. *Am J Med* 1976;61:333–345.
4. Krogstad DJ, Juranek DD, Walls KW: Toxoplasmosis. *Ann Intern Med* 1972;77:773–778.
5. Jordan MC, Rousseau WE, Steward JA, et al: Spontaneous cytomegalovirus mononucleosis: Clinical and laboratory observations in nine cases. *Ann Intern Med* 1973;79:153–160.
6. Lukes RJ, Tindle BH: Immunoblastic lymphadenopathy. *N Engl J Med* 1977;292:1–8.
7. Greenfield S, Komaroff AL, Anderson H: A headache protocol for nurses: Effectiveness and efficiency. *Arch Intern Med* 1976;136:1111–1116.
8. Greenfield S, Anderson H, Winickoff RN: Nurse-protocol management of low back pain: Outcomes, patient satisfaction and efficiency of primary care. *West J Med* 1975;123:350–359.
9. Greenfield S, Friedland G, Scifers S, et al: Protocol management of dysuria, urinary frequency, and vaginal discharge. *Ann Intern Med* 1974;81:452–457.
10. Komaroff AL, Black WL, Flatley M, et al: Protocols for physician assistants: Management of diabetes and hypertension. *N Engl J Med* 1974;290:307–312.
11. Sox HC, Sox CH, Tompkins RK: Training of physicians' assistants by a clinical algorithm system. *N Engl J Med* 1973;288:818–824.
12. Greenfield S, Komaroff AL, Pass TM, et al: Efficiency and cost of primary care by nurses and physician assistants. *N Engl J Med* 1978;298:305–309.

Chapter 19

Sudden Unexpected Death in Adults

George D. Lundberg, MD
Gerhard E. Voigt, MD

The value of autopsy performance in establishing a cause of death, assisting in the determination of the manner of death, comparing the premortem and postmortem findings, producing vital statistics, and monitoring the public health, among other things, has been documented for many decades.[1]

In all legal jurisdictions of the United States and most other countries of the world, autopsy is not performed after every death. In some hospitals in the United States and in some other countries, autopsy is routine after almost every death. Since the Joint Commission on Accreditation of Hospitals recently eliminated its requirement of a certain fixed percentage of autopsies on deaths occurring in the hospital, many now believe that the American autopsy percentage has dropped to new modern lows. In these days of compulsory peer review, government involvement in quality of medical practice, frequent liability suits, questions of industrial health and environmental epidemiology, and the like, one more than ever needs comprehensive valid data gathered from autopsy to evaluate these factors.

One circumstance in which the autopsy can be of great value is sudden death. Much has been written recently about the importance of autopsy in sudden infant death syndrome.[2] Less attention has been paid to its value in sudden unexpected death in adults, which we have termed "SUDA."

Patients and Methods

Because of the authors' knowledge that in many areas of the United States and much of the remainder of the world an autopsy is not performed routinely in SUDA victims, a study was performed at Lund University in Sweden to test the

From: Reliability of a Presumptive Diagnosis in Sudden Unexpected Deaths in Adults. The Case for the Autopsy. *JAMA* 1979;242:2328–2330. Copyright 1979 by the American Medical Association.

validity of whether autopsy is desirable in SUDA. Cases were chosen in the following manner: (1) man or woman older than 18 years, (2) died in Sweden in July or August 1976, (3) no suspicion of unnatural cause or manner of death present after careful police investigation, (4) no evidence at the scene suggesting unnatural cause or manner of death, (5) no hospitalization immediately before death, although patient may have been seen at an emergency room, (6) patient may or may not have had a history of a disease and physician treatment in the past, but no physician of record was willing to sign the death certificate based on his or her medical knowledge of the patient, (7) no evidence of trauma by external examination of the body, (8) no notable postmortem decomposition, and (9) consecutive autopsies were performed or supervised by one of us (G.D.L.).

These nine case criteria were selected to conform to those that often would lead to a diagnosis of ischemic heart disease, heart attack, myocardial infarction, coronary artery insufficiency, occlusive coronary artery atherosclerosis, or similar term as a cause of death without autopsy in much of the United States. The autopsy rate in Sweden is high, exceeding 90% of all deaths in some locales. Routine autopsy is the norm in all cases of SUDA.

In every instance, a complete autopsy was performed, including examination of the brain, tongue, and neck organs and complete opening of the bowel. In many instances, toxicologic analyses of tissues or fluids and microscopic examination of many organs was performed at the discretion of the pathologist. All autopsies were performed either at Lund University or at Malmö General Hospital as the responsibility of the Department of Forensic Medicine.

Results

The results are listed in Table 19–1.

Comment

An autopsy can be viewed as simply another laboratory test or cluster of tests. As such, it is subject in theory to all of the factors that affect other laboratory tests. These include ordering, collection, transportation, identification, preparation, analysis, reporting, interpretation, sensitivity, specificity, false-positives and false-negatives, predictive values, quality control, laws and regulations, data handling, cost accounting, and others.

In assessing the value of performing a laboratory test, eg, an autopsy, a number of factors should be considered. Sensitivity is defined as the percent of positive laboratory results in patients with a specific disease. Specificity is defined as the percent of negative laboratory results among patients who do not have the disease. A sensitive test is positive in patients with the disease. A specific test is negative in patients without the disease. If a test has 90% sensitivity, it will be

Table 19–1.

Autopsy Causes of Sudden Unexpected Death in Adults at Lund University.

Coronary artery disease (n = 49)	
Arteriosclerotic heart disease or old myocardial infarction	22
Recent myocardial infarction	22
Ruptured heart with cardiac tamponade	5
Pulmonary embolism	8
Intoxication—overdose	5
Cardiac hypertrophy	4
Bronchopneumonia	4
Bronchial asthma	4
Intracerebral hemorrhage	3
Aortic stenosis	3
Hepatic cirrhosis	3
Dissecting aortic aneurysm	2
Subarachnoid hemorrhage	2
Acute subdural hematoma	2
Ruptured aortic aneurysm	1
Cardiac amyloidosis	1
Mitral stenosis	1
Hepatitis with massive necrosis	1
Acute pancreatitis	1
Perforated duodenal ulcer with peritonitis	1
Hepatocellular carcinoma	1
Leukemia—lymphoma	1
Carcinoma of the pancreas	1
Fractured cervical spine	1
Aspiration of meat	1
Undetermined	0
Total	100

positive in 90 cases in which the disease is present (true-positives) and negative in ten such cases (false-negatives). If a test has 90% specificity, it will be positive in 90 cases in which the disease is absent (false-positives) and negative in 810 such cases (true-negatives) (see also Chapter 28).

How good should a laboratory test be? In perfection, sensitivity and specificity are each 100%, with a sum of 200%. Pure chance may have any sensitivity or specificity, but the sum is always 100%. Silverstein and Gambino[3] have stated that an ideal sum for laboratory test sensitivity and specificity is greater than 190%. The fabled "sink" test is a test in which a hypothetical laboratory pours a specimen down the sink drain without analysis and produces a fictitious report. It may have either 100% sensitivity or 100% specificity or any number in between, but the sum is always 100%.

Had the test been "cause of death assigned without autopsy" in these 100 cases of SUDA and had there been subsequent verification by autopsy if one had diagnosed the cause of death as some form of coronary artery insufficiency, one would have been correct 49% of the time and incorrect 51% of the time. The sensitivity of that diagnostic approach (cause of death without autopsy) would have been 100%, since all cases of coronary artery disease would have been correctly diagnosed. The specificity, however, would have been 0%, since no cases without that cause of death were considered negative. Thus, the sum would have been 100% or pure chance. We conclude that a diagnosis of coronary artery disease as a cause of death without autopsy in these cases of SUDA in this series would have been the anatomic and forensic pathology counterpart of a sink test, ie, throwing the specimen (body) away without performing the laboratory test (autopsy).

Sweden is an advanced country in terms of social structure, wealth, transportation, health, education, and science. Full access to advanced preventive and therapeutic medical care through socialized medicine has been available to all inhabitants for decades. Yet, even under these circumstances, medical information was not available to clinicians to the extent of being able to sign death certificates in many instances of death. That fact suggests that a wide variety of undiagnosed fatal diseases that present surprisingly as SUDA is even more likely to occur in settings with less fully developed and less freely accessible medical care.

We have alluded only to causes of death. Forensic autopsies, of course, are performed for many other reasons. These include an interest in justice being done as regards homicide detection and documentation, insurance claims being adjudicated fairly, industrial accident documentation, body identification, correct determination of manner of death, and family or friend counseling.

Homicide in Sweden is rare. The jurisdiction involving Lund covers 2.5 million inhabitants but expects only 11 to 15 homicides per year. Although there were examples of suicide and accident in this series of 100, there were disclosed no unsuspected homicides. However, in those parts of the world where homicide is much more prevalent, the influence of that prevalence in the interaction of sensitivity and specificity would cause one to anticipate discovering unsuspected homicide more commonly.

The predictive value of a positive result defines the percentage of positive results that are true-positives, ie, those that correlate perfectly with the presence of the disease being tested for. The predictive value varies with sensitivity, specificity, and prevalence. If a test with 100% sensitivity and 0% specificity is applied to a disease with a prevalence of 50% as a valid cause of death, the predictive value of a positive result would be 50%. The data presented here suggest that 50% is the predictive value of a diagnosis of coronary artery insufficiency as a cause of death without autopsy in SUDA under the circumstances described.

The predictive value of a negative result defines the percent of negative results that are true-negatives, ie, those that correlate perfectly with the absence of the diagnosis. With a prevalence rate of 12 homicides in 26,000 total deaths per year (0.0005%) as seen in Lund, one would expect to find homicide at autopsy as a surprise finding only rarely. However, the population base that one deals with in urban America in this decade is one with as many as 1,600 homicides per 80,000 total deaths (2%). If the sensitivity of a nonautopsy in detecting homicide were 90% in a population death base of 100,000 in which the prevalence of homicide were two percent, 1,800 homicides would be correctly called positive, but there would be 200 false-negatives. These calculations based on the prior assumptions suggest that for every nine homicides identified without autopsy in urban America, an additional one would be missed.

It is not certain what number of deaths in the United States may be classified as SUDA, but it is large. What is the final diagnosis in the absence of autopsy? It is usually some variant of coronary artery disease. If the limited data here could be extrapolated to this country at large, one could anticipate that death certificate figures in regard to this entity frequently would be in error. Other studies do corroborate that view.[4-7]

Why is not autopsy always performed in cases of SUDA in the United States? The answers include ignorance, law, politics, and alleged lack of funds and personnel. None of these factors must be. In this decade in this country, there always seem to be resources for those needs that are truly justified as requirements. Does it matter whether these frequent errors continue? If the medical profession, the public at large, government, and others are concerned about why people die, it matters a great deal from a general point of view. It also may matter individually in regard to justice, disease prevention, and economic fairness.

What is optimal laboratory use in the investigation of SUDA? It is complete gross autopsy by a competent person in every instance with further microscopic, toxicologic, and microbiologic study as deemed appropriate on an individual basis.

References

1. Williams MJ, Peery TM, Dorsey DB, et al: The autopsy: A beginning, not an end. *Am J Clin Pathol* 1978;69(suppl):215–266.
2. Raven C, Maverakis NH, Eveland WC, et al: The sudden infant death syndrome: A possible hypersensitivity reaction determined by distribution of IgG in lungs. *J Forensic Sci* 1978;23:116–128.
3. Silverstein M, Gambino SR: How good should a lab test be? *Lab Med Pract Physician* 1978;1:17–21.
4. Briggs RC: Quality of death certificate diagnosis as compared to autopsy findings. *Ariz Med* 1975;32:617–619.
5. Gwynne JF: The unreliability of death certificates. *NZ Med J* 1974;80:336.
6. Najem GR, Riley HD, Najem LI: Reliability of heart disease diagnosis. *Okla State Med Assoc J* 1975;68:452–457.
7. Moriyama IM, Baum WS, Haenszel WM, et al: Inquiry into diagnostic evidence supporting medical certification of death. *Am J Public Health* 1958;48:1376–1387.

Problems Observed in Laboratory Results

Chapter 20

Maternal-Fetal Incompatibility

Aaron Lupovitch, MD

Ofelia J. Centeno, MD

The increased volume and variety of clinical laboratory tests require new approaches in presenting data to the physician so that reports are clear, concise, and informative. In addition, the need for a logical series of data to answer a physician's query has induced us to assemble laboratory tests into studies geared to a specific purpose. As an example, we present a study to determine maternal candidacy for anti-Rho immune globulin serum after pregnancy to prevent Rho-sensitization, with data plus interpretation reported via a programmable calculator.[1] The study also checks for maternal-fetal ABO incompatibility, and, if present, for homologous antibodies in the infant's cord blood.[2]

Programmable Calculator

Two major problems arise from this approach to laboratory testing. First, since the study is based on a variable sequence of tests from which subsequent tests are selected according to the result of a preceding test, the series must be monitored for adequacy and relevance. Second, since physicians do not order each test individually, they must receive a detailed report of the test data to verify the reported interpretation. Both can be solved with a programmable calculator, which has features resembling a computer but is less costly. These calculators can control a variety of output devices and can be programmed by and accept data from a keyboard, paper tape, or marked cards. They have internal memory of up to several thousand words, with additional memory available on magnetic cards, tape, or disk.

From: Postpartum Assessment of Maternal-Fetal Incompatibility. Use of a Programmable Calculator for Interpretive Reporting of Laboratory Data. *JAMA* 1976;235:2530–2534. Copyright 1976 by the American Medical Association.

The calculator we have used is programmed in BASIC, a conversational-type language, so that our laboratory personnel are readily able to write and alter programs.

With this device, we are able to (1) prepare comprehensive, concise, and clearly formatted reports of the data, (2) monitor input of the variable sequence of tests for logic and completeness, and (3) provide programmed interpretation of the data for their clinical significance (see Table 20–1 on p 166).

The Study and Data

Assessment of the mother's postpartum need for immune anti-D serum or for determining maternal-fetal ABO incompatibility usually begins when we receive cord blood specimens from babies of all mothers who are ABO-group O or Rho-negative. The technologist's bench-manual instructions for the sequence of

Figure 20–1. Patient data input.

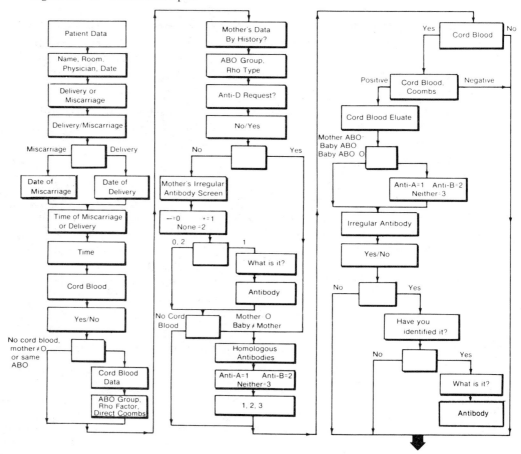

tests to be done parallel the data input section of the program in the programmable calculator and can be best followed by analyzing the program itself (Figure 20–1). This parallelism between analysis at the bench and the calculator's control of data input is the quality control mechanism that prevents errors of omission and eliminates unnecessary tests.

The interaction between calculator and technologist takes place in a conversational mode. The calculator requests the patient's name, room number, physician's name, date of report, and whether the mother had a delivery or miscarriage and its date and time. The calculator asks whether the technologist received a cord blood specimen—"Cord Blood?" If "Yes," cord blood ABO and Rho types and direct Coombs' reaction are requested. If "No," this sequence is bypassed. Next, the calculator requests maternal ABO group and Rho type, if done now or by history. Then, there is the "Anti-D Request?," ie, has the doctor requested an evaluation for giving immune anti-D antiserum? If so, the technologist's bench manual has required that a maternal serum specimen be typed and also screened for irregular antibodies, and that they be identified if present. These answers are requested at this point. If there has been no request for the anti-D serum evaluation, this sequence is bypassed, and the calculator asks for "Homologous Antibodies in Cord Blood." If the immune anti-D evaluation has been requested and there is also maternal-fetal ABO incompatibility (mother = O and baby ABO not same as mother's), both routines are accessioned and must be answered by the technologist.

If there is no need for maternal-fetal ABO incompatibility evaluation or no cord blood specimen was obtained, as with miscarriage or abortion, the "Homologous Antibody" routine is bypassed.

Next, if there is a cord blood specimen and the direct Coombs' reaction is positive, the calculator will request data on antibody in the eluate and its identity. This includes irregular, ie, non-ABO-related, antibody, and if maternal-fetal ABO incompatibility is present, homologous antibodies.

Data entry by the technologist is now complete.

Printing the Report

Data

The calculator proceeds to the second phase of the program and begins printing the report (Figure 20–2). The patient's identifying features are followed by a title selected according to whether the immune anti-D serum was requested by the physician. Next, pertinent tests with corresponding maternal and cord blood results are listed. In doing this, the calculator repeatedly checks for presence or absence of a cord blood specimen so that, if absent, the irrelevant column is omitted. The logic used here parallels the calculator-controlled data input

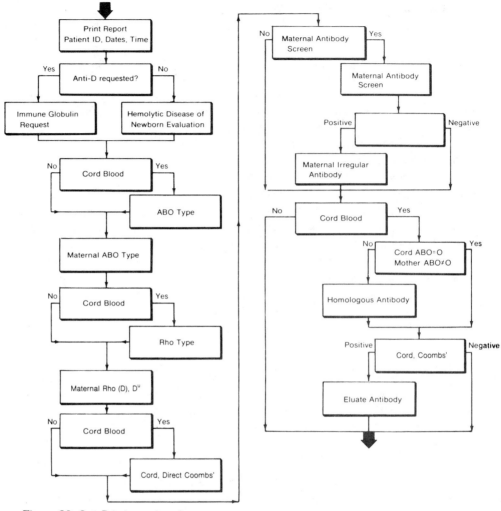

Figure 20–2. Printing patient data.

so that the report contains only data that are pertinent to the study and their interpretation. In addition, other antibodies when present are identified in the report.

Interpretation

The last part of the calculator's program reviews the data for significance according to preprogrammed logic (Figure 20–3). If an evaluation for administering immune anti-D serum has been requested, the calculator checks the mother's Rho type. If Rho-positive, the serum is contraindicated and corresponding com-

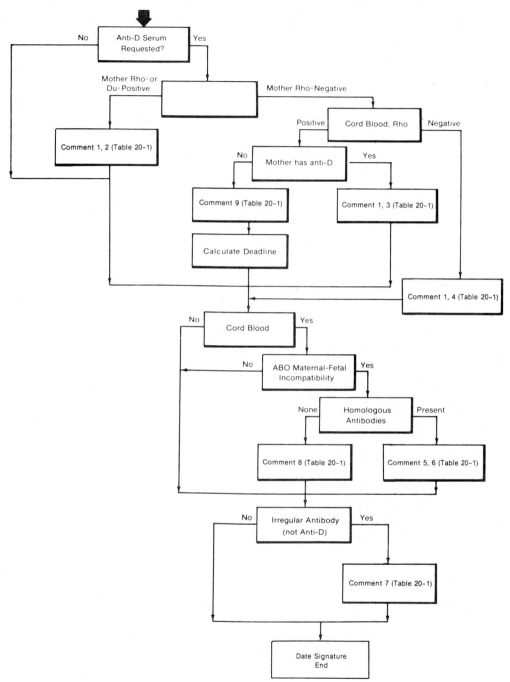

Figure 20–3. Printing interpretive review of patient data. Please refer to Table 20–1 on the following page.

Table 20–1.

Preprogrammed Comments After Interpretive Review of Maternal or Neonate's Data.

---

1. Anti-Rho immune serum is not indicated.
2. Mother is Rho(D) positive.
3. Mother is already sensitized (has anti-D).
4. Infant lacks the Rho(D)(D^u) antigen.
5. Hemolytic disease of the newborn is present due to ABO incompatibility (A, anti-A).*
6. Severity of involvement is best determined by further clinical evaluation.
7. Irregular red blood cell antibody present identified as anti-_____.*
8. ABO maternal-fetal incompatibility is present but there is no evidence of hemolytic disease of the newborn.
9. Serum is indicated and compatible. Administer intramuscularly before _____.

*Specific antigen and antibody are designated according to data input.

Figure 20–4. Fictionalized patient evaluation for anti-Rho immune human globulin administration. Lot no. to be filled in since serum is indicated. Maternal-fetal ABO incompatibility present and evaluated as potential cause of hemolytic disease of newborn.

```
MARY JONES                    3122-2              DR. J. SMITH


DATE OF REQUEST        10/1/83
DATE OF DELIVERY       9/ 30 TIME: 11:00PM


                       ANTI-RHO(D) IMMUNE HUMAN GLOBULIN REQUEST
                                    (RHOGAM)

                       CORD BLOOD        MATERNAL BLOOD
ABO TYPE               A                 O
RHO(D) (D")            POSITIVE          NEGATIVE
DIRECT COOMBS'         POSITIVE          -----
ANTIBODY SCREEN        -----             NEGATIVE
HOMOLOGOUS ANTIBODY    ANTI-A            -----
ELUATE ANTIBODY        ANTI-A            -----

                       RHOGAM SERUM IS INDICATED AND COMPATIBLE
                             (LOT #        )
                       ADMINISTER IM BEFORE 10/  3,  11:00PM


                       HEMOLYTIC DISEASE OF THE NEWBORN IS PRESENT
                       DUE TO ABO INCOMPATIBILITY (A,  ANTI-A)

                       SEVERITY OF INVOLVEMENT IS BEST DETERMINED
                       BY FURTHER CLINICAL EVALUATION.



     TECH:     DATE:        PATHOLOGIST:
```

ments are printed—"Anti-Rho immune serum is not indicated. Mother is Rho-positive" (Table 20–1, comments 1 and 2). When occasional agglutinated clumps of red cells are noted during the microscopic phase of D^u typing, the laboratory will usually perform an acid-elution procedure for fetal red cells. This data can be commented on at this point.

If the mother is Rho-negative, the calculator checks the infant's Rho type. If negative, the serum is not indicated, and corresponding comments are printed (Table 20–1, comments 1 and 4). If the infant has the D or D^u antigen, the calculator next checks for maternal anti-D. If present, the serum is not indicated since the mother is already sensitized, and corresponding comments are printed (Table 20–1, comments 1 and 3). Beyond this point, the mother is not sensitized, is Rho-negative, and has an Rho-positive infant; the calculator concludes that the serum is indicated and calculates the 72-hour deadline for its administration from the data and time of delivery.

In those communities where antipartum injection of anti-Rho immune serum may have been given, the testing and program sequences will have to be modified to account for this possibility (Figure 20–4).

Following this, or after bypassing the previous routine if the immune anti-D serum evaluation was not requested, the calculator checks for presence or absence of a cord blood specimen. If "Yes," it will check for possible ABO-related maternal-fetal incompatibility, ie, a group O mother with a group A or B baby. If this situation exists, the calculator will check for homologous antibodies in the infant's serum or on its cells; if present, it will print comments indicating that hemolytic disease of the newborn is present and the involved antigen and antibody. A cautionary note regarding severity is added, since this type of hemolytic disease of the newborn is usually mild (Table 20–1, comments 5 and 6). If homologous antibody is not present, the calculator prints the conclusion that there is maternal-fetal ABO incompatibility without evidence of related hemolytic disease (Table 20–1, comment 8).

The calculator next checks for data of an irregular antibody, not anti-D and not ABO-related, and, if present, prints it (Table 20–1, comment 7).

The final line is for dating the report and for signature by the technologist and pathologist (Figure 20–4). This serves as the official order to the nurse to give the antiserum when indicated.

References

1. Pollack W. German JG, Freda VJ: Prevention of Rh hemolytic disease. *Progr Hematol* 1969;6:121–147.
2. Mollison PL: *Blood Transfusion in Clinical Medicine*, ed 4. Philadelphia, FA Davis Co, 1972, pp 696–706, 711.

Chapter 21

Anemia

Ralph O. Wallerstein, MD

Anemia is a common clinical finding that can be assessed by a systematic use of the laboratory. More than 30 tests dealing directly with the cause of anemia are available in good hospital laboratories (Table 21–1). Problems with anemia can usually be solved by a few judiciously selected procedures. The tests can be separated into screening and specific classifications (Table 21–1). The screening tests can establish the category in which the anemia belongs, and the specific tests enable further study of the anemia in that category.

It is convenient to begin the workup by considering the four categories of anemia: (1) iron deficiency, (2) megaloblastic, (3) hemolytic, and (4) bone-marrow failure, which has four subcategories—absolute (eg, aplastic anemia, leukemia, myeloma), relative (anemia associated with chronic disease, eg, infection, azotemia, liver diseases), ineffective erythropoiesis (eg, intramedullary hemolysis or refractory normoblastic anemia), and pure red blood cell (RBC) anemia. The most common anemias are iron deficiency and relative marrow failure.

Initial Studies

The following studies should be carried out first before ordering other tests: (1) RBC indexes (obtained by an electronic counter), (2) examination of the blood smear, (3) reticulocyte count, (4) platelet count, (5) serum iron level and total iron-binding capacity (TIBC), and (6) some routine chemical screening.

RBC Indexes. Red blood cell indexes sometimes enable an immediate diagnosis. Mean corpuscular volume (1) less than 80 μm^3 (80 fL) is either iron deficiency or thalassemia minor, (2) less than 100 μm^3 (100 fL) is *not* pernicious

From: Role of the Laboratory in the Diagnosis of Anemia, *JAMA* 1976;236:490–493. Copyright 1976 by the American Medical Association.

Table 21–1.
Standard Laboratory Tests for the Diagnosis of Anemia.

All Tests*	Tests for Megaloblastic Anemia	Specific Tests for Hemolytic Anemia	Tests for Anemia Due to Marrow Failure
Antinuclear antibody	Folic acid, serum	Antinuclear antibody	Bence Jones protein
Bence Jones protein	Gastric analysis	Chromium 51 RBC survival	Cryoglobulin
Bilirubin, serum†	Schilling or other tests of vitamin B_{12} absorption	Cold agglutinin	Immunoelectrophoresis
Blood smear (O)	Vitamin B_{12} serum	Complement	^{111}In-indium chloride scan
Blood urea nitrogen†		Coombs'	Protein electrophoresis, serum
Chromium 51 RBC survival		Fetal hemoglobin	Technetium Tc 99m sulfur colloid scan
Cold agglutinin		Glucose-6-phosphate dehydrogenase	
Complement (R)		Ham	
Coombs'		Haptoglobin	
Cryoglobulin		Heinz bodies	
Fetal hemoglobin		Hemoglobin electrophoresis	
Folic acid, serum (R)		Lead in blood	
Gastric analysis (O)		Methemoglobin	
Glucose-6-phosphate dehydrogenase		Osmotic fragility	
Haptoglobin		Plasma hemoglobin	
Heinz bodies		Sickle cell	
Hemoglobin electrophoresis			
Immunoelectrophoresis			
^{111}In-indium chloride scan			

Iron/TIBC,
  serum
Lactic
  dehydroge-
  nase, serum†
Lead in blood (R)
Methemoglobin (R)
Osmotic fragility
Plasma hemoglobin
Platelet count (O)
Protein
  electrophoresis
Protein, total,
  serum†
RBC indexes
Reticulocyte
  count (O)
Schilling or other
  tests of vitamin
  B_{12} absorption
Sickle cell
Stool for blood
  (guaiac)
Technetium Tc 99m
  sulfur colloid
  scan
Vitamin B_{12}
  serum (R)

*Basic screening tests are boldfaced. TIBC = total iron-binding capacity. O = office laboratory; R = reference laboratory; all others, community hospital laboratory.
†Part of routine chemical screening.

171

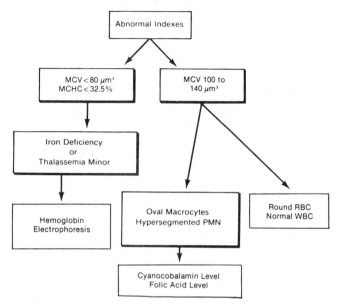

Figure 21–1. Low mean corpuscular volume (MCV) means either iron deficiency or thalassemia minor. Oval macrocytes usually mean megaloblastic anemia; round macrocytes are of little diagnostic value. MCHC = mean corpuscular hemoglobin concentration; PMN = polymorphonuclear cells.

anemia, (3) more than 120 μm^3 (120 fL) usually means liver disease or megaloblastic anemia, and (4) more than 110 μm^3 (110 fL) is strong evidence against anemia of chronic disease or acute blood loss. Mean corpuscular hemoglobin concentration (1) more than 36% means hereditary spherocytosis, and (2) less than 32.5% usually means iron deficiency or thalassemia minor (Figure 21–1).

Blood Smear. Examination of the blood smear should include a search for the following cells or bodies that may lead to the diagnosis: (1) Spherocytes indicate hereditary spherocytosis or autoimmune hemolytic anemia. (2) Schistocytes (contracted cells, helmet cells, triangular cells) suggest mechanical damage to blood vessels by fibrin or cancer. (3) Oval cells suggest congenital elliptocytosis, megaloblastic anemia, and occasionally refractory normoblastic anemia or myelofibrosis. (4) Prominent basophilic stippling (young cells whose RNA is precipitated by Wright stain; these cells are differentiated from reticulocytes whose RNA is precipitated only by supravital stain) suggests lead poisoning or thalassemia minor. (5) Target cells are seen in patients after splenectomy, with jaundice or liver disease, and in many hemoglobinopathies. (6) Howell-Jolly bodies (nuclear remnants) are present after splenectomy and frequently in megaloblastic anemia (Figure 21–2).

Reticulocyte Count. The percentage of reticulocytes may contribute to the diagnosis: (1) Fifty percent or more indicates autoimmune hemolytic anemia

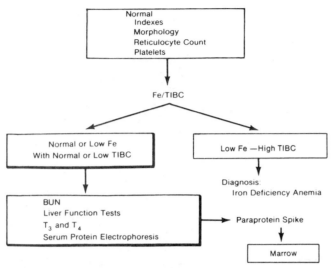

Figure 21–2. When indexes, red blood cell morphology, reticulocytes, and platelets are normal, differential is frequently between iron-deficiency anemia and anemia of chronic disease. Multiple myeloma frequently appears as an unexplained anemia with normal white blood cells and platelets. TIBC = total iron-binding capacity; T_3 = triiodothyronine; T_4 = thyroxine.

(positive Coombs' test) or RBC pyruvate kinase deficiency (negative Coombs' test). (2) Persistence of 10% to 20% usually means hemolysis. Occasionally, acute blood loss can raise the count to this level, and specific therapy for pernicious anemia or folic acid deficiency may result in high counts, but the reticulocytes show an orderly rise, peak at one week, and decline two weeks after initiating therapy. (3) Less than 5% indicates that hemolytic anemia is probably *not* present. (4) Less than 1% suggests aplastic anemia, pernicious anemia, and pure RBC anemia (Figure 21–3).

Platelet Count. (1) A low platelet count ($< 100,000/\text{mm}^3$) with anemia but no frank thrombocytopenic purpura indicates that the marrow is the site of disease and that aplastic anemia, possibly leukemia, or some other malignancy is present. (2) Low platelet count, leukopenia, and moderate anemia are also present in hypersplenism.

Serum Iron Level and TIBC. Serum iron and TIBC should be measured early in the workup. However, they should not be measured in a patient with fever or infection because the values are always low, in patients with a high reticulocyte count because they do not have iron-deficiency anemia, or in patients with pernicious anemia treated with cyanocobalamin because serum iron falls to a low level and stays low for weeks even if body stores of iron are ample. (1) A low serum iron level ($< 35\ \mu\text{g/dL}$ [6.3 $\mu\text{mol/L}$]) with a high TIBC ($> 350\ \mu\text{g/dL}$ [62.6 $\mu\text{mol/L}$]) means iron deficiency, whereas a normal serum iron level excludes iron deficiency. (2) A low serum iron level and a low TIBC are not diag-

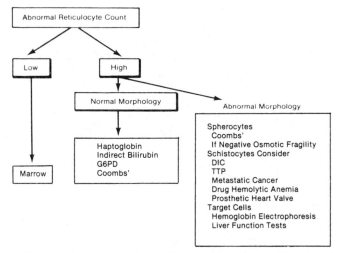

Figure 21–3. Most hemolytic anemias have a high reticulocyte count. Some hemolytic anemias have their specific morphologic abnormalities. If they do not, glucose-6-phosphate dehydrogenase deficiency or autoimmune hemolytic anemia without spherocytes may be the problem. A low reticulocyte count with moderate-to-severe anemia implies some form of marrow failure. G6PD = glucose-6-phosphate dehydrogenase; DIC = disseminated intravascular coagulation; TTP = thrombotic thrombocytopenic purpura.

nostic; the serum iron level in many of the anemias associated with chronic disease may be as low as 10 μg/dL. Percent saturation is not very helpful.

Routine Chemical Screening. Routine chemical screening may provide useful information for determining the cause of anemia. (1) The serum lactic dehydrogenase level may be elevated in megaloblastic anemia, myelofibrosis, or hemolytic anemia with intravascular hemolysis. (2) Blood urea nitrogen level of more than 50 mg/dL (17.9 mmol/L) suggests anemia with decreased RBC production in azotemia. (3) A very low serum total bilirubin level (< 0.4 mg/dL [6.8 μmol/L]) may indicate iron-deficiency anemia. (4) A greatly elevated serum total protein level but a normal albumin level suggest the possibility of myeloma.

Secondary Studies

Helpful Tests. Serum vitamin B_{12} and folic acid measurements, gastric analysis, and the Schilling test are helpful only in differentiating vitamin B_{12} deficiency from folic acid deficiency after megaloblastic anemia has been established by the characteristic morphology of RBCs and white blood cells (WBCs), oval macrocytes, and a high level of serum lactic dehydrogenase.

Marrow aspiration or biopsy is particularly helpful in detecting the presence or absence of iron; in confirming the presence of megaloblastic anemia; and in determining the exact cause of marrow failure, ie, aplastic anemia, leukemia, lymphoma, myeloma, macroglobulinemia, refractory normoblastic anemia, and

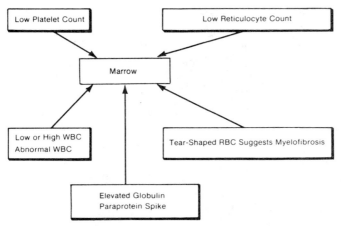

Figure 21–4. Thrombocytopenia, reticulocytopenia, abnormal white blood cells (WBCs), paraprotein, and tear-shaped red blood cells (RBCs) call for examination of marrow.

pure RBC anemia. Marrow analysis is usually unnecessary if iron deficiency anemia has been established by characteristic serum iron values, and it adds little to the diagnosis of hemolytic anemia (Figure 21–4).

Misapplied Tests. Some hematologic tests are frequently misapplied. The Schilling test is noncontributory in patients with a mean corpuscular volume less than 100 μm^3, with elevated WBC count ($>11,000/mm^3$) or reticulocyte ($>3\%$) counts, or with spherocytes. Serum vitamin B_{12} should, of course, not be measured immediately after a Schilling test has been carried out.

Hemoglobin electrophoresis is noncontributory in patients with low platelet ($<100,000/mm^3$) and WBC ($<3,000/mm^3$) counts or normal-appearing RBCs.

Approximately half of the available laboratory tests for the diagnosis of anemia are pertinent only to the furter study of hemolytic anemia. Coombs' test, cold agglutinin, hemoglobin electrophoresis, osmotic fragility, and RBC enzyme studies are useful only to define the cause of hemolytic anemia more precisely. They are noncontributory in patients with a normal reticulocyte count or with hypochromic microcytic anemia.

The diagnostic procedures of nuclear medicine are rarely needed in the initial diagnosis of anemia but may help in quantitating certain defects. Shortened RBC survival can almost invariably be predicted by persistent anemia despite an elevated reticulocyte count and adequate number of marrow erythroblasts, but survival studies with radioactive chromium (^{51}Cr) may be needed to demonstrate sequestration in the spleen. A technetium Tc 99m sulfur colloid scan may show an enlarged but nonpalpable spleen when hypersplenism is suspected. It may also "visualize" splenic cysts. In myelofibrosis, this isotope may highlight areas of remaining reticuloendothelial activity. Similarly, ^{111}In-indium chloride, which attaches to transferrin, may show residual erythroblast activity, but it is not entirely specific.

Hematologic Patterns of Anemias

Iron-Deficiency Anemia. Iron-deficiency anemia is characterized by a mean corpuscular hemoglobin concentration less than 32.5%, a mean corpuscular volume usually less than 80 μm^3, a serum iron level less than 35 $\mu g/dL$, TIBC more than 350 $\mu g/dL$, and absence of hemosiderin in the marrow. These abnormal deviations may not be apparent until four weeks after onset of the blood loss.

Thalassemia Minor. Thalassemia minor, a mild form of anemia, has a similar hematologic pattern as described in iron-deficiency anemia, but must be differentiated from it for therapeutic reasons. The incidence of thalassemia minor is particularly high in areas where many people of Mediterranean, especially Italian, or Cantonese-Chinese origin reside. Unlike iron-deficiency anemia, the hemoglobin value is more than 9 g/dL and usually between 10 and 13 g/dL, but the RBC count is often higher than the normal count. The mean corpuscular hemoglobin concentration is only slightly low, but the mean corpuscular volume is well below 80 μm^3 and may be less than 60 μm^3. The diagnosis of thalassemia minor may be established definitely by finding an elevated concentration of hemoglobin A_2 or F determined by hemoglobin electrophoresis.

Megaloblastic Anemia. This type of anemia is easily recognized by large oval macrocytes, hypersegmented polymorphonuclear cells, characteristic bone-marrow findings, and appropriately low serum levels of vitamin B_{12} (<100 $\mu\mu g/mL$) or folic acid (<2 ng/mL).

Hemolytic Anemia. In most long-term hemolytic anemias, the reticulocyte count is elevated (>5%), and the indirect serum bilirubin level is slightly elevated (>1 mg/dL); the serum lactic dehydrogenase level may be elevated and the haptoglobin absent. After these general signs of hemolysis are established, specific tests to establish the type of hemolysis should be carried out: osmotic fragility to establish hereditary spherocytosis, Coombs' test to establish autoimmune hemolytic anemia, hemoglobin electrophoresis to diagnose hemoglobinopathy, and enzyme studies to diagnose hereditary nonspherocytic hemolytic anemia.

The hemoglobinopathies occur mostly in the black population; target cells are common to all populations. Red blood cell indexes are usually within normal limits. Sickle-cell anemia is the most common hemoglobinopathy, but other variants (eg, SC and CC disease) must be considered.

Absolute Marrow Failure. The normal myeloid tissue has been replaced by fat (aplastic anemia), fibrosis (myelofibrosis), or malignancy (lymphosarcoma, multiple myeloma, or leukemia). The platelet count and absolute reticulocyte count are usually low. Morphologically abnormal WBCs help to make the diagnosis. A bone-marrow aspirate or biopsy specimen is essential for specific diagnosis.

Relative Marrow Failure. This type of anemia is usually found in patients with the anemias of chronic disease. In general, RBCs have normal morphology, and WBC, platelet, and reticulocyte counts are within normal limits.

The serum iron level is low (<50 µg/dL), and the TIBC may be low. This type of anemia is characterized by a moderately shortened RBC survival, with only suboptimal compensatory increase in marrow activity; the RBC survival time is often 85% shorter than in normal subjects, but the marrow activity only compensates for 25% to 35% of this. In contrast, marrow in patients with chronic blood loss or with an uncomplicated hemolytic anemia, such as hereditary spherocytosis, can increase its output by six to ten times. Other abnormal findings are related to impaired protein synthesis and include low levels of transferrin, erythropoietin, and albumin. The relative unavailability of iron accounts for the increase in RBC protoporphrin in these conditions. There are some subtle differences between the anemias caused by relative marrow failure. Anemia associated with cirrhosis of the liver is primarily hemolytic; target cells are frequently present, spur cells are seen occasionally, and the reticulocyte count is usually slightly elevated. Anemia associated with azotemia is primarily hypoplastic; erythropoietin levels are decreased, and sometimes a few burr cells are found in the blood smear. Anemia associated with cancer is sometimes complicated by blood loss, and contracted cells and schistocytes are occasionally present.

Ineffective Erythropoiesis. In this type of anemia or intramedullary hemolysis, production and destruction of erythroblasts are greatly increased in the marrow, permitting only few and often misshapen and poorly made RBCs to reach the bloodstream. Pernicious anemia is the best-known example of this mechanism; the thalassemias also show this form of dyserythropoiesis. In the so-called refractory normoblastic anemias or sideroachrestic anemias, intramedullary hemolysis is a prominent feature and is associated with characteristic ring sideroblasts in the marrow.

Pure RBC Anemia. In this peculiar form of marrow failure, the diagnosis is suspected in patients with profound anemia with very low reticulocyte counts (<1%) but normal WBC and platelet counts and normal RBC morphology. Bone-marrow aspiration or biopsy is essential for diagnosis.

Hypersplenism. This syndrome is usually secondary to some other disease, eg, cirrhosis of the liver, rheumatoid arthritis, or Gaucher's disease. It is characterized by a large spleen, pancytopenia, and cellular marrow without morphologic abnormalities of the RBCs and WBCs or platelets.

Chapter 22

Positive Serologic Test for Syphilis

Terrence J. Lee, MD

P. Frederick Sparling, MD

Since the development of the Wassermann complement-fixation test in 1906, laboratory tests have been invaluable aids in the diagnosis of syphilis. The use of these tests continues on a large scale, but their utility and interpretation are not always clear to the physician, who is the one who must make the critical decisions concerning treatment. The two basic types of serologic tests currently available are nontreponemal and treponemal.

The standard nontreponemal test used in the United States is the VDRL slide test. Other related tests include the rapid plasma reagin and unheated serum reagin tests. Since the antibody measured (reagin) can also be present transiently after immunizations or various febrile illnesses and chronically in conditions such as collagen vascular disease, leprosy, and drug addiction, VDRL test reactivity is not specific for syphilis. On the other hand, the VDRL test is easily quantitated, and serial titers are helpful in following the response to therapy and in assessing the possibility of reinfection. In addition, the VDRL test is practical, inexpensive, and widely available; it remains the test of choice for screening purposes.

To make a serologic diagnosis of syphilis, patients with a positive VDRL test should be tested for presence of specific antitreponemal antibodies. The most widely used treponemal test is the fluorescent treponemal antibody absorption (FTA-ABS) test. The incidence of false-positive FTA-ABS tests is low (1% to 2%) when it is used to confirm a positive VDRL test. Another treponemal test, the microhemagglutination-*Treponema pallidum* (MHA-TP) test, may become more commonly used in the future. Its sensitivity and specificity are nearly identical to the FTA-ABS test, except for patients with primary syphilis (Table 22–1). Both

From: Syphilis. An Algorithm. *JAMA* 1979;242:1187–1189. Copyright 1979 by the American Medical Association.

┌──── **Table 22–1.** ──
│ Percentage of Positive Serologic Tests in Untreated Syphilis.

	Test		
Disease Stage	*VDRL*	*FTA-ABS*	*Microhemagglutination Treponema pallidum*
Primary	70	85	50–60
Secondary	99	100	100
Latent or late	70	98	98

the FTA-ABS and MHA-TP tests are positive in almost all patients with secondary syphilis and in 95% or more of patients with latent syphilis.[1]

We present an algorithm stemming from a positive VDRL test and offer a systematic approach to the clarification, interpretation, and logical consequence of the results. The algorithm will be divided into three main branches—suspicious lesions (Figure 22–1), keys within history (Figure 22–2), and pregnancy (Figure 22–3).

Suspicious Lesions

Suspicious lesions (Figure 22–1), which are important in assessment of a patient with a positive VDRL test, are considered in blocks 1 and 2. The necessity of a careful and complete physical examination cannot be overstressed. This examination should include the anogenital region, the entire skin surface, hair, mucous membranes, and lymph node areas.

The demonstration of treponemes in suspected syphilitic lesions allows the physician to make an absolute diagnosis of syphilis. Although darkfield microscopy is relatively simple to do, many clinics and physicians lack the equipment or experience or both needed for this method. Local, state, and public health officers may be of assistance in this event. The darkfield examination is almost always positive in primary syphilis and in the moist mucosal lesions of secondary and congenital syphilis. Since saprophytic, nonpathogenic treponemes are common around the gingival margins, a darkfield examination of intraoral lesions may be difficult to interpret. If the examination of a lesion is found initially to be negative, darkfield microscopy should be repeated 24 hours later. The patient should be instructed not to use antibiotics and not to wash the lesion with soap or antiseptic solution in the interim.

If the darkfield examination is negative, the VDRL test should be repeated within the week. If the VDRL is positive and a specific treponemal test (FTA-ABS) confirms the result, treatment is begun. The presence of a positive VDRL test but a negative FTA-ABS test suggests a biologic false-positive reaction. A negative VDRL test on repeated examination suggests a technical false-

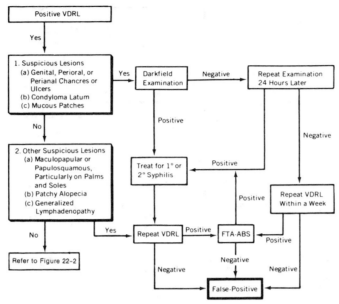

Figure 22–1. Suspicious lesions (positive VDRL). FTA-ABS = fluorescent treponemal antibody absorption.

positive or an acute biologic false-positive. Acute biologic false-positive reactions may occur with atypical pneumonia, vaccinations, malaria, and other bacterial and viral infections. Chronic biologic false-positive reactions may occur with systemic lupus erythematosus (SLE), thyroiditis and other autoimmune disorders, narcotic addiction, lymphoma, leprosy, and also in the elderly.[2]

False-positive reactions are not uncommon. Most false-positive results are, however, in the low titer range (1:1 to 1:4). Moore and Mohr[3] made a clinically useful distinction between various types of false-positive reactions. They defined acute reactors as anyone whose test for reagin reverted to normal in less than six months. Those whose positive tests persisted for more than six months were termed "chronic reactors." Most of the acute false-positive reactions occurred after a variety of infections or immunizations and were of little importance. A long-term false-positive VDRL test, on the other hand, especially in young women, carries a substantive risk that SLE, thyroiditis, or other autoimmune disorders will turn up in the future. Such patients should be followed up carefully for at least a 24-month period.[4]

The other suspicious lesions listed in block 2 are not generally amenable to darkfield examination, although aspiration of a lymph node may occasionally be positive in patients with secondary syphilis. If darkfield examination is not feasible, serologic confirmation will be required for diagnosis.

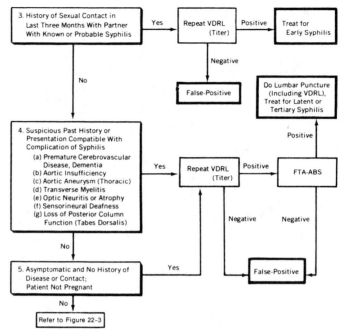

Figure 22–2. Keys in history (positive VDRL). FTA-ABS = fluorescent treponemal antibody absorption.

Keys Within History

Approximately 16% of the named recent contacts of patients with early-stage syphilis will be found to have active untreated syphilis; a similar percentage of persons named as suspects or associates will also have active syphilis. These data emphasize the importance of historical information in assessing the importance of a positive VDRL test and in staging the phase of disease so that appropriate therapy may be designated (Figure 22–2). In patients with a recent positive history (block 3), a repeated VDRL test with titer should be obtained. No single titer is in itself diagnostic, but notable rises (fourfold or greater) in paired sera are strongly indicative of acute primary syphilis.

Patients with a suspicious history and a presentation compatible with complications of syphilis (block 4), as well as those with a negative history (block 5), should have repeated VDRL testing and confirmation with FTA-ABS testing before initiation of treatment. Lumbar puncture should be performed in patients with late or tertiary syphilis to rule out the possibility of asymptomatic neurosyphilis.[5] Spinal-fluid examination is not necessary in patients with early-stage (primary or secondary) syphilis. The cerebrospinal fluid (CSF) serologic test of choice is the quantitative VDRL test.[6] The diagnostic value of the CSF FTA-ABS test in patients with syphilitic neurologic disease remains unproved. The CSF cell count and total protein content should also be determined.

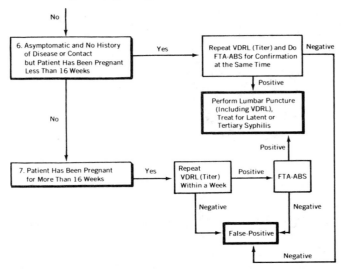

Figure 22–3.   Pregnancy (positive VDRL). FTA-ABS = fluorescent treponemal antibody absorption.

Pregnancy

The pregnant patient represents a special problem because of the risk of infection to the fetus (Figure 22–3). All pregnant women should have the benefit of a VDRL test during pregnancy, and if at high risk of syphilis (young, unmarried, low socioeconomic status, or numerous sexual contacts), a second test should be done before delivery. There has been a widespread belief that the spirochetes of syphilis are unable to cross the placenta and infect the fetus until sometime after the fourth month of gestation. However, Harter and Benirschke[7] recently demonstrated spirochetes in two abortuses (of nine and ten weeks' gestational age) from mothers with serologic and clinical evidence of recent syphilitic infection. Although this work indicates that spirochetes may cross the placental barrier before 16-weeks' gestation, therapy given before the fifth month of pregnancy probably prevents the late sequelae of congenital syphilis.

In general, the pregnant patient should be examined as soon as possible because of the risk of concomitant fetal infection. Patients pregnant less than 16 weeks with a confirmed positive VDRL test and historical or clinical evidence of untreated syphilis should be treated immediately. In other patients who are VDRL-positive but who have no clinical or historical evidence of syphilis and are FTA-ABS-negative, treatment may be withheld temporarily. In such patients a quantitative VDRL test and another FTA-ABS test should be repeated in four weeks. If after the repeated examination, the diagnosis remains equivocal, the patient should be treated to prevent possible disease in the fetus.

Because the intent of this chapter is the clarification of the interpretation and utilization of diagnostic serologic tests for syphilis stemming from a positive screening nontreponemal test (VDRL), we have omitted specific comments concerning therapy. The reader is referred instead to the recent Public Health Service recommendations.[8, 9]

This investigation was supported by fellowship grant AIO5216 from the Public Health Service and grant AI10646 from the National Institute of Allergy and Infectious Diseases.

Martin Siegel, MD, and his colleagues at the Center for Disease Control, Atlanta, reviewed the manuscript and provided helpful comments.

References

1. Jaffe HW: The laboratory diagnosis of syphilis. *Ann Intern Med* 1975;83:846–850.
2. Sparling PF: Diagnosis and treatment of syphilis. *N Engl J Med* 1971;284:642–653.
3. Moore JE, Mohr CF: Biologically false positive serologic tests for syphilis: Type, incidence, and cause. *JAMA* 1952;150:467–473.
4. Catterall RD: Systemic disease and the biological false positive reaction. *Br J Vener Dis* 1972;48:1–12.
5. Sparling PF: Current problems in sexually transmitted diseases, in Stollerman GH (ed): *Advances in Internal Medicine*. Chicago, Year Book Medical Publishers, 1979, vol 24, pp 203–228.
6. Jaffe HW, Larson SA, Peters M, et al: Tests for treponemal antibody in CSF. *Arch Intern Med* 1978;138:252–255.
7. Harter CA, Benirschke K: Fetal syphilis in the first trimester. *Am J Obstet Gynecol* 1976;124:705–711.
8. Syphilotherapy 1976: Position papers for the current USPHS recommendations. *J Am Vener Dis Assoc* 1976;3:98.
9. Venereal Disease Control Division, Center for Disease Control: *Recommended Treatment Schedules for Syphilis—1976*. Atlanta, Center for Disease Control, 1976.

Chapter 23

Suspected Gonococcal Infection

Nicholas B. Riccardi, PhD
Yehudi M. Felman, MD

Gonorrhea is still the most commonly reported infectious disease both on the national and local levels. To control the gonorrhea epidemic, proper laboratory detection of the causative organism from clinical isolates is essential. This chapter discusses the proper diagnostic techniques involved in collecting specimens from primary sites of infection, the sensitivity of Gram-stained smears, and the development of gonorrhea transport systems and selective media. An evaluation of culturing systems intended for the private practitioner is also presented.

Methods of Obtaining the Specimen

The laboratory diagnosis of uncomplicated symptomatic gonococcal urethritis in the man is performed by obtaining specimens from the anterior urethra with an applicator and performing a Gram-stained smear. The finding of typical Gram-negative intracellular diplococci within the pus cells of the urethral discharge is sufficient for a laboratory diagnosis. This test ranges in sensitivity from 93% to 99%.[1] If the Gram's stain is negative in symptomatic men or where history indicates the possibility of asymptomatic urethral infection, ie, known sexual contacts to infected persons, a urethral culture should be obtained and inoculated on gonorrhea selective medium. This is accomplished by inserting a fine calcium alginate swab for approximately 2 cm into the anterior urethra.

In the woman, the endocervix is the site that is most often positive. A direct smear examination of exudates from this site is too insensitive to exclude the diagnosis of gonorrhea. The range of sensitivity for this test is in the area of 38% to 69%.[1-4] Thus, it is necessary to obtain cervical cultures. By culturing the rectum simultaneously, the diagnostic yield can be increased from 3% to

From: Laboratory Diagnosis in the Problem of Suspected Gonococcal Infection. *JAMA* 1979; 242:2703–2705. Copyright 1979 by the American Medical Association.

7%.[2, 5] Cervical specimens are obtained by inserting a bivalve vaginal speculum so as to expose the cervix. The speculum may be moistened only with warm water if a lubricant is necessary. Commercial lubricants should not be used, as they may be toxic to the gonococcus. The area is cleansed of any cervical mucus with a cotton ball, and a sterile cotton-tipped swab is inserted into the endocervical canal, twirled in a ringing motion for a few seconds before removal, and then inoculated immediately onto a gonorrhea-selective medium.

Rectal culturing should be done on all persons who engage in rectal sexual activity. Blind rectal smear examinations have a sensitivity range of about 30% to 48%.[1, 6] The cultures are obtained by inserting a cotton-tipped applicator approximately 2.5 cm into the anal canal. Care should be taken not to contaminate the swab excessively with feces. The specimen should be inoculated onto a gonorrhea-selective medium.

The direct smear examination in pharyngeal gonorrhea is both insensitive and nonspecific. Specimens are obtained by swabbing areas of inflammation in the tonsils and posterior pharynx, which are then inoculated directly onto a gonorrhea selective medium. Since the sensitivity and specificity for pharyngeal cultures are not known, it is advisable to perform several repeated cultures on specimens from this site.

Development of Media

The cultivation of the gonococcus on artificial media was performed a few years after its discovery. The primary cultivation from clinical sources on laboratory media is difficult, because the organism is not only fastidious but is also exceedingly susceptible to the toxic effects of a variety of substances commonly present in media. Gonococci are aerobic organisms but require 2% to 10% atmosphere of carbon dioxide for growth at 35 to 37°C.

Thayer and Martin[7] in 1964 described a selective medium for the growth of pathogenic *Neisseria*. This medium (TM) contained the antibiotics polymyxin B sulfate and ristocetin. The addition of the antibiotics allows for the isolation of the gonococcus from sites highly contaminated with other bacteria.

In 1966, Thayer and Martin[8] changed their original medium. Polymyxin and ristocetin were replaced by vancomycin hydrochloride, colistimethate sodium, and nystatin. The addition of trimethoprim lactate to TM for the suppression of *Proteus* sp is referred to as modified TM (MTM) medium.

In 1973, Faur et al[9] developed NYC medium. This medium contains the following antimicrobial agents: vancomycin, colistin, amphotericin B, and trimethoprim. The medium is transparent and provides for easy colony indentification.

Development of Nonnutritive Transport Systems

Stuart's Medium. Stuart[10] in 1946 described a nonnutritive, semisolid, buffered agar medium to preserve *Neisseria gonorrhoeae* for shipment to the laboratory for culturing. The organism is transported on a swab inside a bottle with a semisolid medium containing a reducing agent. The medium contains no nutrients, thus maintaining the organism without growth potentials until subcultured. The reducing agent is sodium thioglycolate. The semisolid agar content is to reduce the oxygen content. The swabs are treated with charcoal to reduce the toxic effect of agar on the gonococci.

Modified Stuart's Medium. This medium (Amies transport medium) was proposed by Amies[11] in 1967. The variation allowed for the addition of charcoal to the medium rather than on the cotton swab. It also uses a phosphate buffer rather than a glycerophosphate buffer to cut down on coliform contamination. This modification greatly improved the survival of 85 strains of gonococci for as long as 72 hours.

After the development of nutritive transport medium (Transgrow), nonnutritive transport media fell into disfavor. Hosty et al[12] compared TM medium incubated immediately to Transgrow, Amies transport, and Stuart's media held for 24 to 48 hours before reculturing. When held for 24 hours before culturing, Transgrow lost 8%; Amies, 28%; and Stuart's, 44%. When held for 48 hours, Transgrow lost 15%, and Amies lost 59.8%.

Development of a Nutritive Transport System

Transgrow Medium. In 1971, Martin and Lester[13] suggested the further modification of MTM medium by increasing the agar content from 1.25% to 1.5%. The resulting medium, called Transgrow, is a transport culture medium for the diagnosis of *N gonorrhoeae and N meningitidis* (Table 23–1). It is prepared in 33-mL screwcap glass bottles as agar slants charged with carbon dioxide at the time of manufacture.

After initial incubation the bottle should be transported to a laboratory for processing. However, the bottle can be processed directly to avoid a delay. Transgrow offers the following characteristics:

1. The size of the bottle is small, thus, somewhat difficult to inoculate.

2. Colony identification is difficult through the glass bottle; thus, it should be transported to a laboratory for reculturing and processing. The gonococci are labile to room temperature. Any transporting system that involves reculturing, even after preincubation at 35 to 37°C, increases the risk of obtaining a false-negative culture.[14] When Transgrow is transported without preincubation, a large percentage of the cultures will be falsely negative.[14]

3. An increased content of agar even though providing for additional gel strength may be toxic to some strains, thereby decreasing the positivity yield.

Table 23–1.
Systems Available for Private Practice for Diagnosing Gonorrhea.

	Transgrow	Neigon JEMBEC	Microcult	Isocult
Shelf life*	6 wk	12 wk	1–2 yr, dehydrated medium	6 mo
Refrigeration required for storage	Yes	Yes	No	Yes
Oxidase reagent has to be purchased separately	Yes	Yes	No	No
Disadvantages	Difficult to inoculate, colony identification difficult, less sensitive than modified Thayer-Martin (MTM) medium, may require reculturing onto MTM and hence increase time for processing, loss of carbon dioxide if not handled properly, and accumulation of condensation inside bottle masking appearance and spreading contaminants.	None	Inoculating area is small, colony identification difficult, less sensitive than MTM medium, and extremely unreliable for detecting pharyngeal and rectal gonorrhea.	Inoculating area is small, colony identification difficult, medium is a modified Transgrow, less sensitive than MTM, and more expensive per plate.

*According to manufacturer's specifications.

4. Concentration of carbon dioxide may be lowered considerably if the bottle is not handled properly.

5. Condensation frequently accumulates inside the bottles, thus masking the appearance of growth and spreading contaminants.

Development of Nontransport Systems Suitable for Office Practice

The Neigon JEMBEC System. In 1974, Martin et al[15] described the use of a carbon-dioxide-generating tablet in a culture plate sealed in a transparent gas-impermeable plastic bag. This led to the development of the JEMBEC plate (John E. Martin Biological Environmental Chamber), which allows the investigator to add the carbon dioxide required for growth after the specimen has been inoculated. The medium is basically MTM with further modifications, ie, less agar content than Transgrow and a higher concentration of nystatin (may vary according to manufacturer).

The Neigon JEMBEC system has the following characteristics:

1. It has a higher percent clinical yield especially in rectal isolates when compared with the Transgrow system.[14]

2. It was found equal to or superior to MTM in conventional petri dishes with candle jar extinction as the source of carbon dioxide.[16]

3. It has a good surface area and maintains a high level of carbon dioxide after incubation.[16]

4. This system can be transported after an incubation of 24 to 48 hours, or it can be easily processed in the office. If sent to the laboratory for processing, no reculturing is necessary.

The Microcult System. The Microcult system, developed by the Ames Company, is a dehydrated test system using MTM medium. It is rehydrated before use and employs a carbon-dioxide-generating tablet as its source of carbon dioxide. After office incubation the oxidase test can be performed by the office personnel without special training. Since colonial identification is difficult with this system, a paper strip coated with the oxidase reagent is applied to the medium 24 to 48 hours after inoculation. It does not require transportation to any laboratory for processing. This system has the following characteristics:

1. It is less sensitive than MTM medium in candle jar extinction.[17]

2. The system is small, and individual colony identification is practically impossible (only the results of the oxidase test can be seen).

3. It is extremely unreliable for detecting pharyngeal and rectal gonorrhea.[18]

The Isocult System. This system was developed by SKF Diagnostics and consists of a glass tube containing an inner paddle coated with modified Transgrow medium. The lower portion of the paddle is inoculated and then reinserted into the tube. A carbon-dioxide-generating tablet is also added to the tube at this time.

The collar of the tube contains streaking tines, which streak the specimen along the culture medium. The tube is incubated, and after the appearance of bacterial growth, the colonies are treated with the oxidase reagent. The characteristics of this system are as follows:

1. It is rather small, and colony identification is extremely difficult.
2. It is considerably more expensive per plate than the other systems.
3. Accurate field studies have not as yet been performed.

Processing the Culture Plate

The plate should be brought to room temperature before inoculation. After inoculation, the plate should be incubated immediately at 35 to 37°C and inspected 24 to 48 hours later for the small, mucoid, translucent colonies of *N gonorrhoeae* (not applicable to Microcult system). Colonies typical of *N gonorrhoeae* are then flooded with the oxidase reagent (dimethyl-p-phenylenediamine hydrochloride) (Caution: this agent is a potent allergen). This reagent combines with cytochrome oxidase present in all *Neisseria* sp to form dark blue to purple. The presence of a bacteria colony containing the enzyme cytochrome oxidase on a gonorrhea-selective medium is suggestive of gonorrhea. Further evidence is obtained by doing a Gram's stain on the bacteria of the colony. The finding of oxidase-positive, Gram-negative diplococci with typical colonial morphological appearance growing on gonorrhea-selective medium can be considered presumptively gonococci. Confirmatory evidence that the organism is *N gonorrhoeae* can be made by sugar fermentation tests (necessary only in oral infection). *N gonorrhoeae* ferments glucose with acid production but fails to produce acid from maltose, sucrose, or lactose. Subculturing must be done before applying the oxidase reagent.

References

1. Rothenberg RB, Simon R, Chipperfield E, et al: Efficacy of selected diagnostic tests for sexually transmitted diseases. *JAMA* 1976;235:49–51.
2. Caldwell JG, Price EU, Pagin GJ, et al: Sensitivity and reproductivity of Thayer-Martin culture medium in diagnosing gonorrhea in women. *Am J Obstet Gynecol* 1971;109:463–468.
3. Thin RNT, Williams IA, Nicol CS: Direct and delayed methods of immunofluorescent diagnosis of gonorrhea in women. *Br J Vener Dis* 1970;47:27–30.
4. Pariser H, Farmer AD: Diagnosis of gonorrhea in the asymptomatic female. *South Med J* 1968;61:505–506.
5. Schmale JD, Martin JE, Domescik G: Observations on the cultural diagnosis of gonorrhea in women. *JAMA* 1969;210:312–314.
6. Bhattacharyya MD, Jephcott AE: Diagnosis of gonorrhea in women: Role of rectal sample. *Br J Vener Dis* 1974;50:109–112.

7. Thayer JD, Martin JE: A selective medium for the cultivation of *N. gonorrhoeae* and *N. meningitidis. Public Health Rep* 1964;79:49–57.

8. Thayer JD, Martin JE: Improved medium selective for cultivation of *N. gonorrhoeae* and *N. meningitidis. Public Health Rep* 1966;81:559–562.

9. Faur YC, Weisburd MD, Wilson ME, et al: A new medium for the isolation of pathogenic *Neisseria* (NYC medium): I. Formulation and comparisons with standard media. *Health Lab Sci* 1973;10:44–54.

10. Stuart RD: Diagnosis and control of gonorrhea by bacteriological cultures, with preliminary report on new methods of transporting clinical material. *Glasgow Med J* 1946;27:131–142.

11. Amies CR: A modified formula for the preparation of Stuart's transport medium. *Can J Public Health* 1967;58:296–300.

12. Hosty TS, Freear MA, Baker C, et al: Comparison transportation media for the culturing of *N. gonorrhoeae. Am J Clin Pathol* 1974;62:435–437.

13. Martin JE, Lester A: Transgrow: A medium for transport and growth of *Neisseria gonorrhoeae* and *Neisseria meningitidis. US Dept of Health, Education, and Welfare Health Services and Mental Health Administration Health Rep* 1971;86:30–33.

14. Riccardi NB: *A Comparative Study of Rectal and Urethral Gonorrhea With Special Reference to Diagnosis and Culturing Techniques,* thesis. Fordham University, Bronx, NY, 1977.

15. Martin JE, Armstrong JH, Smith PB: A new system for the cultivation of *Neisseria gonorrhoeae. Appl Microbiol* 1974;27:802–805.

16. Martin JE, Jackson RL: A biological environmental chamber for the culture of *Neisseria gonorrhoeae. J Am Vener Dis Assoc* 1975;2:28–30.

17. Lewis JS: Evaluation of a new gonorrhea culture detection system—Microcult GC. *Health Lab Sci* 1976;14:22–25.

18. Neilsen AO, Andersen KE: An evaluation of Microcult GC in venereal disease clinics. *Sex Trans Dis* 1977;4:15–17.

Chapter 24

Hematuria

Eileen D. Brewer, MD
George S. Benson, MD

Hematuria, either gross or microscopic, in any patient warrants laboratory investigation. The direction and magnitude of this evaluation is dependent to a large extent on the age and sex of the patient and the presence or absence of a urinary tract infection. For example, hematuria in an otherwise asymptomatic 70-year-old man requires a significantly different evaluation than does hematuria in a 20-year-old woman with symptoms of cystitis or in an 8-year-old child with increased blood pressure. In this chapter, algorithms for the evaluation of hematuria are presented. The chapter addresses the problem of hematuria in the child, hematuria in the adult, and hematuria secondary to trauma.

Hematuria in the Child

In children, the laboratory investigation of hematuria begins with a urinalysis and urine culture. Further evaluation depends on the results of these tests. If the child has hematuria as well as a positive urine culture and symptoms of a urinary tract infection (which in the infant or younger child may be only fever or lower abdominal pain), the infection should be treated and a follow-up urinalysis and culture obtained (Figure 24–1). If these test results are negative, no further investigation may be needed. However, an infant girl or any boy with a first urinary tract infection, a child whose stature is less than the standards for age, or a girl with a second urinary tract infection should have an intravenous pyelogram (IVP) and voiding cystourethrogram (VCUG) to look for congenital anomalies, stones, or a foreign body in the bladder or urethra that might have predisposed the child to infection. A negative urine culture should be obtained before

From: Hematuria: Algorithms for Diagnosis. I. Hematuria in the Child. *JAMA* 1981;246:877–880. Hematuria: Algorithms for Diagnosis. II. Hematuria in the Adult and Hematuria Secondary to Trauma. *JAMA* 1981;246:993–995. Copyright 1981 by the American Medical Association.

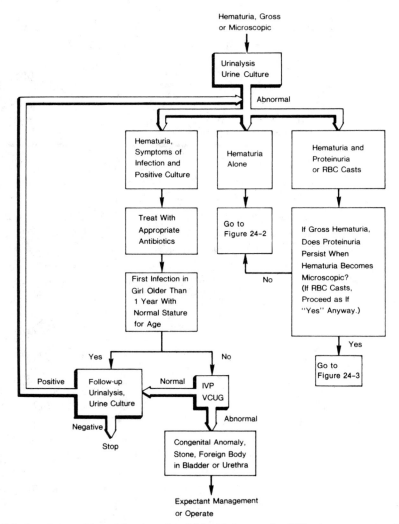

Figure 24—1. Approach to evaluation of a child with hematuria. IVP = intravenous pyelogram; VCUG = voiding cystourethrogram; RBC = red blood cell.

a VCUG is performed. If results of the IVP and VCUG are normal and hematuria persists after treatment of the infection, the evaluation of hematuria should continue.

Hematuria without other abnormalities on urinalysis (Figure 24–2) may be explained by bleeding from lesions of the external genitalia, but these will be obvious on physical examination. A follow-up urinalysis should be obtained when the lesion heals. If hematuria persists, the evaluation should proceed. A careful history will disclose whether the child has been taking a hematuria-causing drug, such as an antibiotic (eg, methicillin sodium), an anticoagulant, or cyclophosphamide. Even in a well-appearing child, the history of a recent upper respiratory tract or skin infection raises the possibility of a mild case of poststreptococcal glomerulonephritis. If there is evidence of a recent streptococcal infection (either a positive culture or rising antistreptolysin O [ASO], antihyaluronidase, or antideoxyribonuclease B titer) and if the serum C3 level is low, a presumptive diagnosis can be made and renal function should be assessed. The child may then be followed up expectantly with appropriate medical treatment. However, if the serum C3 level remains low after one or two months, another form of glomerulonephritis must be considered and further laboratory evaluation pursued.

The child with persistent hematuria (present on three urinalyses on different days) or recurrent hematuria without other abnormalities on urinalysis should have his or her renal function assessed by a serum creatinine level determination. In children, normal values for serum creatinine are lower than the usual adult normal values, and will vary with age, sex, and muscle mass.[1] A number of other blood tests may also provide useful information. Early membranoproliferative glomerulonephritis or lupus nephritis may be suspected by finding a low serum concentration of C3 or C4. A positive antinuclear antibody titer (ANA) will help make the diagnosis of lupus nephritis. Complete evaluation for diagnosis of these entities requires renal biopsy. In black children, a sickle cell screening test is necessary, since hematuria may be associated with sickle cell trait, and sickle cell crisis may present with hematuria, gross or microscopic. Rarely, hematuria will be caused by a coagulopathy (hemophilia, thrombocytopenia, disseminated intravascular coagulopathy), renal tuberculosis, or renal venous thrombosis, and appropriate investigation for these possibilities should be pursued.

An IVP may disclose hydronephrosis, Wilms' tumor, bladder rhabdomyosarcoma, hemangioma, polycystic kidney disease, stones, or a foreign body in the bladder or urethra as the cause for hematuria alone. A VCUG may provide additional information and should be considered in each individual case. An IVP is almost always necessary for evaluation of hematuria, but cystoscopy is rarely necessary in children.[2, 3] Bladder tumors are rare in this age group and are not likely to be missed by roentgenographic studies. Posterior urethritis is usually symptomatic, and cystoscopy does not change therapy.[2] When bright-red gross hematuria persists or recurs, cystoscopy may be helpful at the time of active

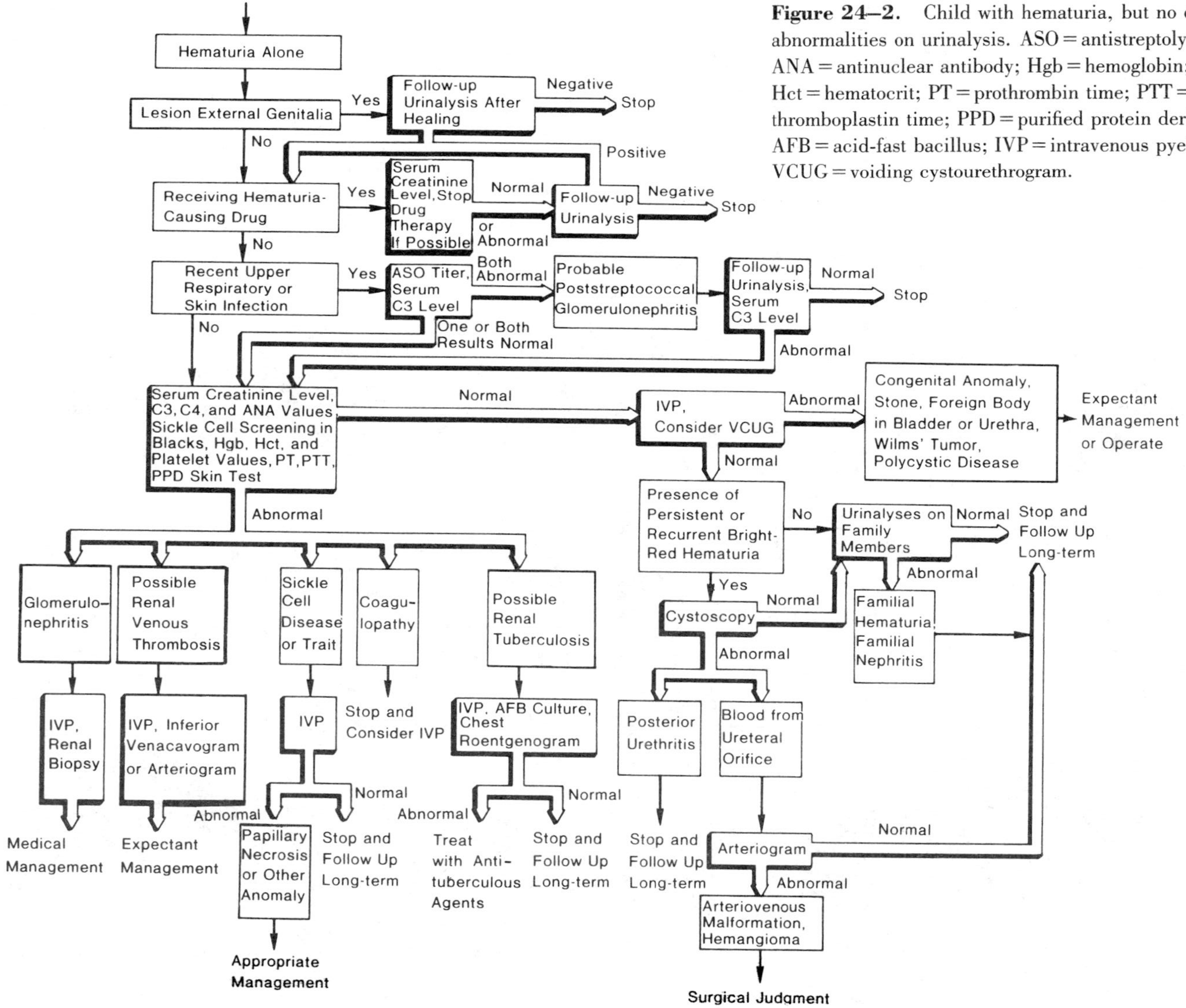

Figure 24-2. Child with hematuria, but no other abnormalities on urinalysis. ASO = antistreptolysin O; ANA = antinuclear antibody; Hgb = hemoglobin; Hct = hematocrit; PT = prothrombin time; PTT = partial thromboplastin time; PPD = purified protein derivative; AFB = acid-fast bacillus; IVP = intravenous pyelogram; VCUG = voiding cystourethrogram.

196

bleeding to localize blood to one or both ureteral orifices. A renal arteriovenous malformation or small hemangioma may be found on an arteriogram.

If results of blood tests and roentgenographic studies are normal, urinalyses of family members may help make the diagnosis of familial hematuria or familial (Alport's) nephritis. When the results of the entire evaluation are normal, hematuria may represent early membranoproliferative glomerulonephritis with normal serum C3, focal glomerulonephritis, IgA nephropathy, the sequelae of Henoch-Schönlein nephritis or poststreptococcal glomerulonephritis, or benign hematuria. Benign hematuria is a diagnosis of exclusion, and long-term follow-up is necessary to comfortably affirm this diagnosis. If the child does not grow normally or has development of increased blood pressure, decreased renal function, low serum C3 or C4 levels, or proteinuria, he or she does not have benign hematuria and should be reevaluated, probably including a renal biopsy. If hematuria alone persists for several years and is a cause of anxiety for parents and child, a renal biopsy to look for glomerulonephritis may be worth the small risk of the procedure to relieve the anxiety.[4]

The child with proteinuria, either in the presence of microscopic hematuria or persisting after gross hematuria becomes microscopic, is likely to have a renal parenchymal lesion. The presence of red blood cell (RBC) casts usually is diagnostic of a glomerular lesion. Laboratory evaluation for these children should include an assessment of filtration function (serum creatinine level and creatinine clearance), serum albumin and cholesterol levels, and quantitative urine protein (Figure 24–3). A positive ASO, antihyaluronidase, or antideoxyribonuclease B titer and a low serum C3 value suggest that poststreptococcal glomerulonephritis is likely. In this case, if the history is also compatible, a renal biopsy is usually not necessary to confirm the diagnosis. However, this child should be followed up, and if hematuria and proteinuria persist for six to 12 months, or if the serum C3 concentration does not return to normal after one to two months, further evaluation, including a renal biopsy, is indicated.

To evaluate for other types of glomerulonephritis (membranoproliferative glomerulonephritis, lupus nephritis, rapidly progressive glomerulonephritis, familial nephritis, chronic glomerulonephritis, focal nephritis, IgA nephropathy) or glomerulopathy (minimal change nephrotic syndrome or focal glomerulosclerosis), percutaneous renal biopsy should be performed after IVP or ultrasound examination has confirmed the presence of two kidneys. Renal biopsy will also be useful for determining long-term prognosis in the child with hematuria and proteinuria attributable to Henoch-Schönlein nephritis, and may be useful in treatment of the child with hemolytic uremic syndrome. Focal nephritis and early focal glomerulosclerosis may be missed on a specimen from a percutaneous needle biopsy, so the child with a normal biopsy result should receive long-term follow-up. Renal venous thrombosis should be considered especially in the infant with preceding diarrhea or a hyperosmolar state (eg, after receiving a large dose of dye for cardiac angiography).

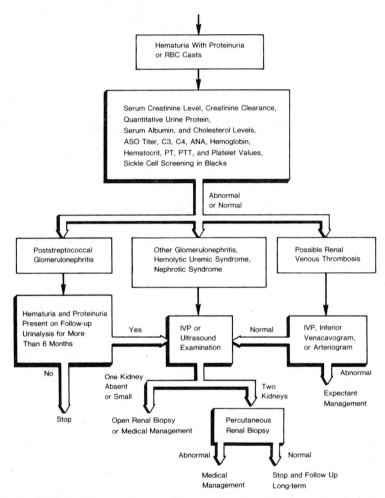

Figure 24–3. Child with hematuria as well as proteinuria or RBC casts on urinalysis. ASO = antistreptolysin O; ANA = antinuclear antibody; PT = prothrombin time; PTT = partial thromboplastin time; IVP = intravenous pyelogram.

Hematuria in the neonate is not considered in this algorithm. Red urine in this age group can be caused by hemoglobin, bile pigments, porphyrins or urate, so a urinalysis on a fresh specimen is mandatory to detect RBCs. When hematuria is present, one must consider the diagnostic possibilities of obstructive uropathy, infection, Wilms' tumor, coagulopathy, congenital nephrosis, infantile polycystic kidney disease, renal venous thrombosis, renal artery thrombosis (especially in the ill neonate with an umbilical artery catheter), cortical or medullary necrosis, or antibiotic-induced nephritis.

Hematuria in the Adult

As in children, the laboratory evaluation of hematuria in the adult begins with a urinalysis and urine culture (Figure 24–4). In most patients, a further evaluation is warranted. The exception to this is the young woman with hematuria, signs and symptoms of uncomplicated cystitis, and a positive urine culture. These patients should be treated for cystitis. If a follow-up urinalysis is normal and culture negative, no further investigation is needed.[5] If, however, the hematuria persists after antibiotic therapy, the evaluation of hematuria should continue. A hemoglobin electrophoresis should be performed for blacks with hematuria to rule out sickle cell disease or trait, a common cause of hematuria in young black adults.

Except in the young woman with cystitis, an IVP is mandatory and usually provides direction for further investigation. If there is clinical doubt concerning the patient's renal function, a serum creatinine measurement should be determined before the IVP. The finding of a congenital anomaly or stone requires surgical judgment as to whether surgical intervention or expectant management is the best course to follow. A filling defect in the renal pelvis or ureter usually represents either a tumor, blood clot, sloughed renal papilla, or nonopaque stone. A retrograde ureteropyelogram is often helpful in delineating the nature of a filling defect. If a renal pelvic or ureteral tumor is suspected, cystoscopy should be performed to rule out a coexistent bladder tumor.

The finding of a renal parenchymal mass on IVP necessitates the determination of whether the mass is a tumor or a benign renal cyst. The radiological evaluation of a renal mass is controversial. In general, we prefer ultrasound as the initial study in the evaluation of a renal mass. If all criteria for a benign cyst are met, the lesion is aspirated. If clear fluid is obtained and the cytological findings are negative, no further evaluation is necessary.[6] A mixed or solid ultrasonic pattern, bloody fluid aspirate, positive cytological findings, or calcification of the mass require surgical exploration. An arteriogram is often helpful before surgery (1) to determine the renal vascular anatomy, (2) to determine renal vein involvement by tumor, and (3) to make an angiographic diagnosis of renal cell carcinoma to allow radical nephrectomy without first inspecting or performing a

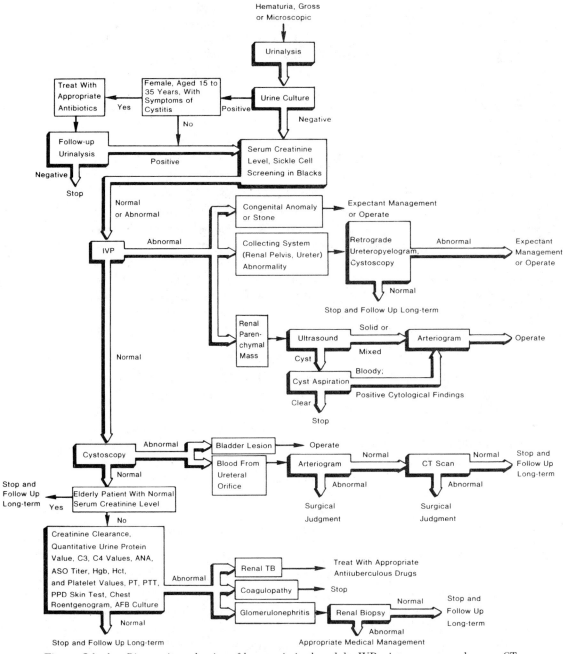

Figure 24—4. Diagnostic evaluation of hematuria in the adult. IVP = intravenous pyelogram; CT scan = computed tomographic scan; ANA = antinuclear antibody titer; ASO = antistreptolysin O; Hgb = hemoglobin; Hct = hematocrit; PT = prothrombin time; PTT = partial thromboplastin time; PPD = purified protein derivative; AFB = acid-fast bacillus; TB = tuberculosis.

biopsy of the lesion. Alternatively, computed axial tomography (CT) scanning may be used to differentiate benign cysts from renal tumors.[7]

Further diagnostic studies are necessary in the evaluation of hematuria in the adult even if the IVP is normal. A bladder tumor must be ruled out by cystoscopy. If no bladder tumor is visualized and the IVP and serum creatinine level are normal, further evaluation depends primarily on the age of the patient and the degree of hematuria. The evaluation of hematuria in an elderly patient with microscopic hematuria can reasonably stop at this point. A young patient or a patient with persistent gross hematuria should have further evaluation. Gross blood seen effluxing from a ureteral orifice can be evaluated by arteriography (to rule out arteriovenous malformation or fistula), CT scan (to rule out anterior or posterior mass lesions that may not be seen on the IVP), or retrograde ureteropyelography (if the ureter is not completely visualized on the IVP).

Glomerular lesions should be considered in younger patients with persistent microscopic hematuria. A creatinine clearance and quantitative urine protein value should be obtained. With reduced creatinine clearance or significant proteinuria, renal biopsy is usually warranted. Rarer causes of hematuria in the adult (coagulopathies and tuberculosis) should also be considered.

Hematuria Secondary to Trauma

Hematuria secondary to trauma (either blunt or penetrating) requires immediate radiological investigation (Figure 24–5). The entire urinary tract can, in general, be visualized with three x-ray studies: (1) retrograde urethrogram (urethra), (2) cystogram (bladder), and (3) IVP (kidneys and ureters). If a urethral injury is suspected in men (blood at the urethral meatus, perineal hematoma, "high-riding" prostate, pelvic fracture, etc), a retrograde urethrogram to rule out injury should be performed before urethral catheterization is attempted. Urethral injuries are rare in women and for the most part can be discounted. If a urethral injury is identified, an operative procedure (either suprapubic cystotomy alone or definitive urethral repair) is indicated after appropriate radiological evaluation of the upper urinary tract (IVP).[8] If the urethrogram is normal, a urethral catheter should be inserted and a cystogram performed. If the cystogram demonstrates a bladder injury, operative repair is generally indicated after an IVP has ruled out significant renal or ureteral injury.

If the retrograde urethrogram and cystogram are normal, or if these studies are not obtained because there is no clinical suspicion of lower urinary tract trauma, an IVP is the initial study of choice to assess renal or ureteral injury. The patient with suspected renal injury and a normal IVP should be treated expectantly. Unilateral nonfunction suggests either a major vascular injury or renal agenesis; the next study of choice to differentiate these two entities is a renal

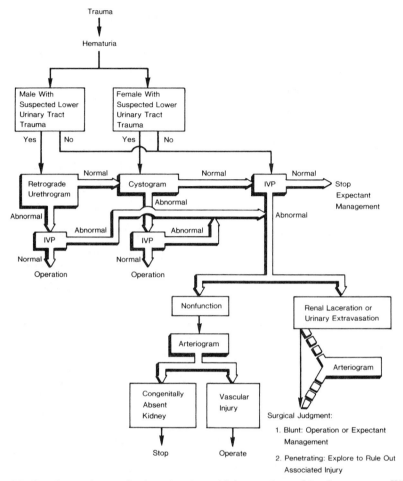

Figure 24–5. Approach to evaluation of patient with hematuria resulting from trauma. IVP = intravenous pyelogram.

arteriogram. A major vascular tear or arterial thrombosis necessitates immediate surgical exploration. The management of renal lacerations or urinary extravasation seen on IVP is somewhat controversial.[9, 10] An arteriogram is usually extremely helpful in assessing the degree of injury and in determining whether immediate surgical exploration is necessary. In general, however, all patients with penetrating renal trauma should have surgical exploration to rule out other associated injuries (pancreas, spleen, liver, or bowel).

References

1. Schwartz GJ, Haycock GB, Spitzer A: Plasma creatinine and urea concentration in children: Normal values for age and sex. *J Pediatr* 1976;88:828–830.

2. Walther PC, Kaplan GW: Cystoscopy in children: Indications for its use in common urologic problems. *J Urol* 1979;122:717–720.

3. Johnson DK, Kroovand RL, Perlmutter AD: The changing role of cystoscopy in the pediatric patient. *J Urol* 1980;123:232–233.

4. West CD: Asymptomatic hematuria and proteinuria in children: Causes and appropriate diagnostic studies. *J Pediatr* 1976;89:173–182.

5. Fair WR, McClennan BL, Jost RG: Are excretory urograms necessary in evaluating women with urinary tract infection? *J Urol* 1979;121:313–315.

6. Pollack HM, Goldberg BB, Bogash M: Changing concepts in the diagnosis and management of renal cysts. *J Urol* 1974;111:326–329.

7. McClennan BL, Stanley RJ, Melson GL, et al: CT of the renal cyst: Is cyst aspiration necessary? *AJR* 1979;133:671–675.

8. Morehouse DD, MacKinnon KJ: Posterior urethral injury: Etiology, diagnosis and initial management. *Urol Clin North Am* 1977;4:69–73.

9. Wein AJ, Murphy JJ, Mulholland SG, et al: A conservative approach to the management of blunt renal trauma. *J Urol* 1977;117:425–427.

10. Carlton CE: Surgery in renal trauma, editorial. *Urology* 1974;3:671.

Chapter 25

Hypercalcemia

Edward T. Wong, MD
Esther F. Freier, MS

The process of diagnosing primary hyperparathyroidism has been one of exclusion of the other causes of hypercalcemia. In the past decade, since the measurement of parathyroid hormone (PTH) by radioimmunoassay became available through commercial laboratories, its use has grown rapidly. Theoretically, PTH levels should be elevated in primary hyperparathyroidism and possibly in malignancies producing PTH ectopically (pseudohyperparathyroidism); in the other causes of hypercalcemia, the levels should be decreased.[1, 2] The number of PTH assays ordered at this hospital has reached 350 per year, whereas during the period of 1970 to 1978 the number of new cases of primary hyperparathyroidism was less than ten per year. This suggested that many physicians were ordering PTH measurements early, if not even first, in the evaluation of hypercalcemia, the expectation being that PTH determinations would separate primary hyperparathyroidism from the other causes of hypercalcemia. Before direct measurements of PTH became available, laboratory tests reflecting a biologic effect of PTH were used to distinguish primary hyperparathyroidism from the other causes of hypercalcemia. These indirect measurements of PTH (urine calcium, urine phosphorus, tubular reabsorption of phosphorus, among others) showed some degree of overlap between the parathyroid and nonparathyroid groups of hypercalcemia.[3] It is not surprising that PTH assays, holding out the promise of a clear separation of primary hyperparathyroidism from the other causes of hypercalcemia, would be adopted with alacrity.

Growth of the array of laboratory tests for the investigation of hypercalcemia did not stop with the advent of PTH assays. More indirect tests of PTH have been introduced, such as the chloride/phosphorus (Cl/P) ratio[4] and urinary cyclic adenosine monophosphate (AMP).[5] Because of its simplicity and ready

From: The Differential Diagnosis of Hypercalcemia. An Algorithm for More Effective Use of Laboratory Tests. *JAMA* 1982;247:75–80. Copyright 1982 by the American Medical Association.

availability and also the reported high sensitivity and specificity of an elevated Cl/P ratio for primary hyperparathyroidism,[4] the Cl/P ratio has been used to determine the direction of further investigation of hypercalcemia. Because finding hypercalcemia is frequent with widespread use of multichannel biochemical screening tests, there is the potential for the expenditure (and perhaps waste) of large sums of money, unless an efficient and cost-effective approach to the investigation of hypercalcemia is developed and followed.

We have examined the recent experience at this hospital with primary hyperparathyroidism and hypercalcemia to assess the contribution of PTH and Cl/P ratio to the other commonly available laboratory tests in the differential diagnosis of hypercalcemia. Based on the clinical as well as the biochemical nature of the problem of hypercalcemia in hospitalized patients, we designed an algorithm that offers an orderly and more cost-effective approach to differential diagnosis.

Algorithm for Hospitalized Patients

Decision 1

Hypercalcemia should first be confirmed to avoid the unnecessary expense of investigating spurious results, such as mislabeling, contamination, and the like. Since proteins, particularly albumin, bind about half the total serum calcium, serum protein electrophoresis should be obtained to assess serum proteins (Figure 25–1). Total serum calcium should be corrected for deviations in albumin levels, because a change of 1 g/dL (10 g/L) in albumin level will change the total serum calcium by 0.8 mg/dL (0.2 mmol/L).[6] Also, an abnormal serum electrophoretic pattern may identify quickly those patients who should be investigated for multiple myeloma (monoclonal gammopathy) or sarcoidosis (increased γ-globulins).

Decision 2

We found, as have others, that the most frequent cause of hypercalcemia in hospitalized patients was carcinoma with metastases to bone.[7–9] Thus, search for metastatic bone lesions should be the most productive way to investigate hypercalcemia occurring in a patient with a present or past history of carcinoma, particularly one with a predilection for bone metastases, such as carcinoma of the breast, lung, or kidney.

Decision 3

If a patient has hypercalcemia documented for more than one year, especially with a history of kidney stones or peptic ulcer, the most likely diagnosis

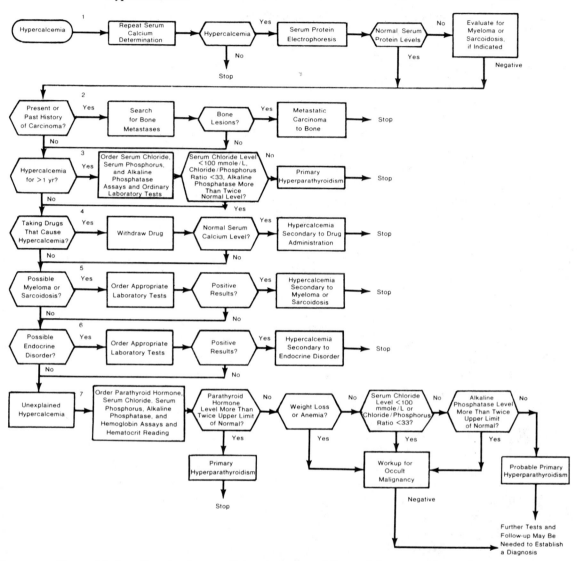

Figure 25–1. Algorithm for use of laboratory tests in differential diagnosis of hypercalcemia. Decision points are in hexagons.

is primary hyperparathyroidism.[1, 7, 10] The duration of hypercalcemia makes malignancy rather unlikely. Sixteen of our 41 patients with primary hyperparathyroidism had hypercalcemia for more than one year before parathyroidectomy. However, in this setting, abnormalities that are inconsistent with primary hyperparathyroidism, such as a serum chloride level of less than 100 mmol/L, a Cl/P ratio of less than 33 (especially a Cl/P <29), and an alkaline phosphatase level greater than 370 U/L, should be a signal that the hypercalcemia is not a result of uncomplicated primary hyperparathyroidism, and that other possibilities must be considered. (Normal range for alkaline phosphatase is 61 to 220 U/L. Because units for alkaline phosphatase are not uniform among laboratories, using twice the upper limit of normal for the decision point would give it more general applicability.)

For patients with simple chronic hypercalcemia, familial hypocalciuric hypercalcemia should be considered.[11, 12] This recently recognized syndrome is rare, so that evaluation of all hypercalcemic patients for it would not be cost-effective. Its importance is that while resembling primary hyperparathyroidism biochemically (chronic hypercalcemia, hypophosphatemia, tendency to hyperchloremic metabolic acidosis, and even, in some instances, elevated PTH levels), it differs in producing serious morbidity rarely, such as peptic ulcer, nephrolithiasis, and other renal damage, and in responding poorly to subtotal parathyroidectomy. The renal calcium:creatinine clearance ratio has been used to separate it from primary hyperparathyroidism, a ratio of less than 0.01 being suggestive of familial hypocalciuric hypercalcemia.

Decision 4

If the patient is taking a drug that can cause hypercalcemia[9] (vitamin D, thiazide diuretics, lithium carbonate, among others), the drug regimen should be stopped to see whether the hypercalcemia resolves before proceeding to investigate hypercalcemia. The "milk-alkali" syndrome should be considered as a type of drug-induced hypercalcemia. History will disclose intake of large amounts of milk and absorbable alkali; nephrocalcinosis and azotemia will be evident.

Decision 5

Hypercalcemia with severe bone pain, bone lesions, abnormal serum protein electrophoresis results, and proteinuria should suggest multiple myeloma. If the clinical findings warrant investigation for multiple myeloma, the appropriate laboratory tests would include a bone marrow biopsy, along with characterization of the monoclonal protein in serum or urine by immunoelectrophoresis and its quantitation. Hypercalcemia with mediastinal and hilar lymphadenopathy on chest roentgenogram and increased γ-globulins should suggest sarcoidosis; the definitive test for sarcoidosis is biopsy of lymph node, skin, or, occasionally, liver, to confirm the presence of noncaseating granuloma.

Decision 6

Certain endocrine disorders may be associated with hypercalcemia, such as hyperthyroidism, Addison's disease, pheochromocytoma, and acromegaly. Nonparathyroid endocrinopathic disorders should be considered among the uncommon causes of hypercalcemia,[6] and laboratory tests for these possibilities should not be ordered unless clinical findings suggest their presence. Hyperthyroidism should be suggested by heat intolerance, weight loss, tremor, tachycardia, sweating, and presence of a goiter. The appropriate laboratory tests would be a free thyroxine index and a free triiodothyronine index. Hyponatremia, hyperkalemia, azotemia, postural hypotension, and increased skin pigmentation would indicate Addison's disease; the appropriate laboratory test is an adrenocorticotropic hormone stimulation test. Hypertension, sustained or paroxysmal, especially with tremor, pallor, palpitations, and tachycardia would suggest pheochromocytoma; appropriate laboratory tests would be measurement of urinary vanillylmandelic acid and metanephrines. Excessive growth of the hands, feet, and jaw would suggest acromegaly; a growth hormone suppression test (measurement of growth hormone levels during a glucose tolerance test) is required either to confirm or to exclude acromegaly.

Decision 7

Having eliminated the causes of hypercalcemia considered in the previous decisions, one is left with unexplained hypercalcemia. In this group, the major problem is to distinguish between primary hyperparathyroidism and pseudohyperparathyroidism because the clinical and biochemical pictures of the two can be strikingly similar. In Lafferty's series,[7] pseudohyperparathyroidism accounted for 15% of the cases of hypercalcemia and was almost as frequent as primary hyperparathyroidism, which accounted for 20% of the cases.

Here, as in decision 3, certain laboratory test results are of value in excluding primary hyperparathyroidism (Table 25–1): a serum chloride level of

Table 25–1.
Sensitivity, Specificity, and Predictive Value of Laboratory Test Results in Diagnosis of Primary Hyperparathyroidism in Hospitalized Hypercalcemic Patients.*

Laboratory Test Result	Sensitivity in No. (%) of Patients	Specificity in No. (%) of Patients	Predictive Value, % Positive	Negative
Chloride, ≥100 mmol/L	40/41 (97.6)	21/41 (51.2)	17.7	99.5
Chloride/phosphorus ratio, ≥33	39/41 (95.1)	22/41 (53.3)	18.1	99.0
Chloride/phosphorus ratio, ≥29	41/41 (100)	16/41 (39.0)	15.0	100.0
Alkaline phosphatase, <370 U/L	37/37 (100)	21/41 (52.5)	18.8	100.0
Parathyroid hormone, >90 μL Eq/mL	18/18 (100)	11/15 (73.3)	28.7	100.0
Parathyroid hormone, >180 μL Eq/mL	10/18 (55.6)	15/15 (100)	100.0	95.4

*Prevalence of primary hyperparathyroidism was 9.7% of all hospitalized hypercalcemic patients.

less than 100 mmol/L, a Cl/P ratio of less than 33 (particularly <29), and an alkaline phosphatase level more than twice the normal value. Lafferty found that pseudohyperparathyroidism was more likely with a short duration of symptoms, rapid weight loss, anemia, chloride level of less than 102 mmol/L, elevation of alkaline phosphatase without bone disease, and calcium level of more than 14 mg/dL (3.5 mmol/L).[7] We did not find a level of calcium that was of particular value in separating the groups. We did not examine the predictive value of either anemia or weight loss for our series. Decision points indicating the need to investigate a possible malignancy (pseudohyperparathyroidism) are based on our findings and those of Lafferty.

Sufficiently high levels of PTH could be used to confirm primary hyperparathyroidism (Table 25–1). Raisz et al[13] showed that PTH assays from three commercial sources had problems of overlap and specificity of normal to slightly elevated values, while a fourth commercial PTH assay had low sensitivity for primary hyperparathyroidism. They found, as we did, that markedly elevated values of PTH confirmed primary hyperparathyroidism. Although all our patients with primary hyperparathyroidism had PTH levels higher than 90 μL Eq/mL suggesting that PTH below this level could exclude primary hyperparathyroidism, we do not recommend this use for PTH. With the PTH assay we used, Potts and Krutzik[2] reported finding values as low as 42 μL Eq/mL in a series of 92 patients with primary hyperparathyroidism. Therefore, the overlap in PTH values between parathyroid and nonparathyroid hypercalcemia extends almost to the limit of sensitivity of the assay (reportedly 20 to 35 μL Eq/mL).

Our algorithm ends with a category called "probable primary hyperparathyroidism" and a note indicating that further testing and follow-up may be needed to establish a definitive diagnosis. The nature of such testing is beyond the scope of this discussion but is well covered in reviews of hypercalcemia.[3, 9, 14]

Evaluation of Laboratory Tests in Differential Diagnosis

The suggested uses of laboratory testing in our algorithm are based in part on the results of a retrospective study of primary hyperparathyroidism and hypercalcemia at this hospital.

Materials and Methods

Clinical Material. The medical record department retrieved the records of 67 patients with diagnoses of hyperparathyroidism during the period of 1970 to 1978. Thirteen records were not available for review. We excluded the records of ten patients who had secondary hyperparathyroidism with chronic renal failure and kidney transplantation. We reviewed the records of 44 patients with a diagnosis of primary hyperparathyroidism. Of these, 41 were proved surgically to have either parathyroid adenoma or primary parathyroid hyperplasia; three patients in whom neck exploration was unsuccessful had probable hyperparathyroidism. The analysis was restricted to the 41 patients with proved primary hyperparathyroidism.

The records of a group of patients with nonparathyroid hypercalcemia were collected by retrieval of 82 patients with a discharge code for hypercalcemia during 1977-1978. Sixty-two records were available for review. Six of the 62 patients had primary hyperparathyroidism, giving an estimate of 9.7% for the prevalence of primary hyperparathyroidism in hypercalcemia of all causes. We excluded the records of 21 patients who had primary or secondary hyperparathyroidism, idiopathic hypercalcemia of infancy, and hypercalcemia of undetermined etiology, leaving 41 patients in the nonparathyroid hypercalcemic group.

In the primary hyperparathyroid group, the mean age was 58.0 years, with a range of 20 to 83 years; 32 of the 41 patients were women. In the nonparathyroid hypercalcemic group, the mean age was 53.5 years, with a range of 15 to 73 years; 25 of the 41 patients were women.

Biochemical Measurements. During 1975 to 1978, PTH assays were sent to the Nichols Institute, San Pedro, California. Before that, we sent PTH to a commercial laboratory now defunct; the small number of PTH data from that laboratory was excluded. Serum chemical examinations were done by standard methods in the clinical chemistry laboratory of the University of Minnesota Hospitals, Minneapolis.

Statistical Analysis. The data were analysed using programs BMDP3D, "Comparison of Two Groups with t-Tests," and BMDP7M, "Stepwise Discriminant Function Analysis."[15]

The concepts of sensitivity, specificity, and predictive value are well described in recent publications, and our use of these terms conforms to their definitions.[16, 17]

Results

Analysis of Single Variables

Table 25–2 shows the biochemical data available for comparison of the hyperparathyroid and the nonparathyroid groups with hypercalcemia. The two groups differed significantly in all 12 laboratory tests.

Discriminant Function Analysis

The program for discriminant function analysis excluded cases with missing data. Being a retrospective study, only 30 cases had sufficient data to be

——— **Table 25–2.** ———
Data for Patients With Primary Hyperparathyroid and Nonparathyroid Hypercalcemia.

| Laboratory Assay | Hyperparathyroid | | Nonparathyroid | | |
	Mean ± SD	Range	Mean ± SD	Range	P
Calcium, mg/dL	11.68 ± 1.05	10.2–15.4	12.76 ± 1.89	10.9–20.9	.002
Phosphorus, mg/dL	2.49 ± 0.48	1.6–3.7	3.26 ± 0.99	1.6–6.2	<.001
Sodium, mmol/L	139.56 ± 2.39	134–143	137.73 ± 3.70	128–148	.009
Potassium, mmol/L	4.30 ± 0.46	3.0–5.3	4.07 ± 0.52	2.9–5.5	.033
Bicarbonate, mmol/L	27.13 ± 3.03	21–35	29.93 ± 3.96	22–39	<.001
Chloride, mmol/L	106.15 ± 4.19	93–113	98.71 ± 5.60	88–117	<.001
Chloride/phosphorus ratio	44.35 ± 9.43	29–66	33.19 ± 10.53	16–64	<.001
Albumin, g/dL	3.66 ± 0.44	2.8–4.6	3.01 ± 0.58	2.0–4.3	<.001
Alkaline phosphatase, U/L	188.84 ± 67.08	69–367	501.70 ± 433.23	102–2070	<.001
Urea nitrogen, mg/dL	16.92 ± 6.33	6–35	28.45 ± 17.56	7–91	<.001
Creatinine, mg/dL	1.02 ± 0.35	0.5–2.2	1.51 ± 0.96	0.6–6.0	.004
Parathyroid hormone, μL Eq/mL	207.56 ± 130.92	92–632	70.80 ± 39.10	22–179	<.001

included in the analysis; of these, 16 patients had primary hyperparathyroidism and 14 had nonparathyroid hypercalcemia.

A linear discriminant function was derived from four laboratory tests:

Discriminant function = (0.40563 × mg/dL of calcium) − (0.10357 × mmol/L of chloride) + (0.00363 × U/L of alkaline phosphatase) − (0.00802 × μL Eq/mL of PTH).

With this discriminant function, the conditions of patients with positive values were classified as nonparathyroid hypercalcemia, while the conditions of those with negative values were classified as hyperparathyroid; 29 of 30 patients (96.7%) were classified correctly into hyperparathyroid and nonparathyroid groups.

Predictive Value Analysis

Table 25–1 shows the predictive value analysis for chloride, Cl/P ratio, PTH, and alkaline phosphatase in diagnosing primary hyperparathyroidism. Laboratory tests are used either to confirm or to exclude a diagnosis; changing the limit for a positive test result to enhance either sensitivity or specificity may make it more useful for these purposes. To confirm a diagnosis, a test should not have any false-positive results and should have specificity of 100% and predictive value positive of 100%. Of these test results, only a PTH level greater than 180 μL Eq/mL could be used to confirm primary hyperparathyroidism. To exclude a diagnosis, a test should not have false-negative results and should have both sensitivity and predictive value negative of 100%. Primary hyperparathyroidism was improbable with either a chloride level less than 100 mmol/L or a Cl/P ratio less than 33, since the predictive value negative was greater than 99% for each test. By lowering the limit for a positive Cl/P ratio to 29, values less than 29 could exclude primary hyperparathyroidism because predictive value negative became 100%. Similarly, an alkaline phosphatase level greater than 370 U/L could exclude primary hyperparathyroidism.

Comment

Univariate analysis of the laboratory tests using the *t* test (Table 25–2) showed highly significant differences between the groups for all 12 laboratory tests. While this type of analysis was useful to describe the biochemical differences between the groups, it did not indicate the optimal use of the laboratory tests in differential diagnosis of hypercalcemia. There were highly significant correlations among many of the tests, but the correlations were no more informative about clinical use of the tests.

Of the techniques of multivariate analysis, the discriminant function analysis was the most relevant to the process of clinical diagnosis because it combined and weighted the laboratory tests into a discriminant function to achieve maximal separation of the groups. A discriminant function derived from just four tests (PTH, calcium, alkaline phosphatase, and chloride assays) was correct in classifying 96.7% of the patients into parathyroid and nonparathyroid groups with hypercalcemia. The other eight tests did not make sufficient independent contributions to the separation of the groups to be included in the discriminant function.

Discriminant function analysis for differential diagnosis of hypercalcemia has been reported previously.[18–21] While attractive in concept, discriminant functions have not gained wide use. Fraser et al,[19] using two discriminant functions derived from five biochemical tests (serum phosphorus, alkaline phosphatase, chloride, bicarbonate, and urea assays), were able to classify correctly 197 of 218 cases of hypercalcemia into diagnostic categories. We had sufficient data to apply their discriminant functions to 70 of our 82 patients. Their discriminant functions were not as effective for classifying our patients as they had been for their patients: 19 of 39 of our nonparathyroid hypercalcemic patients had values that overlapped with the values for our primary hyperparathyroid group. Of their two discriminant functions, their first discriminant function was the basis for the separation of the parathyroid from the nonparathyroid cases of hypercalcemia; serum phosphorus level was heavily weighted in this function.

While hypophosphatemia is frequent in primary hyperparathyroidism, and normal to high phosphorus levels are frequent in nonparathyroid hypercalcemia, hypophosphatemia has low specificity for primary hyperparathyroidism. In patients hospitalized because of hypercalcemia or its precipitating cause, poor dietary intake of phosphate because of anorexia or vomiting can produce hypophosphatemia, regardless of the parathyroid status of the patient. Furthermore, hypophosphatemia is a feature of pseudohyperparathyroidism of malignancy. Therefore, laboratory tests based on serum phosphorus such as the discriminant functions of Fraser et al[19] or the Cl/P ratio are of limited value in the differential diagnosis of hypercalcemia in hospitalized patients.

Developing a discriminant function to be used literally as a diagnostic test was not our intent. Such use of a discriminant function would require extensive validation with a prospective series of hypercalcemic patients. We used discriminant function analysis to identify the combination of laboratory tests leading to maximal separation of the groups. The predictive value analysis indicated clinical uses for the laboratory tests. Our algorithm integrated the laboratory tests with the clinical nature of the problem of differential diagnosis of hypercalcemia.

Use of PTH level as the first step to investigate hypercalcemia would be wasteful. Often the cause of hypercalcemia will be evident from history and physical examination, and extensive laboratory investigation, including PTH assay, will be unnecessary. Furthermore, a PTH determination was only partially effective in separating hyperparathyroid from nonparathyroid causes of hypercalcemia, because PTH levels were not always decreased in the latter. We found normal to elevated PTH levels in patients with malignant neoplasms, perhaps due to ectopic PTH production. However, Habener and Segre[1] state that ectopic PTH production is an infrequent cause of pseudohyperparathyroidism. We found normal to slightly elevated PTH levels even with nonmalignant causes of hypercalcemia (immobilization, use of vitamin D plus thiazide diuretic, or steroid withdrawal) or with malignancies rarely, if ever, associated with ectopic PTH production (carcinoma of the breast or histiocytic lymphoma).[22, 23] The predictive value of a positive PTH value (>90 μL Eq/mL) was only 29%. Therefore, if PTH assays were ordered for all hypercalcemic patients, 71% of the positive values would be false-positive results, and the correct etiology of the hypercalcemia would have to be established on other grounds despite the positive PTH values. Reserving PTH for unexplained hypercalcemia would be more effective use of laboratory technology than using PTH first or even early in the differential diagnosis of hypercalcemia.

We have seen elevated Cl/P ratios interpreted as indicators of primary hyperparathyroidism, which led to the ordering of PTH assay, even though the patient had clear evidence of some other etiology for the hypercalcemia (most often carcinoma metastatic to bone). The specificity and predictive value of a Cl/P ratio greater than 33 were far too low for this practice to be justifiable. Rather, its principal value is that a Cl/P ratio lower than 33, and especially lower than 29, is evidence against primary hyperparathyroidism and indicates a need to pursue some other diagnosis.

We conclude that PTH determination can contribute to the differential diagnosis of hypercalcemia, but that its use is most cost-effective when reserved for cases of unexplained hypercalcemia. Considerable information is available from the clinical database (the history and physical examination) and from simple laboratory test results, and the information should be carefully considered before obtaining a PTH assay. The availability of the PTH assay has not altered the basic process of diagnosing primary hyperparathyroidism: it has been and continues to be one of exclusion of the other causes of hypercalcemia.

References

1. Habener JF, Segre GV: Parathyroid hormone radioimmunoassay. *Ann Intern Med* 1979;91:782–785.
2. Potts JT Jr, Krutzik SR: Parathyroid hormone (PTH), in Nichols AL, Fisher DA (eds): *Radioimmunoassay Manual*, ed 3. San Pedro, Calif, The Nichols Institute, 1976, pp 209–220.
3. Strott CA, Nugent CA: Laboratory tests in the diagnosis of hyperparathyroidism in hypercalcemic patients. *Ann Intern Med* 1968;68:188–202.
4. Palmer FJ, Nelson JC, Bacchus H: The chloride-phosphate ratio in hypercalcemia. *Ann Intern Med* 1974;80:200–204.
5. Kaminsky NI, Broadus AE, Hardman JG, et al: Effects of parathyroid hormone on plasma and urinary adenosine 3′,5′-monophosphate in man. *J Clin Invest* 1970; 49:2387–2395.
6. Scholz DA, Purnell DC, Goldsmith RS, et al: Diagnostic considerations in hypercalcemic syndromes. *Med Clin North Am* 1972;56:941–950.
7. Lafferty FW: Pseudohyperparathyroidism. *Medicine* 1966;45:247–260.
8. McLellan G, Baird CW, Melick R: Hypercalcemia in an Australian hospital adult population. *Med J Aust* 1968;2:354–356.
9. Lee DB, Zawada ET, Kleeman CR: The pathophysiology and clinical aspects of hypercalcemic disorders. *West J Med* 1978;129:278–320.
10. Heath H III, Hodson SF, Kennedy MA: Primary hyperparathyroidism: Incidence, morbidity and potential economic impact on a community. *N Engl J Med* 1980;302:189–193.
11. Marx SJ, Spiegel AM, Brown EM, et al: Divalent cation metabolism: Familial hypocalciuric hypercalcemia versus typical primary hyperparathyroidism. *Am J Med* 1978;65:235–242.
12. Marx SJ: Familial hypocalciuric hypercalcemia. *N Engl J Med* 1980;303:810–811.
13. Raisz LG, Yajnik CH, Bockman RS, et al: Comparison of commercially available parathyroid hormone immunoassays in the differential diagnosis of hypercalcemia due to hyperparathyroidism or malignancy. *Ann Intern Med* 1979;91:739–740.
14. Singer FR, Bethune JE, Massry SG: Hypercalcemia and hypocalcemia. *Clin Nephrol* 1977;7:154–162.
15. Dixon WJ, Brown MB (eds): *BMDP-79: Biomedical Computer Programs, P-series*. Berkeley, Calif, University of California Press, 1979, pp 170–184, 711–733.
16. Feinstein AR: Clinical biostatistics: XXXI. On the sensitivity, specificity, and dis-

crimination value of diagnostic tests. *Clin Pharmacol Ther* 1975;17:104–116.

17. Galen RS, Gambino SR: *Beyond Normality: The Predictive Value and Efficiency of Medical Diagnosis*. New York, John Wiley & Sons Inc, 1975.

18. Amenta JS, Harkins ML: The use of discriminant functions in laboratory medicine: Evaluation of phosphate clearance studies in the diagnosis of hyperparathyroidism. *Am J Clin Pathol* 1971;55:330–341.

19. Fraser P, Healy M, Rose N, et al: Discriminant functions in differential diagnosis of hypercalcemia. *Lancet* 1971;1:1314–1319.

20. Transbol I, Jorgensen FS, Hornum I, et al: Hypercalcemia discrimination index: A multivariate analysis of parathyroid function in 107 hypercalcemic patients. *Acta Endocrinol* 1977;86:768–783.

21. Watson L, Moxham J, Fraser P: Hydrocortisone suppression test and discriminant analysis in differential diagnosis of hypercalcemia. *Lancet* 1980;1:1320–1325.

22. Gordan GS: Hyper- and hypocalcemia: Pathogenesis and treatments. *Ann NY Acad Sci* 1974;230:181–186.

23. Singer FR, Powell D, Minkin C, et al: Hypercalcemia in reticulum cell sarcoma without hyperparathyroidism or skeletal metastases. *Ann Intern Med* 1973;78: 365–369.

Chapter 26

Positive Urinary Sugar Test

Harvey C. Knowles, Jr, MD

Often the practicing physician is faced with the problem of one of his or her patients unexpectedly showing a positive urine test for sugar. This may occur in a routine office checkup, during hospitalization, or perhaps during an examination performed elsewhere, such as for life insurance or employment. To solve the diagnostic aspect of the problem, I would use the approach shown in Figure 26–1. Before discussing the steps involved, however, certain definitions and laboratory methods must be given.

Mellituria. A condition in which any type of sugar is excreted in the urine.

Glycosuria. A condition in which glucose is excreted in the urine.

Copper Sulfate Tablets. Tablets (Clinitest [Ames Co]) containing copper sulfate, which acts as an oxidizing agent. Sugars having a keto- group will be reduced. The only sugar appearing abnormally in the urine that has no keto- group and thus cannot reduce copper or other oxidizing agents is sucrose. A series of graded readings by color change occurs with use of either a 5-drop or 2-drop Clinitest system.

Glucose Oxidase Paper Materials. Certain paper or stick materials (such as Clinistix, Diastix, or Testape) prepared with glucose oxidase enzyme, which, acting on glucose, produces a color change specific for glucose.

Blood, Serum, or Plasma Glucose Level. Circulating levels of glucose determined with enzymes (glucose oxidase, hexokinase) or in some laboratories (about 15%) by reduction methods. Serum and plasma values are similar and are about 15% higher than those of whole blood. For present purposes, the term "plasma glucose" will indicate either serum or plasma glucose.

From: Evaluation of a Positive Urinary Sugar Test. *JAMA* 1975;234:961–963. Copyright 1975 by the American Medical Association.

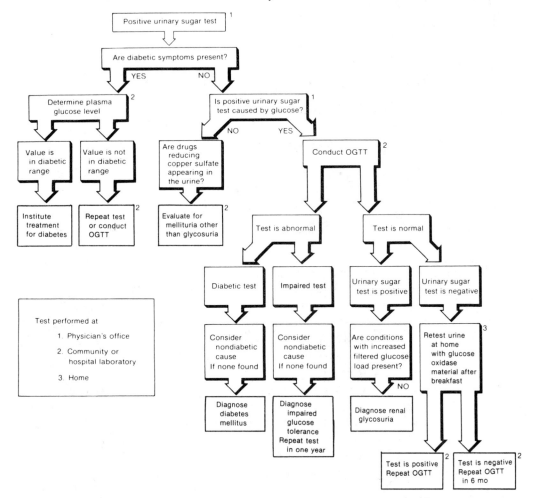

Figure 26–1. Algorithm for the evaluation of a positive urinary sugar test. OGTT = oral glucose tolerance test.

Oral Glucose Tolerance Test (OGTT). The test conducted as described by the National Diabetes Data Group.[1] The results may be interpreted as diabetic, impaired, or normal glucose tolerance.

Diabetes Mellitus. A metabolic disorder, usually aggregated in families, with two groups of characteristics: (1) the chemical consequences of insulin insufficiency, and (2) the risks of angiopathy, neuropathy, and other complications.

Urine Test

To return to the positive test for urinary sugar, steps given in the algorithm may be followed for diagnosis. First, inquiry should be made about symptoms of uncontrolled diabetes. Their presence would require investigation without delay, for all too often uncontrolled diabetes progresses to acidosis or hyperosmolar coma before the diagnosis is made. If no symptoms are present, inquiry might be made as to how the test was made, since the substance in question might not be glucose. If glucose oxidase materials were used, glucose was the offending substance. But if a copper sulfate tablet was used, certain medications taken or sugars other than glucose might have reduced the copper sulfate. Glucose oxidase materials will give a negative test in these circumstances. If in this instance there is no history of drug ingestion, study should be made for aberrant urinary sugars such as fructose, lactose, galactose, and pentose, which would react with a copper sulfate tablet but not with glucose oxidase materials.

If it is found that the positive urine test is due to glucose, it is very likely that the cause is diabetes. The presence of gross symptoms of uncontrolled diabetes such as polyurea, polydypsia, weight loss, and in women pruritis vulvae, along with elevation of a random plasma glucose level in excess of 200 mg/dL (11.1 mmol/L), usually are sufficient to diagnose diabetes. Two fasting plasma glucose levels of 140 mg/dL (7.8 mmol/L) or more also establish the diagnosis. Any urine tested when random samples of blood are obtained for glucose analysis should be tested for ketones (acetoacetic acid with nitroprusside) as well.

Oral Glucose Tolerance Test

In the event diabetic symptoms are not present, it will in all likelihood be necessary to carry out a glucose tolerance test. The patient should not be receiving hormonal or drug therapy nor be under a state of stress such as infection or injury. Urine samples for glucose analysis are obtained simultaneously with blood samples. Though many approaches to conduction and interpretation of the OGTT have been proposed, the current recommended approach is that described by the National Diabetes Data Group.[1] The patient should have an intake of at least 150 g of carbohydrate daily, and this can be assured by an ingestion of an extra serving of starch at each meal for three days preceding the test. The test must be conducted in the morning, and the patient should have been fasting for ten to 12 hours. The oral loading dose is 75 g of glucose usually taken in the form of 75 g of commercially available hydrolyzed cornstarch (Glucola). After a fasting blood sample is obtained for glucose determination, the glucose load is ingested over about a five-minute period. Zero time is at the start of drinking, and blood samples for glucose analyses are obtained thereafter at 30-minute intervals for two hours. The samples should be placed in tubes containing a proper antiglycolytic preservative. Urine samples for sugar measurement are obtained at the same times as the blood samples.

Interpretation of the OGTT results is shown in Table 26–1.[1,2] Diabetes is diagnosed in the face of fasting plasma glucose (FPG) levels less than or equal

—————— **Table 26–1.** ——————
Criteria for Diabetes Mellitus, Impaired Glucose Tolerance, and Normal Glucose Tolerance. *

Diabetes mellitus
   Symptoms of uncontrolled diabetes with unequivocal elevation of plasma glucose
   Fasting plasma glucose level is ≥140 mg/dL (7.8 mmol/L) on two occasions
   Glucose tolerance test values listed below when fasting plasma glucose level is ≤140 mg/dL (7.8 mmol/L)
      One value at ½, 1, or 1½ hours is ≥200 mg/dL (11.1 mmol/L)
      Two-hour value is ≥200 mg/dL (11.1 mmol/L)

Impaired glucose tolerance
   Fasting plasma glucose level is ≤180 mg/dL (10.0 mmol/L)
   One value at ½, 1, or 1½ hours is ≥200 mg/dL (11.1 mmol/L)
   Two-hour value is 140 mg/dL (7.8 mmol/L) to 199 mg/dL (10.9 mmol/L)

Normal glucose tolerance
   Fasting plasma glucose level is ≤115 mg/dL (6.4 mmol/L)
   Values at ½, 1, and 1½ hours are ≤200 mg/dL (11.1 mmol/L)
   Two-hour value is ≤140 mg/dL (7.8 mmol/L)

Test values above normal but below those of impaired glucose tolerance or diabetes are nondiagnostic of these conditions.

*Analyses made on venous blood.

---

to 140 mg/dL (7.8 mmol/L) when the level at two hours and at one point from one-half, one, or 1½ hours is 200 mg/dL (11.1 mmol/L) or greater. If the tolerance test is positive for diabetes, specific causes such as pancreatic disease or endocrinopathies (adrenal or pituitary hyperactive states) should be considered. These specific causes are infrequent, however, and familial diabetes will most likely be present. Treatment for diabetes should be instituted. The National Diabetes Data Group recommends that the test be positive twice to diagnose diabetes, but the American Diabetes Association Statistics Committee accepts one positive test as sufficient.[2]

   Impaired glucose tolerance is diagnosed if the FPG is less than 180 mg/dL (10.0 mmol/L), the two-hour level is between 140 mg/dL (7.8 mmol/L) and 199 mg/dL (10.9 mmol/L), and a level at one-half, one, or 1½ hours is equal to or greater than 200 mg/dL (11.1 mmol/L). Specific conditions commonly causing impaired tolerance are endocrine disorders, pancreatic disease, liver disease, and renal failure. If these conditions are not apparent, a repeat test should be performed in six to 12 months. The patient is instructed in the achievement of a normal nutritional state and advised concerning the development and symptoms of overt hyperglycemia.

   Glucose may appear in the urine while plasma glucose levels in the OGTT are in normal range. This may occur under conditions of an increased filtered load or a decreased rate of tubular reabsorption of glucose. In pregnancy there may be increased filtered glucose caused by marked elevation of renal blood flow. The filtered load may exceed tubular reabsorption capacity with small amounts of sugar appearing in the urine. An OGTT should always be performed in patients with asymptomatic glycosuria of pregnancy because of the high prevalence of gestational diabetes.

Two uncommon situations that result in increased filtered load of glucose are adrenocortical steroid treatment and heavy urinary proteinuria. With adrenocortical steroid treatment, the glomerular filtration rate is increased, and, combined with the mild hyperglycemia of steroid therapy, this may cause mild glycosuria. With heavy proteinuria, hexosamines may be transported with protein into the urine and glucose be liberated. In these two conditions, glycosuria is usually minimal (less than 100 mg/dL), however, and may be apparent only with testing by glucose oxidase materials. The oxidase materials give a color change at a glucose level of 10 mg/dL (0.6 mmol/L) to 100 mg/dL (5.6 mmol/L), whereas copper sulfate tablets rarely give a color change with a glucose level of less than 150 mg/dL (8.3 mmol/L). Finally, if none of the conditions listed is met, a diagnosis of renal glycosuria can be made. This is an inherited disorder in which tubular reabsorptive capacity is decreased; it is often familial. The condition is usually judged benign though it has been suggested as a possible precursor to diabetes. It may be more common than appreciated.

If the OGTT result is normal and no glycosuria results, the patient may be instructed to test urine with glucose oxidase materials on random urine specimens passed after breakfast. In the event of a positive urine test, the OGTT should be repeated. If no positive urine tests occur, a two-hour postprandial plasma glucose level can be determined. If it is 140 mg/dL (7.8 mmol/L) or more, a repeat OGTT should be done.

Glycosuria is an important sign, and the probability of diabetes is great. It behooves the physician to keep this cause in mind when other possibilities have been eliminated. In particular, the patient should be made aware of the possibility of diabetes and educated concerning the symptoms of uncontrolled diabetes.

References

1. Classification and diagnosis of diabetes mellitus and other categories of glucose intolerance, National Diabetes Data Group. *Diabetes* 1979;28:1039–1057.
2. Shuman CR, Spratt IL: Office guide to diagnosis and classification of diabetes mellitus and other categories of glucose intolerance, American Diabetes Association Statistical Committee. *Diabetes Care* 1981;4:335.

Chapter 27

The Centinormalized Unit for Reporting Enzyme Results

Joseph E. Buttery, PhD
Peter R. Pannall, MBBCH, FRCPath, FRCPA

From time to time, the suggestion is made that laboratory results be expressed as a percentage of the upper limit of the "normal" or reference range rather than as absolute concentrations. The understandable aim of this is to eliminate the need to memorize reference ranges and to promote uniformity of results from different laboratories using different methods. The major disadvantage is the obscuring of relationships between different substances. Absolute concentrations, especially when expressed in molar terms as in the International System of Units (SI), enables us to appreciate such relationships and can lead to better understanding of physiology and pathology.[1]

The same argument cannot, however, be applied to the results of enzyme assays. Most enzymes are measured by their activity in an assay system, and this measured activity not only reflects enzyme concentration but is influenced by activators or inhibitors, any of which may vary in pathological states. The result is an empirical figure, and it is interpreted in the light of past experience.

While mass concentrations of some enzymes can be measured by immunological methods, it is likely that activity will remain the basis of most assays because it is convenient and easily measured. This being so, there is no valid reason to report in defined units, as there is no true physiological basis for them. The question is: Would the use of a centinormalized unit (CU), where results are expressed as a percentage of the upper limit of the reference range, achieve the dual purpose of promoting uniformity between laboratories and eliminating the need to remember reference ranges, as is suggested by several authors?[2–4]

There is a further, stronger reason why enzyme results have been considered suitable for such a method of reporting. In no field of clinical chemistry is there such a welter of different methods and units. It is, however, unfair to blame

From: The Centinormalized Unit for Reporting Enzyme Results. A Note of Caution. *JAMA* 1981;245:2431–2432. Copyright 1981 by the American Medical Association.

the SI,[3] as the recommendations for reporting enzyme results have not been generally adopted. Indeed, the confusion is only partly due to units and the SI could not correct the main problem, which is methodological.

The preparation of reagents for enzyme analyses requires time and great care. Many laboratories, including our own, prefer to purchase reagents, often in kit form, from reputable commercial companies. Since absolute standards are rarely available, quality control is achieved by using commercially available serum specimens. The information supplied with such serum specimens includes the value expected using different, but commonly used, assay methods and often provides a reference range for each method. We will use the information from one such control serum (Ortho Abnormal Control Serum, lot No. 5S110, Ortho Diagnostics) to illustrate the problem further. There are 20 listed methods for alkaline phosphatase (ALP), 22 for lactic dehydrogenase (LDH), and 21 for aspartate transaminase (AST or SGOT). The expected values for LDH on the same specimen, quoted variously as U/L, IU/L, or mU/mL, range from 227 to 1,110. The accompanying reference ranges vary from 34 to 72 and 120 to 366. We recognize that many laboratories establish their own reference ranges and that these may differ from those quoted. Nevertheless, the variation is apparent. These differences are due to different reagents and, more particularly, to the different temperatures at which the analyses are performed.

Would the concept of the CU eliminate these differences? The answer, unfortunately, is no, not completely. The calculated value of CUs, obtained on this single sample but by different methods, ranges from 160 to 374, or from the clinician's point of view, from a mild to significant elevation. In patient specimens, there is an additional problem. Lactic dehydrogenase, for example, is not a single enzyme but a composite of several isoenzymes. Some isoenzymes react better in one assay system than in another. A sample from a patient with myocardial infarction (predominantly LDH_1 and LDH_2) may react differently than one from a patient with an increase in the liver isoenzyme (LDH_5), even though the amount of enzyme present was the same. It would still be necessary for clinicians to learn by experience what the value actually means for the assay performed in the laboratory they use. This experience may not be valid for (apparently) the same assay performed in another laboratory. This problem is not restricted to LDH, and Table 27–1 outlines the more divergent results quoted on the information sheet. Data sheets from other quality control serum samples provide similar information. Validate-A (General Diagnostics) lot 0194126, for example, provides values for ten methods for ALP with calculated CU ranging from 151 to 321. The CU ranges for LDH (13 methods) and AST (SGOT) (13 methods) are 101 to 196 and 160 to 419. Again we stress that all these results refer to the same sample.

All that has happened in calculating CU values is that yet another variable—the upper limit of the reference range—has been introduced. It is clear that the clinician using several different laboratories would not benefit from CUs

—— **Table 27–1.** ——
Examples of Different Enzyme Results on the Same Sample. *

Test	Method	Value, Units	Upper Limit of Normal	CU
Acid phosphatase	Eskalab	24	12	200
	KDA	7	0.57	1,228
Alkaline phosphatase	BMC (30°C)	290	280	104
	ABA	296	92	332
Amylase	Coleman 91	327	200	164
	Beckman (Enzymatic)	294	21	1,400
	Beckman (Enzymatic DS)	251	110	228
Creatine kinase	Hycel 17	85	52	163
	Clinicard	423	100	423
Lactic dehydrogenase	Calbiochem (Wacker) (30°C)	234	138	170
	Calbiochem (Wroblewski) (30°C)	653	278	235
	BMC (Wacker) (30°C)	277	74	374
	BMC (Wroblewski) (30°C)	546	334	163
Aspartate transaminase	Coulter Chemistry (25°C)	54	31	174
	Beckman TR	133	27	493

*The figures represent some of the expected values by different methods on a quality control serum (Ortho Abnormal Control Serum lot 5S110). The centinormalized units (CU) are calculated on the upper limit of the reference (normal) range provided for each method. All assay temperatures are 37°C unless otherwise indicated.

if the laboratories used different methods. With different units and different reference ranges for different methods, no assumption of comparability is justified.

We may now examine the second quoted advantage of CUs. Can clinicians using a single laboratory dispense with the need to remember reference ranges? In many cases this would be true, and they could assess a value or follow a trend of results adequately using such units. There are pitfalls, however. Reference ranges for enzymes, as for several other substances in the blood, may be dependent on age or sex. The upper limit of the range for γ-glutamyl-transferase (GGT) activity measured in our laboratory is 70 IU/L for men and 35 IU/L for women. A result of 350 IU/L would then be reported as 500 CU for a man, but 1,000 CU for a woman. This is misleading, since it is probable that normal men have values about 35 IU/L higher than, rather than double, those of women and that 350 IU/L would be expressed more appropriately as $[(350 - 35)/35] \times 100$, or 900 CU.

Age dependency is particularly evident in the case of serum ALP estimations. Levels before puberty are two to three times higher than those of adults, but there is a wide variation of values at the time of the pubertal growth spurt, which may itself vary in the age at which it occurs. Reference ranges, however, are necessarily arbitrary and must be recognized as such. If the quoted upper limit of the reference range before the age of 14 years is 250 IU/L and thereafter 100 IU/L, a patient with a value of 200 IU/L could be reported on as 80 CU immediately before his or her birthday and 200 CU immediately afterward. The use of CU has obscured the true meaning of the value, which in the case of ALP does have a physiologic basis.

We must conclude that the introduction of CUs would not solve the problems of enzyme reporting but may create an unwarranted and dangerous assumption of comparability of results within and between laboratories. This is not to deny the deplorable confusion that exists at present. The only solution lies in the adoption of standardized methods, such as those being recommended by the International Federation of Clinical Chemistry. It is likely that, as such methods are approved, manufacturers of reagents will produce kits to comply with them. Until such time, it is imperative that all laboratory reports of enzyme results provide reference ranges. It is not sufficient to provide a separate list of such ranges. Furthermore, clinicians must interpret results against the stated range only and not use that of another laboratory.

References

1. Young DS: SI units for clinical laboratory data. *JAMA* 1978;240:1618–1621.
2. Gerstbrein HL, Lederer WH: Uniform presentation of enzyme determinations. *JAMA* 1974;227:325.
3. Langdon DE: SI units and enzyme levels. *JAMA* 1979;241:1229.
4. Burkart TJ: Uniform presentation of enzyme determinations. *JAMA* 1979;242:1362.

Organizing the Laboratory to Benefit the Patient

Chapter 28

Why Clinical Laboratory Tests Are Performed and Their Validity

Arthur F. Krieg, MD
S. Raymond Gambino, MD
Robert S. Galen, MD

Today, several billion medical laboratory tests are performed each year in the United States, at an annual cost of many billions of dollars. Does this high utilization indicate better patient care at lower cost through modern medical science? And will the projected increases represent further progress toward better health? The answer is, not necessarily.

Why do physicians request laboratory tests? Some results—of blood gas, glucose, and electrolyte determinations—are needed to monitor and guide treatment of critically ill patients. Other results—as from creatinine and thyroxine tests—help us to detect early renal or thyroid disease. Still other tests appear to be done primarily because they are available. But in all cases, the usefulness of a positive test result will vary with the *sensitivity* and *specificity* of the test, and with the *prevalence* of the disease in the population tested.[1]

Sensitivity

Sensitivity means percent of positive results in patients with the disease. The test for phenylketonuria is highly sensitive: In all patients with the disease, a positive result is obtained (100% sensitivity). In contrast, the carcinoembryonic antigen (CEA) test for colon carcinoma has a relatively low sensitivity: Only 72% of patients with the disease are found to have a positive result.[2] In addition, the sensitivity of the CEA test varies with the severity of the disease. The sensitivity is less than 20% for early colon carcinoma, but a much greater sensitivity is found in cases of extensive carcinoma with metastases.

From: Why Are Clinical Laboratory Tests Performed? When Are They Valid? *JAMA* 1975;233:76–78. Copyright 1975 by the American Medical Association.

The serum thyroxine (T_4) value is a highly sensitive indicator of severe hypothyroidism—100% of hypothyroid patients will have low levels. However, of patients who are "borderline" hypothyroid (nonspecific symptoms plus an elevated level of thyroid-stimulating hormone), fewer than 80% will show a low level of serum T_4. Reports in the literature often are misleading or contradictory where sensitivity is concerned: A test that is 100% positive in advanced disease may be only 20% positive in early stages of the same condition. Thus, a negative result on a laboratory-screening test may provide a false sense of security, or even lead to neglect of findings on history and physical examination. Sensitivity in early disease seldom equals that reported in studies based on "proved cases."

Specificity

Specificity means percent of negative results among people who do not have the disease. The test for phenylketonuria is highly specific: 99.9% of "normal" individuals give a negative result (99.9% specificity). In contrast, the CEA test has variable specificity: About 3% of "normal" nonsmoking individuals give a false-positive result (97% specificity); whereas in smokers, the specificity falls to about 80%, since 20% of smokers give a false-positive result. Although serum T_4 value is highly specific in distinguishing "normals" from "hyperthyroid," there is much overlap between "normal pregnancy" and "hyperthyroid" because of variations in levels of thyroxine-binding globulin. Thus, specificity will vary with the "control group" used. Physicians usually do not have difficulty in discriminating between health and disease, but do find it essential and more difficult to discriminate between disease A and disease B, C, or D. Specificity in actual practice is less than in literature reports based on "normal control groups."

Predictive Value

The *predictive value* of a positive result defines the percentage of positive results that are true positives. The predictive value will vary with sensitivity, specificity, and prevalence. It is easy to understand how sensitivity and specificity affect predictive value. However, the important role of prevalence often is not fully appreciated. We will illustrate this by applying a test with 95% sensitivity and 95% specificity to two different populations, one with a disease prevalence of 10% and the other with a disease prevalence of 1%.

If a test with a specificity of 95% and a sensitivity of 95% is applied to a population with 10% prevalence, and we collect data on 10,000 subjects, the data will look like those in Table 28–1. Of the 1,400 positive results, 450 are false-positives. Thus, the predictive value of a positive result is only 68% since only 950 of the 1,400 positive results were true positives.

However, if disease prevalence is 1% instead of 10%, the predictive

Table 28–1. Data for Disease With 10% Prevalence.		
Subjects	No. With Positive Test	No. With Negative Test
1,000 Diseased	950	50*
9,000 Nondiseased	450	8,550†
Total	1,400	8,600

*Sensitivity, 95%
†Specificity, 95%.

value is much worse. In Table 28–2, of the 590 positive results, only 95 are true positives. Thus, the predictive value of a positive result is only 16%. Subjects whose test specimens give a positive result have only one chance in six of having the disease.

The effect of prevalence on the predictive value of a positive result is summarized in Table 28–3 for a test with 95% sensitivity and 95% specificity. Serum creatinine level will have a higher predictive value in a group of patients on the urology service than in the general population because of the higher prevalence of renal disease on the urology service. Likewise, the two-hour postprandial glucose determination will have a higher predictive value in subjects with a family history of diabetes than in those without such a history. Serum T_4 value will have a higher predictive value in women with weakness, dry skin, lethargy, slow speech, and cold intolerance than in the general population.

In the previous examples, clinical data are used to increase the likelihood of the disease and thus to increase the likelihood that a positive test result is a true positive. This effect is understood intuitively by most physicians. Therefore, they usually expect the laboratory result to agree with their clinical diagnosis, and if it does not, they often assume that the laboratory is in error. But the problem often is not "lab error"; rather, it is the complex interaction of sensitivity, specificity, and prevalence.

Table 28–2. Data for Disease With 1% Prevalence.		
Subjects	No. With Positive Test	No. With Negative Test
100 Diseased	95	5*
9,900 Nondiseased	495	9,405†
Total	590	9,410

*Sensitivity, 95%.
†Specificity, 95%.

—— **Table 28–3.** ——————

Effect of Prevalence on Predictive Value of Positive Result.

Prevalence, %	Predictive Value of a Positive Result, %
0.1	2
1.0	16
2.0	28
5.0	50
10.0	68
50.0	95

Other Factors

In addition to seeking confirmation of a clinical impression, what other factors motivate physicians to request laboratory services? Are tests sometimes requested to show the patient or professional associates we are doing something—even if an abnormal result will never lead to any change in diagnosis or therapy? Are requests occasionally based on a desire to do a complete work-up, for benefit of the chart, rather than the patient? How often are requests made on the basis of a recent journal article that does not include a critical analysis of the sensitivity, specificity, and predictive value of the proposed test?

Which Tests to Order

Too often clinical laboratory studies are neither carefully planned nor thoroughly studied. Williamson[3] found that "physicians did not always pay attention to reports of pyuria and albuminuria. Many abnormal reports were ignored." Griner and Liptzin[4] suggest that

patterns of laboratory use may bear little relation to the needs of the patient for optimal care. The data suggest that . . . laboratory studies are excessive . . . Further studies are necessary to determine how often the results of laboratory tests influence diagnostic or therapeutic decisions or affect the outcome of care.

Schneiderman et al[5] found that "physicians tended to pay little attention to 'abnormal' results of screening . . . laboratory tests." Edwards et al[6] reported: "There was no consistent logical approach to the use of bacteriological culture results." Schroeder et al[7] found that "variations in costs of laboratory . . . use . . . among 33 faculty internists . . . at a university clinic was 17-fold. Distribution of the results of the cost audit was followed by a 29.2% decrease in laboratory . . . expenditures." Kelley and Mamlin[8] concluded: "The frequency that abnormal test results were unknown to physicians . . . ranged from a low of 28%

for chest roentgenograms to a high of 93% for urine colony counts." Apparently, laboratory studies are not always selected with care, and results are not always used to benefit the patient. How can we as physicians improve our performance?

Before ordering a test, we should

• attempt to determine whether test sensitivity, specificity, and predictive value are adequate to provide clinically useful information, and

• ask ourselves the three questions suggested by LaCombe[9]:

1. Will results of this test change the diagnosis, prognosis, or therapy?

2. Will results of this test provide a better understanding of the disease process in this patient?

3. What am I looking for and why? Will the patient benefit if I find it?

Physicians should request laboratory services with an understanding of the inherent statistical limitations of all procedures, including history and physical diagnosis. Few medical schools provide formal education in this area, and there is little applied research on the clinical value of our multi-billion annual expenditure on laboratory tests. Unless physicians regard the ordering of laboratory tests as a serious responsibility, worthy of the same thoughtful consideration as a history and physical examination, the privilege to select such services freely may not remain unrestricted in the future.

References

1. Vecchio TJ: Predictive value of a single diagnostic test in unselected populations. *N Engl J Med* 1966;274:1171–1173.

2. Hansen HJ, Snyder JJ, Miller E, et al: Carcinoembryonic antigen (CEA) assay. *Hum Pathol* 1974;5:139–147.

3. Williamson JW: What questions to ask? The answer may tell. *Hosp Pract* 1969;4: 113–115.

4. Griner PF, Liptzin B: Use of the laboratory in a teaching hospital. *Ann Intern Med* 1971;75:157–163.

5. Schneiderman LJ, DeSalvo L, Baylor S, et al: The 'abnormal' screening laboratory result. *Arch Intern Med* 1972;129:88–90.

6. Edwards LD, Levin S, Balagtas R, et al: Ordering patterns and utilization of bacteriologic culture reports. *Arch Intern Med* 1973;132:678–682.

7. Schroeder SA, Kenders K, Cooper JK, et al: Use of laboratory tests and pharmaceuticals. *JAMA* 1973;225:969–973.

8. Kelley CR, Mamlin JJ: Ambulatory medical care quality determination by diagnostic outcome. *JAMA* 1974;227:1155–1157.

9. LaCombe MA: A six-point test ban treaty for house staff. *Resident Staff Physic* 1973;19:47–48.

Chapter 29

Why Physicians Order Laboratory Tests

Bradley G. Wertman, MD
Stuart V. Sostrin, MD
Zdena Pavlova, MD
George D. Lundberg, MD

The number of clinical laboratory tests performed has increased greatly in recent years in nearly all health centers in the United States. This rise in laboratory use has been a major factor contributing to escalating health care costs.[1] The need for so large a number of laboratory tests has quite reasonably been questioned.[2] Several authors[3-6] have offered reasons for the increased number of tests. These include overzealous documentation, medicolegal considerations, building of a personal database, public relations, and profit, in addition to valid clinical indications.

Little hard data are available in print to document why physicians order laboratory tests or to indicate what percentage of tests is ordered for the various reasons cited (see also Chapter 30).[5,6] This study collected such information by asking physicians directly why they ordered laboratory tests and whether and how the results influenced their diagnostic and therapeutic decisions.

Methods

The Los Angeles County–University of Southern California Medical Center is a 2,100-bed general teaching public hospital, with a physician population drawn from more than 75 medical schools, providing a broad cross section of educational background and philosophy.

The Section of Laboratories and Pathology at the Medical Center performed more than 16 million tests in 1976 to 1977. For this study we chose the 11 most frequently requested laboratory tests or panels: electrolyte-renal-bone panel (serum sodium, potassium, bicarbonate, calcium, inorganic phosphorus, glucose, urea nitrogen, uric acid, creatinine, and alkaline phosphatase—four-

From: Why Do Physicians Order Laboratory Tests? A Study of Laboratory Test Request and Use Patterns. *JAMA* 1980;243:2080–2082. Copyright 1980 by the American Medical Association.

hour turn-around time [TAT]); liver-cardiac panel (serum total protein, albumin, total and direct bilirubin, alkaline phosphatase, creatine phosphokinase, lactic dehydrogenase, aspartate aminotransferase, and alanine aminotransferase—24-hour TAT); glucose—one-hour TAT; and hematology profile and leukocyte differential count, VDRL, prothrombin time, arterial blood gases (P_{O_2}, P_{CO_2}, pH), bacterial culture and sensitivity, mycobacterial culture and urinalysis. These tests accounted for 52% of the total number of tests performed in these laboratories and 33% of the work load, based on College of American Pathologists work-load unit values.

For each of these 11 tests or panels, 100 result report sheets were selected randomly around the clock over a two-week period. A multiple-choice questionnaire was constructed to inquire about the following points: status of the physician ordering the test; primary reason for ordering the test; actions taken on the basis of the result; whether the result of this test was substantially different from the immediately preceding test; the interval between this test and the preceding test of the same type; whether the physician planned to repeat the test; who obtained the specimen; length of patient hospitalization; whether additional tests would be ordered because of this result; and whether the physician would have ordered the test if the patient had had to pay for it without reimbursement. The questionnaire and a self-addressed envelope were attached to a result report sheet and were distributed through the usual laboratory reporting channels. Physicians were asked to complete the questionnaire and return it via the intrahospital mail. It was emphasized that the questionnaire answers were to apply only to the single attached report.

The results of each laboratory test were classified as normal or abnormal based on the hospital's identified "normal range"; in the case of cultures, whether the flora was abnormal for the location in which it was found. Chemistry test panels were classified as abnormal only if three or more results were outside the normal limits defined for the test.

Results

A total of 310 questionnaires were returned by 111 physicians from 63 different nursing units. Medicine, surgery, obstetrics and gynecology, and pediatrics were represented, as well as many specialties within those areas. The physicians were practicing in acute care wards, intensive care units, outpatient clinics, emergency rooms, and long-term care wards.

Table 29–1 shows that diagnosis, screening, and monitoring were the most frequent reasons given by physicians for ordering laboratory tests. Education, medicolegal aspects, presentation to senior staff, and nonavailability of previous results only rarely were reasons for ordering tests. Positive bacteriology and mycobacterial cultures were more frequently ordered for diagnosis than were other tests. Serology and urinalysis were more often ordered for screening. The tests

Table 29-1.
Physicians' Reasons for Ordering Laboratory Tests.

Test	Frequency Ordered, %								
	Diagnosis	Screening	Prognosis	Monitoring	Previous Abnormal Result	Education	Medicolegal	For Presentation to Senior Staff	Previous Result Not Available
Glucose	31	8	8	44	11	6	3	0	0
Potassium and sodium	44	6	6	44	38	0	0	0	0
Electrolyte-renal-bone panel	8	11	6	53	31	3	0	0	6
Liver-cardiac panel	46	49	21	26	15	0	0	0	0
Hematology profile	48	48	9	35	0	4	0	0	0
Serology	21	88	0	0	0	0	0	0	0
Prothrombin time	3	11	8	76	11	3	0	0	0
Blood gas	57	0	14	50	14	7	0	0	7
Routine culture	86	9	5	9	5	0	0	0	5
Tuberculosis culture	90	20	5	0	5	0	0	0	0
Urinalysis	36	69	0	12	5	0	3	0	0
All tests	37	32	7	33	12	2	1	0	1

more frequently ordered for monitoring were prothrombin time, electrolyte panel, sodium, potassium, glucose, and blood gases.

Table 29–2 denotes the assessment of the recipient physicians of the importance of the test result and what action came from it. In 32% of the cases there was no change in diagnosis, prognosis, therapy, or understanding of the patient's condition. The tests most frequently used for screening were most likely to result in no change and were least likely to be changed appreciably from the previous result. The tests that were most frequently ordered for monitoring were also more likely to (1) have an abnormal result, (2) show an important change from the previous result, (3) lead to a change in therapy, and (4) be repeated in the future.

Most requests were initiated by the house staff (80%). Senior staff physicians initiated 15% and medical students, 3%. In 2% the origin could not be ascertained.

Comment

In this study we found no clear most common reason for ordering a laboratory test. Rather, three reasons contributed almost equally to the ordering of laboratory tests. These were diagnosis (37%), screening (32%), and monitoring (33%). These were far more common than the next most frequent reason, a previously abnormal result (12%).

Professional and lay literature frequently mentions fear of malpractice litigation as a reason for the increasing use of laboratory tests by physicians. In this study we found that medicolegal considerations were cited as a contributing factor for only 1% of all tests ordered, and even in those it was not necessarily the sole factor. This is especially interesting since this study was conducted shortly after a large increase in professional liability insurance costs in California, which was accompanied by extensive public and professional debate on the problem of malpractice litigation. Residents and interns were aware that a malpractice suit during their years of training could affect their future insurability.

Several reasons frequently discussed as a cause of increased laboratory use in teaching hospitals were infrequently reported as reasons for ordering tests. Educational considerations were mentioned in only 2% of the cases, and the need to have a result to present to a senior staff member or on rounds was not mentioned as a contributing factor in a single response.

As one measure of the benefit of laboratory tests, we attempted to assess what action was taken because of the specific test result reported. Two thirds of all the responses indicated that some change in diagnosis, therapy, prognosis, or understanding of disease came about because of the report of this particular result. This indicates that, in the opinion of the physician using the report, most hospital laboratory tests contribute appreciably to the management of the case.

More objective data show us that the results of laboratory tests were ab-

Table 29-2.
Action Brought About by Test Report.

Test	Change in Diagnosis	Change in Therapy	Change in Prognosis	Better Understanding of Disease	No Change	Result of This Test Was Abnormal	Important Change From Previous Result	This Test Will Be Repeated	Additional Tests Will Be Ordered Because of This Test	Would Not Have Ordered if Patient Had Had to Pay
						Frequency of Action, %				
Glucose	22	78	14	14	11	67	50	64	53	14
Potassium and sodium	13	88	6	13	13	87	56	81	69	0
Electrolyte-renal-bone panel	14	58	6	22	20	89	36	72	39	3
Liver-cardiac panel	51	28	23	28	33	35	23	44	44	5
Hematology profile	26	35	22	26	35	61	13	65	48	8
Serology	8	13	4	13	68	8	0	0	13	13
Prothrombin time	0	71	13	18	18	82	32	74	50	3
Blood gas	29	88	21	14	14	86	29	64	43	0
Routine culture	18	59	0	18	27	14	18	32	27	5
Tuberculosis culture	45	40	25	20	40	0	10	15	35	0
Urinalysis	21	31	12	21	60	28	5	21	26	12
All tests	22	51	13	20	32	55	25	48	40	6.5

normal in 55% of all cases. This percentage of abnormalities was even greater for those tests not ordered primarily for screening. In addition, one third of the physicians reported that, in their opinion, the tests that were being repeated showed a noteworthy change from the previous result reported. Since changes in diagnosis, therapy, prognosis, or understanding of disease can be a product of a normal test result, or one that does not change importantly from a previous result, these data support the view that a large percentage of laboratory tests result in some direct benefit to the patient and physician. The usefulness of these tests to the physician is further indicated by the fact that 48% of the respondents intended to order the same test again on the same patient.

As an evaluation of how important physicians thought the laboratory test was to the care of their patients, 6.5% of the respondents indicated that they would not have ordered this laboratory test if patients had had to pay for it themselves. This figure could be interpreted in the obverse—that 6.5% of the tests were unnecessarily ordered because of liberal third-party payment. However, since the patient population in the study was composed primarily of low-income groups for whom personal payment for even vital laboratory procedures would constitute a hardship, this figure of 6.5% seems low.

A closer examination of the actions brought about by the test reports shows that by far the most common action was a change in therapy (51%). This indicates that physicians are using laboratory tests to monitor and control therapy. Further examination shows that the tests that resulted in a change in therapy were primarily those that were reported as a quantitative result, such as glucose, sodium, potassium, prothrombin time, and blood gases. It seems that many laboratory tests are ordered in an attempt to quantify the disease process. A numerical quantity can be used to monitor the patient's course.

We can develop a profile of the way tests are used for monitoring. Such a test result is generally abnormal (82%) and often shows an important change from a previously ordered test (52%), even though the tests are being repeated daily in 55% of the cases. Tests ordered for monitoring were reported to result in a change in therapy 71% of the time. Only 17% of the time was there no change in therapy reported on the basis of such a result. Nearly one half of the patients for whom a test was requested for monitoring had been in the hospital longer than one week (48%), and monitoring contributed to the reason for ordering 60% of all these laboratory tests for patients who had been in the hospital longer than one week.

Thus, the use of laboratory tests to follow the progress of and to control therapy for patients who have important biochemical abnormalities and long hospitalization represents a major use of laboratory resources.

The data reported here contradict the popular notion that a large percentage of laboratory tests are ordered for medicolegal or educational purposes or that the results are often useless. In fact, they indicate the opposite: that almost all of these tests are ordered for realistic medical purposes and that a surprisingly large percentage of laboratory results lead directly to modification in patient care.

The data may be somewhat biased by the selection of the tests included in the study. However, even if the test group is biased as a sample of the total population of laboratory tests, these tests alone represent over one half of all tests ordered in our laboratory and one third of its work load. As such, their contribution to the cost of patient care and laboratory services is noteworthy in its own right.

Most of these data are limited to the subjective opinions of the physicians who ordered and used the laboratory tests. We have made no attempt to determine objectively whether these tests were actually necessary for the decisions and actions reported to take place. Such an evaluation was beyond the scope of this study. However, these results do represent the professional judgment and opinion of a large cross section of medical school teaching faculty and physicians in training. The pattern of test ordering and result use they reported in this study will, in all probability, continue to be used by them for many years of their professional lives and undergo only gradual modification.[7] As a result of the wide diversity of backgrounds and large number of physicians involved, it seems unlikely that these patterns reflect bias that can be attributed to any one school or region.

Conclusion

The results of this study show that diagnosis, screening, and monitoring are the most common reasons given by physicians for ordering hospital laboratory tests. Other often-mentioned reasons, such as medicolegal considerations and education, contribute little to test ordering.

The physicians reporting in this study indicated that two thirds of these laboratory tests contributed to a change in diagnosis, therapy, prognosis, or understanding of disease, and one third of repeated laboratory test results showed an important change from the previous result.

The use of laboratory tests for monitoring abnormal values and controlling therapy emerges as a major reason for using laboratory tests equal to the more widely discussed reasons of diagnosis and screening.

References

1. *The Problem of Rising Health Care Costs*, Council on Wage and Price Stability. Washington, DC, Executive Office of the President, 1976.
2. Benson ES: Strategies for improved use of the clinical laboratory in patient care, in Benson ES, Rubin M (eds): *Logic and Economics of Clinical Laboratory Use*. New York, Elsevier/North Holland Biomedical Press, 1978, pp 245–258.

3. Krieg AF, Israel M: Why physicians order too many tests. *Med Lab Observ* 1977;9: 46–51.

4. Swisher SN: Lab utilization—the profit motive. *Hospital Practice* 1976;11:19.

5. Griner PF, Liptzin B: Use of the laboratory in a teaching hospital. *Ann Intern Med* 1971;75:157–163.

6. Schroeder SA, O'Leary DS: Differences in laboratory use and length of stay between university and community hospitals. *J Med Educ* 1977;52:418–420.

7. Eisenberg JM: An educational program to modify laboratory use by house staff. *J Med Educ* 1977;52:578–581.

Chapter 30

How Physicians Use Laboratory Tests

Laurence P. Skendzel, MD

The medical community knows more about the quality of laboratory testing than they do about the use of diagnostic tests by physicians. This neglect is unfortunate, for the reaction of physicians to laboratory data is as important as accuracy in testing. The way a test is applied in patient care has a bearing on the precision needed in laboratory assays.

Following the introduction of quality control systems 25 years ago, clinical laboratories have been striving to improve the reliability of the testing process. The College of American Pathologists (CAP) has collected volumes of data that describe the accuracy and precision of assay methods commonly used in laboratories across the nation. Data from CAP's national laboratory surveys and regional quality control programs show a pattern of gradual improvement in the precision of testing.

Now that laboratory precision has been defined, physicians in laboratory medicine are focusing attention on what happens after the test is completed. Cole[1] reviewed patients' records to decide how test results aid the attending physician in diagnoses and treatment. Barnett,[2] using the expert opinion approach, assigned estimated precision needed in laboratory testing for medical decisions. To my knowledge, no one has investigated the reaction of a group of physicians to laboratory tests. How does the clinician apply test results in the treatment of patients? What precision is required to meet clinical needs? Reliable answers to these complex questions were not easy to come by, but I believed that someone should study the physician's use of laboratory tests in the same fashion as we would evaluate laboratory precision. A study of this nature, however, requires the application of a method of accounting that goes beyond the recording of facts and undertakes measurements of the ways in which the physician perceives and

From: How Physicians Use Laboratory Tests. *JAMA* 1978;239:1077–1080. Copyright 1978 by the American Medical Association.

reacts to a test result. This study attempted to answer these questions from a questionnaire distributed to physicians engaged in clinical practice.

Questionnaire Design and Distribution

The questionnaire consisted of ten brief, simulated clinical resumes describing a patient's history and laboratory findings. Laboratory values slightly above or below the normal ranges were generally selected, since in borderline cases, the clinical findings are likely to be ambiguous and the test should be most helpful. The physicians were asked to decide the change in results that would alter the diagnosis and treatment or prompt further assessment of the patient's condition. A range of possible responses was listed on the questionnaire, and the respondents recorded their opinions by circling one of the values. The physicians were asked questions like these:

Q. The patient is a well-controlled diabetic in the hospital with a myocardial infarction. The laboratory reports a fasting plasma glucose level of 110 mg/dL. The test is reordered the next day. Which of the following values indicates a clinically important change, ie, the value that alters the diagnosis or treatment or prompts further evaluation of the patient's condition: 115, 120, 125, 130, 140, 145 mg/dL?

Q. The patient receives gentamicin sulfate daily. The serum urea nitrogen level is 21 mg/dL. The test is reordered the next day. Which value indicates a clinically important change: 23, 25, 27, 29, 31, 33, 35, 37, 39, 41, 43, 45 mg/dL?

Q. The patient receives gentamicin sulfate daily. The serum creatinine level is 0.8 mg/dL. The test is reordered the next day. Which value indicates a clinically important change: 1.0, 1.2, 1.4, 1.6, 1.8, 2.0, 2.2, 2.4, 2.6, 2.8 mg/dL?

Q. The patient is having a routine physical examination and does not have any complaints. A battery of tests is ordered. Assume that the tests are reordered at the time of the next office visit. Which value indicates a clinically important change? The results are as follows:

Test	Initial result, mg/dL	Retest result, mg/dL
Uric Acid	7.2	7.4, 7.6, 7.8, 8.0, 8.2, 8.4, 8.6, 8.8, 9.0, 9.2
Calcium	10.3	10.5, 10.7, 10.9, 11.1, 11.3, 11.5, 11.7, 11.9
Triglycerides	160	165, 170, 175, 180, 185, 190, 195, 200, 205, 210
Cholesterol	240	245, 250, 255, 260, 265, 270, 275, 280, 285, 290

Q. The patient adheres to a salt-restriction diet and regularly takes a diuretic. The plasma sodium concentration is 130 mEq/L. The test is reordered at the time of the next office visit. Which value indicates a clinically important change: 128, 126, 124, 122, 118, 116, 114, 112, 110 mEq/L?

Q. The patient adheres to a salt-restriction diet and regularly takes a diuretic. The plasma potassium concentration is 3.6 mEq/L. The test is reordered at the time of the next office visit. Which value indicates a clinically important change: 3.4, 3.2, 3.0, 2.8, 2.6, 2.4, 2.2, 2.0, 1.8, 1.6 mEq/L?

Q. The patient has had a resection of the large intestine three days ago. The plasma potassium concentration is 5.0 mEq/L. The test is reordered the next day. Which value indicates a clinically important change: 5.2, 5.4, 5.6, 5.8, 6.0, 6.2, 6.4, 6.6, 6.8, 7.0 mEq/L?

Q. The patient has had a resection of the large intestine three days ago. The plasma sodium level is 140 mEq/L. The test is reordered the next day. Which value indicates a clinically important change: 142, 144, 146, 148, 150, 152, 154, 156, 158, 160 mEq/L?

Q. The hemoglobin level of a patient who has had a bowel resection three days ago is 10 g/dL. The test is reordered the next day. Which value indicates a clinically important change: 9.8, 9.6, 9.4, 9.2, 9.0, 8.8, 8.6, 8.4, 8.2, 8.0 g/dL?

Q. The patient has had a thyroidectomy four days ago. The calcium concentration is 8.5 mg/dL. The test is reordered the next day. Which value indicates a clinically important change: 8.3, 8.1, 7.9, 7.7, 7.5, 7.3, 7.1, 6.9, 6.7, 6.5 mg/dL?

Questionnaires along with a note explaining the scope of the study were sent to 300 internists selected at random from a membership roster furnished by the central office of the American College of Physicians. Responses were received from 125 physicians.

Design of Study

Two variables in this study are the precision of laboratory testing and the physician's opinion of a clinically important change in test results. Even under ideal conditions, a laboratory assay does not give the same result each time it is repeated. The unavoidable change, frequently called imprecision of laboratory assay, inherent variability, inherent analytical variation, or unavoidable laboratory error, must be considered when deciding whether the day-to-day change in a patient's test result is clinically important (ie, the change stems from physiologic or pathologic events and not laboratory testing factors).

The CAP provides estimates of the inherent variability of assay procedures in laboratories across the nation. More than 1,000 participants in their Quality Assurance Service (QAS) analyze aliquots of a serum pool every day with each batch of laboratory assays. The results are sent to the CAP Computer Center, where the inherent analytical variation is calculated and expressed as the 95% range of repetitive assays. Table 30–1 lists the average analytical variation from CAP/QAS laboratories during November 1976 for commonly tested constituents.

Table 30–1.
Estimated Analytical Variation of Laboratory Tests.*

Tests	No. of Labs	Analytical Variation % Estimate†	Estimate Applied to Specific Test Result
Glucose, mg/dL	1,539	6.1	110 ± 7
Urea nitrogen, mg/dL	1,312	8.1	21 ± 2
Creatinine, mg/dL	950	8.0	0.8 ± 0.1
Sodium, mEq/L	1,190	2.1	140 ± 3 130 ± 3
Potassium, mEq/L	1,194	3.4	5 ± 0.2 3.6 ± 0.2
Osmolality, mOsm/kg	111	2.1	270 ± 6
Hemoglobin, g/dL	421	4.5	10 ± 0.5
Calcium, mg/dL	920	4.2	8.5 ± 0.4 10.3 ± 0.4
Uric acid, mg/dL	892	5.6	7.2 ± 0.4
Triglyceride, mg/dL	304	12.8	160 ± 20
Cholesterol, mg/dL	766	7.8	240 ± 19

*Based on data from regional quality control program.
†Estimate of limits of analytical variation based on average coefficient variations for all assay methods. College of American Pathologists data, December 1976.

In my experience, pathologists select the method used for testing after reasonable assurance that it is accurate, precise, and practical, but we seldom solicit the clinician's view of how well the laboratory performs. Responses to the question of a clinically important change in test results are indicators of the physician's appreciation for unavoidable laboratory error. The approach I used in this study was to apply limits of analytical variation from the CAP/QAS to the test results included in the patient resumes sent to physicians. The range of values listed in Table 30–1 served as a guideline for separating unavoidable laboratory error from a clinically important change.

Individual answers from each physician were placed into three groups: agreement, disagreement, and borderline. A physician group was in agreement when the value selected as an indicator of a clinically important change exceeded the limits of inherent analytical variation. The clinical and laboratory views of a clinically important change were in agreement. Conversely, a group was in disagreement when the selections were within the estimated range of inherent analytical variation. From the viewpoint of the laboratory, the change was not clinically important. A group was defined as borderline when values selected by the physicians coincided with the upper or lower limits of the analytical variation range.

Results

Of all the study's results, none are more fascinating than the differences in attitudes toward laboratory tests. At one extreme there are physicians who rely on small changes to signal a need for patient reevaluation. At the other extreme there are physicians who apparently react only to wide swings in values. Responses to the question of a clinically important change in plasma glucose ranged from 5 mg/dL (0.3 mmol/L) to 35 mg/dL (1.9 mmol/L) above the initial test result. In the management of the condition of a patient receiving gentamicin, opinions of a clinically important change in urea nitrogen levels varied from 2 mg/dL (0.7 mmol/L) to 24 mg/dL (8.6 mmol/L).

The three most frequent values selected as indicators of a clinically important change (Table 30–2) account for an average of three fourths of all re-

Table 30–2.
Distribution of Opinions of Physicians About a Clinically Important Change.*

Clinical Setting	Tests	Initial Result	Physician Selection of Clinically Important Change		
			First Frequency Value (%)	Second Frequency Value (%)	Third Frequency Value (%)
Well-controlled diabetic	Glucose, mg/dL	110	145(42)	140(22)	130(17)
Daily dose of gentamicin sulfate	Urea nitrogen, mg/dL	21	27(31)	25(28)	31(17)
	Creatinine, mg/dL	0.8	1.2(41)	1.4(30)	1(11)
Third day after operation for large-bowel resection	Potassium, mEq/L	5	5.6(37)	5.4(35)	5.8(11) 5.2(11)
	Sodium, mEq/L	140	146(36)	148(26)	150(25)
	Osmolality, mOsm/kg	270	281(20) 285(20)	276(12)	288(10) 294(10)
	Hemoglobin, g/dL	10	9(30)	9.4(21)	9.6(18)
Strict adherence to salt restriction diet and daily dose of diuretics	Sodium, mEq/L	130	126(40)	124(26)	128(16)
	Potassium, mEq/L	3.6	3.2(50)	3(23)	3.4(20)
Fourth day after thyroidectomy	Calcium, mg/dL	8.5	8.1(39)	7.9(29)	8.3(20)
Routine physical examination	Uric acid, mg/dL	7.2	8(25)	9(21)	7.8(13)
	Calcium, mg/dL	10.3	10.7(28)	10.9(20)	10.5(14)
	Triglyceride, mg/dL	160	180(23)	200(21)	190(14)
	Cholesterol, mg/dL	240	260(22)	290(20)	280(15)

*In successive laboratory assays.

sponses (range, 60% to 90%). Opinions generally centered around the most frequently selected value. In clinical situations involving cholesterol and triglyceride assays, a convergent trend toward one value did not occur, and choices were roughly equally divided among the three values. When examined by the type of clinical setting, slight differences occurred in physicians' attitudes on sodium and potassium assays. They apparently expected greater precision in the low-normal ranges for both tests. Although a wide range of opinions was recorded, the first frequency value offers an estimate of the thinking of physicians who took part in this study on the issue of a significant change in laboratory values in specific clinical situations.

Table 30–3 separates the opinions of the respondents by the limits of inherent laboratory variability. In this population sample, 80% were in the agreement group. A relatively small proportion, one of ten of those questioned, selected values that fell with the range of inherent analytical variation (disagreement group). The best rating was seen in questions involving glucose, creatinine, sodium, and potassium; nine of ten responses were in the agreement group. At least 70% of the responses for urea nitrogen, osmolality, hemoglobin, uric acid, and cholesterol were in the agreement group. Major disagreements occurred in the interpretation of a clinically important change in calcium and triglyceride results.

——— **Table 30–3.** ———
Physicians' Opinions vs Estimates of Laboratory Reproducibility.

Tests	Initial Result and Estimate of Analytical Variation	125 Physicians' Opinions			
		Agree	Disagree	Borderline	No Response
Glucose, mg/dL	110 ± 7	103	1	. . .	21
Urea nitrogen, mg/dL	21 ± 2	115	. . .	9	1
Creatinine, mg/dL	0.8 ± 0.1	125	. . .	. . .	. . .
Sodium, mEq/L	140 ± 3	123	. . .	. . .	2
	130 ± 3	104	20	1	. . .
Potassium, mEq/L	5 ± 0.2	111	. . .	14	. . .
	3.6 ± 0.2	124	. . .	. . .	1
Osmolality, mOsm/kg	270 ± 6	94	4	13	14
Hemoglobin, g/dL	10 ± 0.5	98	27	. . .	. . .
Calcium, mg/dL	8.5 ± 0.4	51	25	48	1
	10.3 ± 0.4	72	18	35	. . .
Uric acid, mg/dL	7.2 ± 0.4	113	4	7	1
Triglyceride, mg/dL	160 ± 20	63	29	28	5
Cholesterol, mg/dL	240 ± 19	107	16	. . .	2
Totals		1,403(80%)	144(8%)	155(9%)	48(3%)

Roughly half of the respondents selected values so close to the original calcium result that it was impossible to separate unavoidable error from a clinically important change. One of four selections of a clinically important change in triglyceride results was in the disagreement group. Judging from this population sample, most internists take inherent laboratory variations into account when making decisions on what is clinically important.

Comment

There is a new sense of awareness that the activities and achievements in laboratory testing have been viewed without enough assessment of how the physician uses the test in patient care. It is no easy task to bring the issues of test result and clinical application into focus.

Many factors affect medical decisions. The inherent analytical variations, activity and posture during testing, physiologic variations, changes in disease and organ malfunction, drug interactions, random errors, and time of day the blood sample is taken all contribute to variations in the test results (see also Chapter 28).[3,4] In addition, the physician's appreciation of these factors varies depending on training or area of particular interest. There are so many variables that it is difficult to isolate one of them and attempt to make simple positive relationships between test result and medical decisions. Given the number of variables, it is still important to obtain information about the physician's reaction to test results.

Physicians' attitudes on clinically important change are indicators capable of guiding us in decisions on laboratory precision. The current analytical variation in clinical laboratories on assay of selected constituents such as glucose, urea nitrogen, sodium, and postassium is adequate for clinical surveillance of the patient. On the other hand, the study's results point out the need for pathologists and primary care physicians to reassess the precisions needed for other assays such as calcium and triglyceride.

The study's results point out areas for improvement in medical education. Responses to the question of a clinically important change in triglyceride values reflect a lack of appreciation for physiologic variation and for the imprecision of current methods of assay. The pathologist's role is in supply of results and opinions. This is no reflection on the clinician's judgment, since no physician has in-depth knowledge of all branches of medicine. The pathologist must inform clinicians of the inherent error of testing and offer opinions of what is a clinically important change in test results.

The study raises several questions. How reliable is the questionnaire technique? What inferences can be drawn from a small sample size? These questions cannot be answered with the information available, but the present data do give an indication that the laboratory is providing test results with sufficient precision and that the physician takes inherent laboratory variation into account when deciding whether a change in test values run on successive days is clinically important.

References

1. Cole GW: Clinical usefulness of multiple result ranges for a laboratory test: the serum urea nitrogen. Report to the Guidelines for Appropriate Utilization of Laboratory Procedures Committee, College of American Pathologists, Skokie, Ill, Sept 16, 1976.
2. Barnett RN: Medical significance of laboratory results: *Am J Clin Pathol* 1968;50: 671–676.
3. Williams GZ, Harris EK, Widdowson GM: Comparison of estimates of long-term analytical variation derived from subject samples and control serum. *Clin Haematol* 1977;23:100–104.
4. Zieve L: Misinterpretation and abuse of laboratory tests by clinicians. *Ann NY Acad Sci* 1966;134:563–572.

Chapter 31

Use of the Microbiology Laboratory

Raymond C. Bartlett, MD

Use of the Laboratory

Unique pitfalls may be encountered by the physician in making optimum use of the microbiology laboratory. A request for a "culture" is nonspecific compared with a request for a blood glucose determination. The request for a culture is an implied request to search for "anything in the specimen that could contribute to the diagnosis and treatment of an infectious disease." Physicians usually do not know exactly how this request will be construed by laboratory personnel. What would happen if blood were submitted to the chemistry laboratory with a comparable request for "chemical abnormalities" that might suggest the presence of disease? What microorganisms will the laboratory seek in a specimen submitted for "culture"? Will a Gram-stained direct smear be performed, and if so, will the results of this examination be reported? The request for culture usually leads to a search for bacteria that would commonly be expected at the site represented. Will *Neisseria gonorrhoeae* be sought in pus from a tubo-ovarian abscess? Will the laboratory culture stool specimens for *Vibrio, Yersinia enterocolitica,* and *Campylobacter,* or will it confine its search to the commonly accepted pathogens *Salmonella* and *Shigella?* Should a request for stool culture in a hospitalized patient with diarrhea include a test for *Clostridium difficile* toxin?

Documentation of infection caused by fungi, mycobacteria, viruses, *Chlamydia,* parasites, and such recently discovered agents as the *Legionella* re-

From: Making Optimum Use of the Microbiology Laboratory. I. Use of the Laboratory. *JAMA* 1982;247:857–859. Making Optimum Use of the Microbiology Laboratory. II. Urine, Respiratory, Wound, and Cervicovaginal Exudate. *JAMA* 1982;247:1336–1338. Making Optimum Use of the Microbiology Laboratory. III. Aids of Antimicrobial Therapy. *JAMA* 1982;247:1868–1872. Copyright 1982 by the American Medical Association.

quires close cooperation between physicians and microbiologists. The diagnosis and treatment of common bacterial infections will be the subject of discussion in this three-part chapter.

More Information Not Necessarily Better

Sporadic reports of infection with microorganisms most commonly representing indigenous or colonizing flora, usually in patients with compromised host defenses, have contributed to a trend toward reporting isolation and antimicrobial susceptibility of increasing numbers of organisms that have no relevance to infection. Proficiency-testing programs intended to improve the quality of work performed in microbiology laboratories have also contributed to the attitude that the physician should be provided with as much information as can be gleaned from a specimen and that it should also be the physician's responsibility to distinguish that which is clinically important from that which is not.

The problem is presented not so much by specimens from normally sterile body sites, such as blood and spinal fluid, but by specimens collected from body sites containing indigenous or colonizing bacteria. These latter are best typified by sputum and urine specimens, which, to compound matters, are usually collected by the patient, with little supervision. The oropharynx, skin, gastrointestinal tract, and vagina contain a plethora of microorganisms; only a minority are capable of causing infection in the uncompromised host. Mixed infections do occur, but the probability that all, or even most, of the isolates in a mixed culture are responsible for such an infection is in inverse proportion to the number of indigenous and colonizing species present and other evidence of superficial contamination, such as the presence of squamous epithelial cells. Ironically, the specimens that contain the largest number of microbial species incur the greatest amount of laboratory cost, yet are less likely to provide useful guidelines for diagnosis and treatment than are specimens that yield fewer types of organisms.

Unfortunately, few quantitative data exist to establish the predictive value of the increasing amount of information that is being produced to guide diagnosis and effective therapy. Galen and Gambino[1] have introduced useful guidelines for the assessment of the medical usefulness of various laboratory tests. However, the many subjective variables that affect specimens submitted for microbiologic examination have made it extremely difficult to compute the usefulness of these procedures. The result has been an escalation in the volume of specimens submitted and information reported, because neither physicians nor laboratories are willing to risk neglecting the possibility that *some* of the information *may* be useful. These practices have followed the "flat of the curve" described by Enthoven,[2] in which an increase in the generation of information through application of more intensive technology does not result in a commensurate increase in the quality of the health care provided.

Establishing a Liaison With the Laboratory

Guidelines have been proposed for use by laboratorians in evaluating the appropriateness of requests received as well as the quality of specimens submitted.[3] Many laboratorians have been reluctant to implement these policies because they fear a lack of support from physicians. Physicians should collaborate with laboratorians through medical staff committees to establish mutual acceptability for such guidelines. It should be established clearly that when specimens are not processed, or are incompletely processed, the physician or patient care unit will be notified promptly; the specimen or cultures will be held in the laboratory at 4°C for several days to provide the physician with an opportunity to request complete processing, if this is clinically preferable to submitting a fresh specimen. Physicians should regard such a practice not as an obstacle to their access to the laboratory, but as an adjunct to improving cost effectiveness and minimizing the production of potentially misleading information.

Site and Time of Collection

The optimum site and time of collection of specimens probably has an important influence on the usefulness of microbiology reports. Material should be collected from as close to the site of infection as possible. Only patient convenience and comfort justify collection of voided urine, sputum, or external drainage from deep infections. Often, meaningful information can be obtained only by aspirating material with a needle inserted into the bladder, lung, or soft-tissue site of infection. Collection from any site administration of antibiotics is usually futile at best and misleading at worst because of the recovery of resistant, indigenous bacteria that are unrelated to infection.

Blood cultures for *Leptospira* and *Salmonella typhi* are likely to be productive only during the first seven to ten days of the illness, when serologic test results are usually negative. Later in the course of these diseases the converse is true. After several weeks, cultures of blood are less likely to be positive than are cultures of urine for *Leptospira* or feces for *S typhi*.

Delay in Transport

Microbiologic specimens are subject to deterioration during transit because of temperature extremes, delay, dehydration, and the presence of nutrients from body fluids. Although refrigeration and the use of specialized transport media can minimize these effects on some specimens, the added expense and delay are not justified in most instances. The death of fastidious microorganisms and the overgrowth of less important but more hardy strains frequently lead to misleading reports when processing is delayed by more than several hours.

Specimens of Dubious Value for Culture

Physicians and laboratorians should establish categories of specimens that should not be processed without a direct consultation from the requesting physician, because certain specimens consistently yield mixtures of bacteria unrelated to infection. These include specimens from most mouth lesions, bowel content, perirectal abscesses, decubiti, vaginal discharge, and Foley catheter tips, as well as material collected from the hospital environment or inanimate objects. In such cases, the computer aphorism "garbage in equals garbage out" applies to the quality of information that would be reported.

For other types of specimens (with the exception of blood), more than one specimen—collected by the same method, from the same apparent site, on the same day—should generally not be processed without a direct consultation to establish unique justifying circumstances.

Use of Gram-Stained Direct Smear

Agreement should be reached on the performance of Gram-stained direct smears and the rapid reporting of results. Although Gram's stain is generally provided for spinal fluid and male genital tract specimens, it is inconsistently performed on exudates from the respiratory tract or wounds, partly because physicians have been skeptical of the significance of the results and have not understood the reporting terminology.

Cells. Gram-stained direct smears should be examined first using a ten times objective with oil on the slide to determine the relative numbers of squamous cells and neutrophils. An abundance of squamous cells and an absence of neutrophils suggest that the material is superficial and does not represent an inflammatory exudate.[4] Bacteria observed in such specimens are not likely to be related to infection, nor will those that will be isolated from culture. Repeated collection, avoiding superficial contamination, should be recommended promptly to the physician or patient care unit by laboratory personnel. Except for sputum, these specimens should be cultured despite request for re-collection, because occasionally *Staphylococcus aureus* or *Streptococcus pyogenes* will be isolated from wounds or superficial sites in patients with infections caused by these organisms despite the superficial appearance of the specimen. Isolation of anaerobic bacteria, *Pseudomonas,* and various Enterobacteriaceae from such specimens is of doubtful clinical significance.

Bacteria. All bacteria seen in direct smears of specimens should be reported, with the exception of those from lower respiratory tract secretions, where the reporting of small numbers, especially when mixtures of types are observed, can be misleading. Unless they are the only morphologic form observed, Gram-negative rods in direct smears of respiratory secretions probably should be reported only when they exceed about ten per field using a 100 times objective, and Gram-positive cocci when they exceed about 25 per field using a 100 times objective.

Physicians should encourage microbiologists to be more specific in the reporting of bacteria observed in smears.[3] For example, when Gram-positive cocci are observed, it would be helpful if the report could indicate whether staphylococci, streptococci, or *Streptococcus pneumoniae* are suggested. The same applies to the reporting of Gram-negative bacilli, which may suggest enteric bacteria, *Pseudomonas*, *Hemphilus*, or *Bacteroides*. In many instances, it will not be possible to speculate on the presence of these genera and species based only on Gram-stain morphology; in such cases, the report should indicate that the distinction cannot be made. In many instances, microbiologists feel confident suggesting the presence of one or the other of these genera or species, but they have been reluctant to put this in writing because they fear that the culture may not support their initial impression. Physicians should reassure microbiologists that the clinical usefulness of the rapid reporting of suggested genera and species is of sufficient clinical value to warrant the risk.

The Anaerobic Culture Dilemma

Great interest has been expressed in recent years in anaerobic infection and in more complete examination of specimens for anaerobic bacteria. Physicians frequently forget to request anaerobic cultures from sites where anaerobic infection may occur. Sometimes they also request anaerobic culture of specimens collected from superficial sites that contain indigenous and colonizing anaerobic bacteria that are unlikely to be related to infection. Physicians should establish appropriate guidelines with laboratory personnel for processing of specimens for anaerobic bacteria. Laboratorians should report that specimens from superficial body sites such as skin, mucous membranes, or urine are not suitable for anaerobic culture. Re-collection should be recommended promptly when other types of specimens purportedly representing deeper sites are submitted for anaerobic culture but demonstrate squamous cells under low-power microscopic examination. On the other hand, criteria should be established to ensure anaerobic culture of specimens that demonstrate a reasonable probability of yielding clinically significant anaerobic bacteria when the physician has not requested it. These include specimens collected from deep body sites such as transtracheal aspirates and aspirations from organs or closed cavities that demonstrate no squamous epithelial cells in Gram-stained direct smears. All currently recommended blood culture systems include culture for anaerobic bacteria. Anaerobic meningitis and septic arthritis are infrequent and do not justify routine anaerobic culture of spinal or joint fluid.

Microbial Identification

Microbial identification that exceeds diagnostic, prognostic, or therapeutic requirements is of little clinical value. Advancing technology permits subdivision of many bacterial species into serotypes and biotypes that are only occasionally of epidemiologic interest. Physicians should review microbial identification practices with laboratory staff to ensure that unnecessary expense is not incurred in microbial identification exceeding clinical requirements. Examples of occasionally performed identifications of doubtful clinical value are serotyping of *Salmonella* species, typing of *Hemophilus influenzae* other than type B, typing of *Neisseria meningitidis*, and typing of *Klebsiella pneumoniae*. Species identification of yeasts isolated in mixed cultures of specimens from superficial body sites is of doubtful clinical value. Laboratorians should be urged to consult with physicians before engaging in time-consuming and expensive identification of isolates of borderline pathogenicity from superficial body sites. In most instances, these isolates are of no clinical importance and may be reported as "atypical Gram-negative rods," "nonlactose-fermenting Gram-negative rods," and the like. If, on the other hand, such atypical organisms are isolated under circumstances that suggest pathogenicity, complete and accurate identification is required.

Confusion may result when microbiology laboratories change nomenclature without notifying physicians. Physicians should review recently abandoned taxonomic terms with microbiologists to minimize confusion. The medical staff should be notified when changes in nomenclature occur.

Urine, Respiratory, Wound, and Cervicovaginal Exudate

As previously discussed, physicians may encounter many pitfalls in the submission of specimens that are commonly contaminated with indigenous and colonizing bacteria. These pitfalls apply especially to specimens from the respiratory tract, superficial wounds, draining lesions, and the female genital tract.

Urinary Tract

Many different types of specimens may be collected from the urinary tract. "Clean-catch" specimens are the most subject to contamination. Specimens collected by straight single catheterization or cystoscopy have a much decreased probability of contamination with urethral flora. Those collected by suprapubic aspiration should contain no contaminating organisms. Specimens collected from closed drainage systems or from ileal bladders are likely to contain mixtures of bacteria representing colonization of those sites.

Direct Examination. Physicians should make greater use of direct examination of urine to evaluate the quality of the specimen and to determine the presence of significant numbers and types of bacteria. This may be done by examining the unstained centrifuged urine sediment with a 40 times objective. The finding of 20 or more bacteria in each random field correlates with cultures showing 10^5 or more bacteria per milliliter.[5] Alternatively, a drop of uncentrifuged urine may be placed on a slide (it should not be spread out), dried, and stained by Gram's method. The finding of one organism in each random field examined with a 100 times objective correlates with cultures showing 10^5 or more bacteria per milliliter.[5]

Significance of Numbers of Bacteria. Physicians should review with laboratory staff criteria for complete identification and antimicrobial-susceptibility testing of isolates from urine specimens, depending on the number of bacteria per milliliter detected and the number of different species observed. Most patients with urinary tract infections will demonstrate at least 10^5 bacteria per milliliter. Emptying of the bladder a short time before collection of a specimen or irrigation of the bladder may reduce these numbers substantially in patients with infections. Unnecessary laboratory expense can be avoided by holding cultures that demonstrate fewer than 10^5 bacteria per milliliter and reporting broad bacterial categories such as "coliform-type bacteria isolated 10^3/mL" on the basis of colonial morphology, with the appended comment that the number is generally insufficient to suggest infection.

Mixed Cultures. In some patients with closed drainage systems, the finding of abundant neutrophils may suggest an active bladder infection. There is ample evidence, however, that antimicrobial therapy is not beneficial and may induce superinfection with more resistant strains. We have found that mixed cultures of clean-catch urine specimens signify contamination 90% of the time (unpublished data). In specimens from Foley catheter drainage systems showing mixed cultures, only 36% showed the same mixture of organisms in a second specimen. Physicians should establish policies with microbiologists to report such mixtures from both clean-catch specimens and from closed drainage systems on the basis of colonial morphology, without application of biochemical tests for identification or antimicrobial susceptibility testing, unless the same mixture of isolates was obtained from a previous specimen.

Gross and colleagues[6] have stated that the risk of bacteremia in patients with closed drainage systems dictates that the antimicrobial susceptibility of all organisms present in the bladder should be known. Physicians should reassess carefully whether empirical antimicrobial therapy would be more appropriate to administer to such bacteremic patients and whether the choice of drugs should be influenced by the susceptibilities of the bacteria that happened to be isolated from one urine specimen several days earlier. One possible exception would be the presence or absence of *Pseudomonas aeruginosa* based on colonial morphologic characteristics supported by a rapid oxidase test. Physicians should appreciate that most laboratories receive more urine specimens than any other type of specimen. We have demonstrated that the largest single source of saving in the expenditure of microbiology resources in a cost-containment program resulted from curtailing the complete identification and antimicrobial susceptibility testing of mixed urine cultures.[7]

Special Procedures. Anaerobic culture should not be performed on urinary tract specimens except by special consultation. Although *Staphylococcus saprophyticus* is a newly recognized cause of cystitis in women, physicians should establish an agreement with microbiologists that all isolates of coagulase-negative staphylococci be reported as such, with the understanding that the physician will specifically request further identification if clinically indicated.

Upper Respiratory Tract

Most throat cultures are submitted in conjunction with the diagnosis of acute pharyngitis. Physicians should support a laboratory policy of seeking and reporting the presence or absence only of group A β-hemolytic streptococci. In specific situations, physicians may want to request isolation and identification of *N gonorrhoeae* or *Corynebacterium diphtheriae*. Other lesions of the mouth and throat may suggest Vincent's infection, peritonsillar abscess, or candidiasis, in which case this should be specifically indicated on the request slip. *S pneumoniae*, *H influenzae*, *S aureus*, Enterobacteriaceae, or *Pseudomonas* should not be reported because of the frequency with which these organisms are isolated from patients in whom they play no infective role. Search for such organisms may be established through special consultation in assessing colonization rates in immunosuppressed patients, for example.

Lower Respiratory Tract

Predictive Value of Sputum Culture. We have found that sputum cultures demonstrate bacteria capable of causing pneumonia in 74% of patients with clinical evidence of pneumonia and in 38% of patients without clinical evidence of pneumonia. Applying the criteria of Galen and Gambino[1] to a population of patients in which the prevalence of pneumonia is 50% suggests that only 54% of positive sputum cultures would be obtained from patients with pneumonia. If the prevalence of pneumonia among patients were only 10%, only 12% of sputum specimens containing pathogens might be obtained from infected patients. If the prevalence of pneumonia were only 1%, only 1% of specimens containing pathogens would represent infected patients. The efficiency of sputum culture for diagnosis of pneumonia is only 56% when the prevalence is 50%. Thus, even in a population of patients with a high prevalence of pneumonia, the sputum culture provides only 6% more assurance than would a coin toss that the presence of pathogens signifies pneumonia. By contrast, transtracheal aspiration demonstrates an efficiency of 91%.[8] The physician must weigh the advantages of this greater diagnostic efficiency against the potential morbidity, expense, and time required for collection. Physicians must realize that the presence of pathogens in a sputum specimen is of no help in establishing a diagnosis of pneumonia. It simply indicates which organisms are present.

A number of measures may be taken to reduce the probability that isolates from sputum represent colonizing or indigenous flora of the upper respiratory tract. Preparation of the patient may be improved, and collection may be supervised or induced. Nasotracheal aspiration often produces a less-contaminated specimen. In other instances, bronchoscopy or direct needle aspiration of the lung may be required to obtain suitable material for microbiologic examination. Culture for anaerobic bacteria is only indicated from transtracheal or direct lung aspirate because of the invariable contamination with anaerobic organisms of all specimens that pass through the oropharynx (including bronchoscopic washings).

Gram-Stained Direct Smear. Physicians should support the laboratory practice of preparing Gram-stained direct smears of all respiratory tract secretions for detection of relative numbers of neutrophils and squamous cells. Numerous quantitative criteria have been recommended, but all dictate that an abundance of squamous cells and a scarcity of leukocytes suggest a high probability that any pathogens that are isolated will represent only pharyngeal flora. In these cases, specimens should be re-collected.

When specimens demonstrate an abundance of neutrophils and an absence of squamous cells in Gram-stained direct smears, reporting of categories of pathogens may provide an early indication of the cause, enabling prompt administration of appropriate therapy. This procedure was reviewed earlier in this chapter.

Mixed Cultures. It is probably not clinically helpful to provide complete identification and antimicrobial susceptibility of more than three pathogens from the best-quality specimen. In such circumstances, it cannot be known whether one or more pathogens represent the causative agent. In such instances empirical therapy is usually indicated, and the substantial expense of the identification and susceptibility testing of multiple isolates is not warranted. On the other hand, correlation of the culture isolates with the morphologic types observed in the Gram-stained direct smear may help to establish that some isolates bear greater relevance to infection than others. In such instances, complete identification and susceptibility testing on only those isolates that are observed in both the direct smear and the culture should be encouraged.

Wounds and Soft-Tissue Infections

Specimens collected from wounds and soft-tissue infection sites are subject to contamination with indigenous and colonizing bacteria from the skin and adjacent mucous membranes. Proper preparation of the skin with antiseptic solutions minimizes this problem. Whenever possible, a small piece of tissue should be submitted instead of a swab containing the material. It is also preferable to aspirate purulent material with a syringe instead of collecting it on swabs. Although swabs are convenient, they are the least desirable means of collecting material for microbiologic examination.

A transport medium that contains nonnutritive stabilizing substances should always be used if swabs are used. Refrigeration or incubation should be avoided; instead, specimens should be processed within one or two hours. Although anaerobic culture may be performed on swab-collected specimens placed in transport medium containing reducing substances, special anaerobic transport containers should be available. Appropriate practices to ensure that anaerobic culture is performed on specimens most likely to be taken from sites of anaerobic infection were described earlier, along with measures to avoid anaerobic culture of specimens with little likelihood of yielding anaerobic bacteria associated with infection.

Genital Tract

Men. Physicians should support the laboratory practice of seeking and reporting only the presence or absence of *N gonorrhoeae* in urethral specimens from men; physicians should consult the microbiologist in individual cases where a search for other organisms, such as *Mycoplasma* and *Chlamydia*, is indicated.

In men, the bacterial cause of prostatitis may be established either by massaging the prostate with culture of any exudate that may be expressed from the urethral meatus or by culture of the last few drops of a voided urine sample.

Women. It is extremely difficult for microbiologists to produce meaningful information from specimens obtained from the female genital tract without knowing whether the problem represents (1) possible gonorrhea, (2) vaginitis, (3) surgical wound infection, or (4) possible endometritis. Without this information, an abundance of bacteriologic media must be employed, and numerous organisms may be identified and reported, many unrelated to the clinical problem. Physicians should indicate on the request slip which of these four conditions applies to the specimen. Specimens from surgical wounds may be treated as previously described for surgical-wound exudates. Specimens from patients with possible endometritis should receive approximately the same treatment except that the presence of squamous cells should be viewed as evidence of cervicovaginal contamination, which would obfuscate the significance of any potential pathogens that might be isolated. Therefore, the presence of squamous cells in such specimens should lead to a request for re-collection. Physicians should realize that demonstration of pathogens in the endometrial cavity post partum does not establish a diagnosis of endometritis. The endometrial cavity becomes contaminated and colonized with vaginal flora after most normal vaginal deliveries. In the case of vaginitis, direct smears and cultures for *Candida*, *Gardnerella* (formerly *Corynebacterium* or *Hemophilus*) *vaginale*, and wet preparations for *Trichomonas* should be employed. The same applies to a search for *N gonorrhoeae* in patients suspected of infection with that organism.

Gram-stained direct smears and cultures of amniocentesis fluid collected by transcervical aspiration provide useful predictive information regarding intrauterine infection. Similarly, culture of amniotic fluid from the endometrial or amniotic cavity or both at the time of cesarean section is useful for establishing the presence and cause of endometritis. Physicians should also consider collecting material by culdocentesis for supporting a diagnosis of pelvic inflammatory disease.

Aids of Antimicrobial Therapy

Physicians and microbiologists must work together to facilitate interpretation of laboratory data used to guide antimicrobial therapy. The techniques used and the mode of reporting information should optimize therapy at minimum cost.

Antimicrobial Susceptibility: 'S-I-R' vs MICs

In recent years, much technological change has occurred in the in vitro testing of antimicrobial susceptibility of bacteria isolated from clinical specimens. The disk method of testing was applied initially in a highly unstandardized manner and led to unreliable results in many instances. More recently, the Kirby-Bauer method has become highly standardized in the majority of laboratories. Still, most physicians are only vaguely aware of how the designations "S," "I," and "R," which stand for *sensitive, intermediately* (or *indeterminately) sensitive,* and *resistant,* relate to achievable antimicrobial levels by various routes of administration. This has been further compounded by the transition in many laboratories toward technology that produces the minimum inhibitory concentrations (MICs) of each antimicrobial tested. If only these MICs are reported, the physician must determine the probability that the concentration of the antimicrobial being administered will adequately exceed the MIC at the site of the infection.

In Vitro Criteria for Antimicrobial Susceptibility

Much disparity will be observed among the values recommended by various authors.[9–13] It is not the purpose here to resolve which of these recommendations is correct, but to emphasize the need for physicians and microbiologists to agree on the criteria to be used and ensure that the medical staff understands them so that antimicrobial therapy will be correctly administered. Physicians should review with microbiologists the implications of the designations S, I, and R if they are to be used. Usually, S indicates that mean peak levels after administration of a conservative oral dose will exceed by two to four times the MIC of the organism. If the drug cannot be given orally, then S applies to the minimum parenteral dose. The designation I usually signifies intermediate susceptibility, or susceptibility to maximum parenteral doses if the testing is done by broth dilution.

When this result is obtained with the Kirby-Bauer disk test, it should be interpreted as an indeterminate result that does not establish susceptibility with sufficient accuracy to ensure a satisfactory therapeutic response.

Dependence on the Kirby-Bauer disk method, or any of several automated instrumental techniques that are calibrated to yield results that agree with the Kirby-Bauer method, may indicate S for susceptibility to ampicillin when concentrations of 8 μg/mL or less are shown to be inhibitory, despite the fact that mean peak levels of this drug after oral administration are only about 2.5 μg/mL.

Implementation of standards tentatively recommended by the National Committee for Clinical Laboratory Standards may cause the majority of isolates of *Pseudomonas aeruginosa* to be reported as I, or moderately susceptible, to aminoglycosides if tests are performed by broth dilution.[11] Many physicians may view this as an increase in resistance to these drugs and a contraindication to their use for the treatment of this organism. Actually, the reduction in the MIC required to classify isolates as S to aminoglycosides simply separates the highly susceptible isolates from those that are somewhat less susceptible but should be readily treatable by maximum parenteral dosage.

Other sources of potential confusion include testing of carbenicillin disodium and cephalosporins (cephalothin being the most common of this group to be tested in vitro). The designation S would signify susceptibility to orally administered indanyl carbenicillin, cephalexin, or cephradine. The designation I, if determined by a dilution method, should indicate a high degree of susceptibility to parenterally administered carbenicillin or cephalothin.

In many instances, agreement may be reached between medical staffs and microbiologists that techniques should be used to enable both MICs and S-I-R data to be reported. If this is the case, agreement should be reached as to what MIC values will cause isolates to be classified into these three categories. Information should be disseminated and made readily available to physicians to enable them to correlate results with the levels that may be achieved by various routes of administration. This may include distribution of tables of levels achieved in various body fluids by various doses and routes of administration of commonly used antimicrobial agents. Such guidelines are already available from commercial suppliers of susceptibility-testing materials and are currently being distributed to medical staffs in some hospitals. Ellner and Neu[14] have recently suggested use of an "inhibitory quotient" to assist physicians in interpreting results of susceptibility testing.

Culture and Sensitivity Requests

In some instances, the physician may have no interest in the results of susceptibility testing. When there is concern about choice of therapy, it is difficult for the physician to anticipate whether isolates will be recovered that require antimicrobial susceptibility testing. In some instances, laboratorians have construed the request for "sensitivities" as an order from the physician. This has resulted in routine testing of such isolates as *Streptococcus pyogenes*, which are uniformly susceptible to penicillin and, in the vast majority of instances, to the most likely alternative drug, erythromycin. The decision to perform susceptibility testing should be based on a previously arranged schedule of bacteria that may be isolated and does not depend on the specific request of the physician. In general, in vitro testing is useful and reliably applied only to common, rapidly growing microorganisms such as staphylococci, enterococci, Enterobacteriaceae, and *P aeruginosa*. More fastidious streptococci, *Neisseria*, and fastidious Gram-negative bacteria are usually treated more reliably empirically on the basis of published guidelines. The same may be said for anaerobic bacteria. All laboratories should be equipped to detect the production of β-lactamase by staphylococci, *H influenzae*, and *N gonorrhoeae* and be able to detect susceptibility of *H influenzae* to chloramphenicol and *S pneumoniae* to penicillin.

A useful guide to empirical therapy can be provided by tabulating and distributing the profiles of susceptibility of species commonly isolated and tested. This information is provided in most hospitals, and commercial systems are available to assist in analyzing and printing the information in a convenient format. Periodic testing of batches of isolates of anaerobic bacteria, *Staphylococcus epidermidis*, and enterococci to develop a profile of susceptibility may serve as an adequate alternative to the individual testing of most clinical isolates of these bacteria. For example, the results of testing individual isolates may be reported as follows: "*S epidermidis*, cefazolin (92%); clindamycin (72%); erythromycin (62%); oxacillin (66%); penicillin (54%)." An explanatory note should be appended to indicate sources of the percentages reported. As in all such instances of incomplete processing, the cultures should be held in the laboratory for completion of testing if clinically indicated.

Which Drugs Should Be Tested?

Physicians should review with laboratorians those organism-antimicrobial susceptibility results that should be tested and reported because they are important for guiding therapy. Many years ago, the Food and Drug Administration restricted the distribution of numerous different antimicrobial disks representing essentially the same generic drug to minimize unnecessary testing in clinical laboratories by the Kirby-Bauer method. The promotional activities of pharmaceutical companies led physicians to request and depend on the results of reports of susceptibility to a multiplicity of commercial analogues of antimicrobial agents, when the reporting of testing with a single generic drug would have been applicable. The current transition toward development of systems that do not depend on FDA-approved materials raises the specter of a new proliferation of testing of multiple antimicrobial agents of essentially identical generic activity.

Physicians also should agree with microbiologists to eliminate the reporting of susceptibility of certain bacteria to antimicrobial agents that would not constitute rational therapeutic choice. For example, it would be inappropriate to report the results of testing the susceptibility of *Citrobacter, Enterobacter,* and *Klebsiella* to ampicillin. The majority of these will be resistant, and the drug should not be used against these organisms even if susceptibility is demonstrated in vitro. Such reporting only creates the risk of misdirecting antimicrobial therapy.

Some laboratories using the broth-dilution test use cefazolin instead of cephalothin in vitro because of its greater activity against Gram-negative bacilli. Criteria for testing other newer cephalosporins such as cefamandole, cefoxitin, moxalactam, cefoperazone, and cefotaxime must be reviewed by physicians with microbiologists to minimize unnecessary testing and to prevent the indiscriminate use of the newer, more effective agents. It may not be practical to eliminate the in vitro testing of some organism-antimicrobial combinations because the identification of the organism frequently is not known when testing is initiated. Reporting the results of testing chloramphenicol may be omitted to discourage its arbitrary choice for therapy when it is infrequently a first-line agent for any of the organisms being reported. It may be decided that this information can be obtained from the laboratory on specific request. Epidemiologists may request the susceptibility testing of numerous agents of no actual therapeutic value for typing purposes. Clearly, reporting the results of such testing may be misleading and should be avoided.

The results of testing susceptibility to antimicrobial agents that are effective only for the treatment of urinary tract infections should be restricted to reporting the results on urinary tract isolates. This will avoid the improper use of an agent such as nitrofurantoin or sulfisoxazole for treatment of an infection outside the urinary tract. These agents have a high degree of predictable activity against certain organisms. For example, nitrofurantoin or sulfisoxazole will effectively inhibit 99% to 100% of isolates of *Escherichia coli* in the urinary tract. This suggests that *E coli* need not be tested and reported, but experience has shown that physicians often neglect the use of antimicrobics for which susceptibility is not determined and reported by the laboratory.

How Often to Test

Physicians should establish an agreement with laboratory staff regarding repetition of testing antimicrobial susceptibility on sequential days. Except for unusual circumstances, which should be based on a consultation between the physician and the microbiologist, there would appear to be no need for testing more frequently than every fourth day.

Inhibitory vs Bactericidal

Determination of the minimum bactericidal concentration (MBC) of an antimicrobic requires an extra day and additional microbiologic effort. Such testing is usually desirable with isolates obtained from patients with bacterial endocarditis but is of unproved value in other types of infections. Testing to establish actual MICs or MBCs when the laboratory uses the Kirby-Bauer or some other procedure that does not establish the precise MIC is occasionally indicated. This is most commonly required in the treatment of endocarditis due to various streptococci but also is usually justified for testing of staphylococci, *P aeruginosa*, and Enterobacteriaceae isolated from such patients. When the MBC is 16-fold or more greater than the MIC, this has been said to express "tolerance" to the antimicrobic. Successful therapy may require levels in vivo that substantially exceed the MBC.

Minimum Antibacterial Concentration

Recent attention has been given to the observation that some antimicrobial agents may be effective against certain bacteria at concentrations below the MIC.[15] These results may be obtained by conventional determination of MICs, but the use of these tests for studying such antibacterial concentrations should be viewed as insufficiently well established to be considered a routine procedure.

Other Tests

Other tests employed to guide antimicrobial therapy include the Schlichter test, or serum inhibition (or serum bactericidal) titer, tests to determine the activity of antimicrobial agents in combination, and assays of antimicrobial concentrations in body fluids. Guidelines should be established that will result in requests for consultations from physicians to explain the clinical value of tests requested under other circumstances. It should also be established whether these procedures should be available in the hospital laboratory or obtained through a referral laboratory.

The Schlichter Test. The Schlichter test is the simplest and most convenient means of establishing adequate antimicrobial therapy in patients with bacterial endocarditis. It has also been used for establishing the adequacy of therapy in osteomyelitis. Application to infections of other types has been described, but the effectiveness of this test for guiding the adequacy of therapy in other conditions is not well established.[16]

It is important that the Schlichter test be performed by serially diluting the patient's serum in pooled normal human serum to maintain the protein-binding relationships. Otherwise, misleadingly elevated titers may be obtained in patients being treated with highly protein-bound antimicrobial agents such as oxacillin or cefazolin. In general, a bactericidal titer of 8 or greater is predictive of an effective and curative therapeutic regimen. The test is usually applied to samples collected within one hour of the administration of the antimicrobial agent.

Antimicrobial Synergy. Certain antimicrobial agent combinations are used empirically with the expectation that synergistic activity against bacteria will be obtained. In other instances, synergistic activity either has not been described or has been reported to be unpredictable. Determination of antimicrobial synergy in vitro is cumbersome and probably should not be performed in laboratories that perform this test infrequently. It should not be the function of the routine diagnostic service laboratory to investigate the potential synergistic activity of drug combinations that have not been shown to have potential synergistic activity. Based on such reports, physicians should establish antimicrobial combinations for which synergy testing could be useful. Requests for evaluation of the activity of drug combinations of unknown potential value should be performed only on consultation between the physician and the microbiologist.

Comment

Clinical pathologists, microbiologists, medical technologists, and other laboratory personnel are becoming increasingly aware of the need to concentrate their resources on specimens that are most likely to produce useful clinical information. Implementation of such practices has in many cases been impeded by fear of adverse reaction from physicians and, in some cases, condemnation of these practices by physicians. Fear of legal liability has played an important role in stimulating requests for laboratory analyses that, otherwise, physicians might not consider essential for patient care.[17] Similarly, it may be questioned whether the laboratory could be held liable if it did not carry the processing of every specimen and the reporting of results to the full extent allowed by modern technology. Traditionally and legally, the attitude has been that no stone should be left unturned in seeking optimum care for the individual patient. Paradoxically, as more information is reported, the risk increases that physicians will overlook the most crucial data and even misinterpret or be misguided by data of lesser relevance to infection. Thus, excessive information may become a liability and not an asset.

Even if it could be assured that unlimited application of technology would not lead to an "information overload," medicine, society, and the legal profession will be forced by economic constraints to compromise between the best interests of the individual and society. Hiatt[18] has drawn attention to the fallacy that the economics of our society can support a health care system based on the traditional view "that one should do everything possible for the individual patient." As more and more practices are developed that may be beneficial to individuals but not to the best interests of society, "we risk reaching a point where marginal gains to individuals threaten the welfare of the whole."[18]

Physicians should appreciate that advancing technology in microbiology enables more complete microbiologic examination but that application of these techniques in an indiscriminate manner wastes resources and produces an abundance of information, much of which may be irrelevant to the clinical problem at hand. A cooperative approach between physicians and laboratory workers will lead to conservation of resources while simultaneously improving the quality of the information produced for patient care.

References

1. Galen RS, Gambino SR: *Beyond Normality: The Predictive Value and Efficiency of Medical Diagnosis*. New York, John Wiley & Sons Inc, 1975.
2. Enthoven AC: Shattuck lecture: Cutting cost without cutting the quality of care. *N Engl J Med* 1978;298:1229–1238.
3. Bartlett RC: How far to go—how fast to go, in Lorian V (ed): *Significance of Medical Microbiology in the Care of Patients*, ed 2. Baltimore, Williams & Wilkins Co, 1981.
4. Barlett JG, Brewer NS, Ryan KJ: *Cumitech 7, Laboratory Diagnosis of Lower Respiratory Tract Infections*, Washington JA (ed). Washington, DC, American Society for Microbiology, 1978.
5. Kunin CM: *Detection, Prevention and Management of Urinary Tract Infections*, ed 3. Philadelphia, Lea & Febiger, 1979, pp 94–97.
6. Gross P, Flower M, Barden G: Polymicrobic bacteriuria: Significant association with bacteremia. *J Clin Microbiol* 1976;3:246–250.
7. Bartlett RC, Rutz C: Processing control and cost in bacteriology. *Am J Clin Pathol* 1980;74:287–296.
8. Bartlett JG: Diagnostic accuracy of transtracheal aspiration bacteriologic studies. *Am Rev Respir Dis* 1977;115:777–782.
9. *Performance Standards for Antimicrobial Disc Susceptibility Tests*, National Committee for Clinical Laboratory Standards. Villanova, Pa, 1976.
10. *Performance Standards for Antimicrobic Disc Susceptibility Tests*, suppl 1, National Committee for Clinical Laboratory Standards. Villanova, Pa, 1981, pp 141–156.
11. *Standard Methods for Dilution Antimicrobial Susceptibility Tests for Bacteria Which Grow Aerobically*, National Committee for Clinical Laboratory Standards. Villanova, Pa, 1980.
12. Witebsky FG, MacLowry JD, French SS: Broth dilution minimum inhibitory concentrations: Rationale for use of selected antimicrobial concentrations. *J Clin Microbiol* 1979;9:589–595.
13. Barry AL: A system for reporting quantitative antimicrobic susceptibility test results. *Am J Clin Pathol* 1979;72:864–868.
14. Ellner PD, Neu HC: The inhibitory quotient: A method for interpreting minimum inhibitory concentration data. *JAMA* 1981;246:1575–1578.
15. Lorian V: Effects of subminimum inhibitory concentrations of antibiotics on bacteria, in Lorian V (ed): *Antibiotics in Laboratory Medicine*. Baltimore, Williams & Wilkins Co, chap 3, pp 342–408.

16. Jordan GW, Kawachi MM: Analysis of serum bactericidal activity in endocarditis osteomyelitis and other bacterial infections. *Medicine* 1981;60:49–61.

17. Eisenberg JM, Rosoff AJ: Physician responsibility for the cost of unnecessary medical services. *N Engl J Med* 1978;299:76–80.

18. Hiatt H: Protecting the medical commons: Who is responsible? *N Engl J Med* 1975;293:235–243.

Chapter 32

Physician-Oriented Data Processing

Samuel Raymond, MD

Patient care as a primary objective of the laboratory computer has often been overlooked by people who design laboratory systems. Clinical pathologists, microbiologists, chemists, hospital administrators, laboratory equipment manufacturers, and especially computer designers have frequently tried to decide what the laboratory itself needs, and what kind of services it will provide, rather than asking what physicians need and want from the laboratory for the care of their patients.

There has been a fairly high degree of agreement within the computer industry as to what the clinical laboratory needs and wants, although in practice their systems have not achieved widespread success (fewer than 3% of clinical laboratories have computer systems[1]). Computer industry proposals usually call for a high degree of automation and for complete computerization of the clinical laboratory. The systems proposed are usually based on large central computers to be used for all hospital data processing needs. In the technically most advanced systems, the laboratory function begins with Direct Order Entry at remote terminals. It ends with direct on-line reporting, also via remote terminals. In between, within the laboratory, there is heavy emphasis on real-time, on-line, direct data acquisition, with closed-loop control of laboratory procedures as an ultimate goal. Such systems provide much in the way of automated standardization, quality control programs, and other intralaboratory processing designed to make life safer, easier, or more comfortable for the laboratory staff. Yet conspicuously missing from this scene is the physician, the essential connecting link between the laboratory and the patient.

From: Physician-Oriented Data Processing. *JAMA* 1975;234:83–85. Copyright 1975 by the American Medical Association.

What Does the Physician Want From the Laboratory?

No one can presume to speak for the entire profession, but the conclusions expressed here are derived from an informal survey among the staff of an active teaching hospital, posing the following question: What do you personally want from the clinical laboratory? The answers ranged from a simple one-word "Help!" to a rather detailed specification for a terminal-based inquiry system. The answers can be reduced to two basic needs: (1) to order tests, and (2) to get reports. From these two needs, properly interpreted, we can derive major insight into the realistic requirements of a laboratory data management system. Let us reconstruct what the physician means about each of these.

Ordering Tests

The first need is to order tests. The physician very strongly expresses that he or she can "never" put in an order for a laboratory test. The physician is, of course, exaggerating to express annoyance and frustration with the usual procedures for laboratory orders. The "never" in this context objectively means that some fraction of laboratory orders do not go through. And most of the failures seem to occur with just those requests that the physician is most concerned about, especially the orders personally filled out and sent to the laboratory.

Here is a valuable clue as to just what is wrong with the system as the physician meets it. But to understand this clue we must make a closer analysis of how a test is ordered. Leaving aside screening procedures and similar "automatic" laboratory orders, the procedure begins when the physician mentally formulates a need for a laboratory test on a specific patient to meet a specific medical need.

The next step is to get that mental formulation into the data processing system. There is no computer than can read a physician's mind (very few can even read a physician's handwriting). Consequently, the system requires that the physician express mental formulations in a form suitable for data entry: *it must be encoded*. This is a rigid technical requirement. Someone has to write out the data in a form suitable for keyboard entry.

We have, then, the physician who has formulated the laboratory order about to write it out or otherwise enter it into the system. And here is the crux of the problem: *All too often, the physician does not have all the information needed to enter the order in a form acceptable to the computer.* For example, the physician may not have the hospital number, the bed location, or even the correct spelling of the patient's name and, therefore, should not have the responsibility for encoding or entering the order. This is a technical job, requiring special mental attitudes and special training. The clinician does not have them and should not be concerned with them.

But if the physician does not have the information necessary to enter the laboratory order correctly, how can we get the clinical laboratory work done? Very often, the laboratory system attempts to provide the necessary information on a patient charge plate or equivalent. Thus the information can normally be transferred to the laboratory order by a simple mechanical imprinting operation. This charge-plate operation is normally done by the ward clerk and rarely by the physician. Consequently, if the charge plate is correct, the ward clerk's orders pass and the physician's often fail.

Good as it is, the charge plate often fails too, in two ways: (1) inaccuracy in the plate itself, and (2) missing charge plate. In our hospital, 1% of charge plates carry errors and 30% of the laboratory orders consistently do not have the charge plate imprint. Very often the missing charge plates represent an essential requirement in any medical system, a requirement for flexibility and adaptability in a well-articulated system. There will always be the emergencies, the ambiguities of information, the decisions related to convenience and efficiency that have to be made in the light of the immediate circumstances surrounding the physician when formulating a need for laboratory work. The data processing system must not interfere with this flexibility.

We must, therefore, find some other way to get the necessary data input. Can the laboratory computer system undertake to retrieve or recreate the missing information? Can the information be found in time to enable the laboratory to complete satisfactorily the laboratory work called for by the order?

The answer to these questions is an unequivocal "yes." Over the last four years, with the conditions just described, with 30% of the initially formulated laboratory orders incomplete or actually carrying inaccurate information, the system in our laboratory has rarely failed to identify the patient properly and to perform the tests called for. We know it can be done.

The system we use[2] (Figure 32–1) is based on a realistic, practical, and economical application of computer technology to do the clerical work that has to be done in getting 100% completion of the laboratory orders. This clerical work is done by trained clerks in the computer area of the laboratory. With use of a small laboratory computer, with programs and data files, including a complete hospital census, they complete every laboratory order, while the laboratory is in process of completing the test itself.

This, then, is our answer to the first of the physician's problems. We offer the facility of ordering tests as the physician sees fit; the physician uses a standard of care that he or she thinks adequate in the circumstances and we guarantee to pick up and to complete every laboratory order written out. We do not demand that the physician go to any particular place in the hospital or use any particular piece of equipment, such as a computer terminal, to enter the order. We do expect the physician to formulate his or her need for laboratory work and to write it down, using, if possible, the patient charge plate. But we accept the physician's decision as to what is possible in the circumstances faced at that time. And our laboratory computer clerks accept the responsibility for completing and verifying the orders.

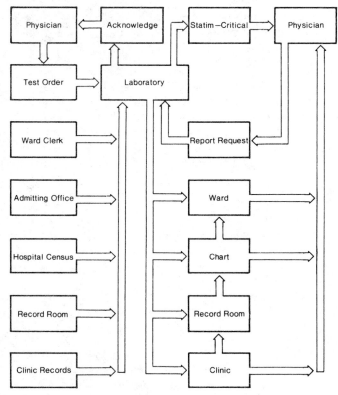

Figure 32–1. Flow chart of pathways of laboratory test requests and results; not particularly the report-request loop.

Physicians in our hospital have accepted this arrangement with gratitude. And we have gone three steps further. First, we notify the physician immediately that we have received the lab order and the specimen to go with it. Second, we offer the facility for telephoning orders in to the laboratory, but this service is rarely used. The physician prefers to order laboratory work through the medium of the written order rather than through the telephone. Finally, we arrange for automatic computer-generated test orders in certain defined situations, especially for routine on-admission tests and for certain kinds of preadmission tests, as specified by the professional staff.

Getting Reports

The second problem is getting reports. The physician complains that reports "never" are received, meaning of course that he or she is frustrated by the difficulties encountered, just as with the test-order entry. But when we investigate *this* problem, we find that even if we make the usual report system work perfectly, the physician will not find it acceptable. The usual system is oriented towards individual patient reports, to be posted in the patient's chart. Instead, the physician needs and wants a physician-oriented report—a summary report each day *for each physician,* containing just today's results on his or her patients only. With adequate computer-system design, we can generate such reports, and we can deliver them when and where the physician uses them. These reports are the equivalent, in information content, of the individual patient reports the physicians were accustomed to, but they offer several attractive features. In the first place, they are not put into the patients' charts. Each physician has a personal copy, each copy carries only that physician's patients, the individual reports are compactly printed (ten per page), and they are delivered at a specified time. They are updated frequently within the laboratory computer, and the physician always receives the latest edition.

Our clinical staff has accepted these reports fully. They find that they can rely on the information as printed—that when the 3 PM report states the result, or notes that it was not ready, they can believe it. Telephone calls to the laboratory have dropped to near zero. Of course, we continue to produce the cumulative record for the patient's chart as a permanent record, but print and post it only once a day. No one objects.

The principles of our system seem to be as follows:

Speed Is Not Essential. Speed is not crucial in reporting except in medical emergencies, which are served outside this system.[3]

Reports on Schedule Are Essential. Predictability is the keynote. The physician is willing to specify a schedule that he or she will follow, based on regular delivery of laboratory reports.

Systematic Rather Than Random Reports. The physician should not have to search through a pile of random reports, delivered at random time, when the computer can so easily provide systematic orderly reports at a scheduled time. This same principle applies to reports delivered via terminals, either on call by the physician or originated by the laboratory. The on-line concept is particularly at fault here. If the laboratory reports a value as soon as it is ready, this means that it will be reporting test results in random order and at random times. This is not a system.

Throwaway Reports. The classical concept of the laboratory report is an official document that is issued once, in response to a specific test request. It is the sole and official report, and it must be preserved carefully as such in the patient's chart; a mere summary or copy is not "legal." We call this the "one-in-one-out system." We replace it with the concept that the laboratory keeps the original report in the computer, and issues copies of it for different purposes, which can be used once and thrown away. It is far more economical for the computer to print the same report four times than to let four physicians leaf through the patient's chart to find it on four separate occasions.

Multiple Copies. In our hospital, the chief medical resident and three of his colleagues make rounds together. Of course, they use their daily report. But we provide four copies, instead of one, so that they do not have to pass it back and forth among themselves. Our printer can print one copy in ten seconds. The extra three copies require 30 seconds, or 5-cents worth of computer time. At the current cost of physician time, each resident would have to save only seven seconds a day by having a personal copy of the report to make it worthwhile. Extra reports certainly save far more time than that.

Reports Direct to User. As an example, our outpatient records were originally sent to the record room to be inserted in the chart. The record room is normally weeks behind in this work. Consequently, the report was not available on the next clinic visit. Then we sent individual reports direct to the clinic to be put in the chart on the next clinic visit. But 40% of the time the chart was missing when the patient came into the clinic. Now we send a copy of the report directly from the computer, where the original report is kept, to the physician who is going to use the report, on the day the patient returns to the clinic. We bypass the record room, the chart, the clinical secretary, and place the report directly in the hands of the person who uses it. This has solved the problem.

Outpatients Are People Too. With a computer and the realization of differences between inpatient and outpatient reports, you can give outpatients just as good service as inpatients.

Interpretation

In the 100 years or so that the clinical laboratory has been a part of the medical care system, it has never been the custom for the laboratory to furnish the kind of interpretative reporting that is used by the radiologist or cardiologist. The physician does not, now, recognize this as a deficiency. In older times any questions raised about the significance of a laboratory test were resolved by a personal conference between the physician and the laboratory. This is no longer possible. There have been recent trends toward interpretation[4] but we have to admit that we still have so much trouble getting the data to the physician that we cannot worry much about interpretation yet. The contribution of the clinical laboratory to the practice of medicine has changed drastically in the last decade. The variety of laboratory tests available has increased beyond our most extreme expectations, and the volume of tests ordered has not lagged behind. In these circumstances we can easily forsee the necessity of evaluating the flood of data on an individual-patient basis in the laboratory before releasing it to the clinician. This does not mean the usual quality control statistics; rather, we must attempt to see if this particular result is valid for this particular patient and if so, what is its medical significance. We must also begin to evaluate whole patterns of laboratory values to extract meaning out of a mere collection of numbers.[5] Finally, we shall have to look forward to problem-oriented laboratory requests, procedures, and reports, rather than individual tests. All this is not to replace the basic report system, but in addition to it.

But, first, let's get the basic report right.

References

1. Sherman WN: Clinical laboratory computerization. *Lab Management*, February 1972, pp 22–24.
2. Hamilton WF, Raymond S: Extended clinical laboratory information processing system. *Comput Biol Med* 1973;3:3–12.
3. Lundberg GL: When to panic over an abnormal value. *Med Lab Observer*, March 1972, pp 2–6.
4. Reece RL: Numbers are not enough. *Med Lab Observer*, Fall 1973, pp 48–53.
5. Grams RR, Johnson EA, Benson ES: Laboratory data analysis system. *Am J Clin Pathol* 1972;58:177–219.

Chapter 33

Interpretive Reporting in Clinical Pathology

Carl E. Speicher, MD
Jack W. Smith, Jr, MD

A good clinical history and physical examination have always been the basis for sound medical diagnosis and management. Modern medicine has extended this data base through a wide variety of techniques, of which clinical laboratory studies play a major role. These studies have grown explosively, and the accompanying paperwork can overwhelm the laboratory and the clinician. Thick patient charts bulging with laboratory reports threaten the ability of busy clinicians to find the information they require. Computer-generated reports have not yet solved the problem. Attempts by the laboratory to assist the clinician in managing these data have included marking abnormal results with asterisks, printing reference values adjacent to test results, grouping of data by system or organ,[1] displaying data in more informative ways,[2] suggesting diagnostic possibilities,[3] making interpretive comments,[4] and suggesting additional studies or performing additional studies automatically.[5]

In this chapter, all of these efforts to reduce laboratory data to clinically useful information have been designated as interpretive reporting. The methods, variety, and scope of interpretive reporting are not well documented in the medical literature. Because this approach constitutes a serious effort to improve the use of laboratory data for patient care, a survey of its prevalence in the practice of pathology in the United States was undertaken. Implicit in the concept of interpretive reporting should be the realization that only thoughtfully designed laboratory strategies lend themselves to effective interpretation.

Methods

The names and addresses of 3,784 hospitals in the United States having more than 100 beds were obtained from the American Hospital Association's

From: Interpretive Reporting in Clinical Pathology. *JAMA* 1980;243:1556–1560. Copyright 1980 by the American Medical Association.

Guide to the Health Care Field,[6] and a form letter was sent to the director of laboratory services of each hospital. The letter requested the directors to forward examples of each kind of interpretive report they generate. The directors were promised an analysis and summary of this material as well as appropriate credit in any publication.

The letters were mailed through February and March 1978, and June 15, 1978, was established as the cutoff date for inclusion of replies in this report.

Results

Replies were received from 183 directors of laboratory services, of whom 146 enclosed examples of their reports. At least 150 of these 183 directors were recognized as pathologists. The 37 directors who did not enclose examples said they were not using interpretive reports but were interested in the study. Of the 183 replies, 150 were from community hospitals, 22 were from university hospitals, and 11 were from federal hospitals. Interpretive reports were organized into 16 categories as given in Table 33–1.

Several kinds of information were included in interpretive reports. The first was the provision of reference values. The second was some type of analogue display where abnormal test results were marked with asterisks or placed in different columns from normal test results or were depicted graphically. The third was the provision of diagnostic possibilities that should be considered when various results occurred. The fourth was the inclusion of an interpretive comment in which the pathologist stated the importance he or she attributed to a given group of studies.

Interpretive reports usually included results from two or more laboratory measurements that were grouped together, eg, an organ panel or a coagulation screen. Occasionally these measurements were performed in a sequential manner, but most of the time they were done in parallel.

Interpretive reports were executed in a variety of ways. Most used pre-printed forms (Figure 33–1). Additional information was either handwritten or typed. Many used a memory typewriter. An example of interpretive reporting by code number using a magnetic card typewriter is as follows:

Serum Protein Electrophoresis. Total protein, 7.6 g/dL. The albumin through beta regions appear nonremarkable. In the mid-gamma region, a narrow zone of restriction is evident. Densitometric quantitation of this restricted zone shows a quantity of 0.6 g/dL protein. The remainder of the gamma zone is nonremarkable.

Immunoelectrophoresis. An IgG kappa monoclonal protein is evident. No free monoclonal light chains are noted in serum. The normal polyclonal immunoglobulins (G, A, and M) appear normal in amount.

Laboratory Impression: IgG kappa minor monoclonal protein.

Suggest:

1. Urine immunoelectrophoresis, if this has not been previously ordered,
2. Hematology consult, and

Table 33–1.
Interpretive Report.

Type of Report	% Using Report	Type of Report	% Using Report
Screening		*Endocrinology and metabolism*	
Multiphasic screening	23	Glucose tolerance	21
Acid-base, water, and electrolytes		Thyroid function panel	20
Blood gases	18	Steroid panel	2
Serum electrolytes and		Hypopituitarism panel	1
osmolality	9	Parathyroid function panel	1
Anion gap	3	Parathyroid hormone	1
Urine electrolytes and		Metabolic panel	1
osmolality	1	Nutritional assessment	1
Cardiovascular disease		*Immunology and rheumatology*	
Lipid panel	46	Serum protein	
Cardiac injury panel	31	electrophoresis	50
Lactic dehydrogenase		Immunology consultation	12
isoenzymes	28	Immunoglobin panel	8
Creatine phosphokinase		Immunoelectrophoresis	5
isoenzymes	18	Arthritis-collagen panel	5
Hypertension panel	3	Febrile agglutinins	5
Cardiac evaluation panel	1	Immune competence panel	2
Pulmonary disease		Antinuclear antibody,	
Cystic fibrosis	2	antimitochondrial antibody, and	
Pulmonary panel	1	antismooth muscle antibody	2
α_1-Antitrypsin	1	*Pediatrics, obstetrics, and gynecology*	
Renal and urinary tract disease		Fetal maturity	10
Renal panel	8	Placental function	5
Urine protein electrophoresis	4	Erythroblastosis panel	3
Urine chemistry	3	Antibody screen	3
Stone analysis	2	Amino acid screen	1
Prostatic panel	1	Chromosome analysis	1
Gastrointestinal disease		*Neuromuscular and bone disease*	
Gastric analysis	11	Bone panel	1
Duodenal analysis	1	Muscle panel	1
Lactose tolerance	1	*Infectious diseases*	
Xylose tolerance	1	Antibiotic sensitivity	13
Malabsorption panel	1	Infection by site	3
Liver, bile ducts, and pancreas		Identification and	
Liver panel	11	interpretation	1
Pancreatic panel	1	Viral hepatitis	1
Cholinesterase	1	Hypersensitivity pneumonitis	1
Hematology and oncology		*Blood bank*	
Coagulation screen	22	Transfusion reaction	29
Hemoglobin identification	16	Antibody identification	6
Bone marrow	12	Rhogam eligibility	1
Peripheral blood	7	Paternity test	1
Anemia study	6	*Body fluid and special topics*	
Serum iron	5	CSF proteins	8
Coagulation consultation	4	Semen analysis	7
Osmotic fragility	2	Joint fluid	5
Schilling test	1	Serous cavity fluid	3
Transition panel	1	*Therapeutic monitoring and toxicology*	
Haptoglobin	1	Therapeutic monitoring	8
		Toxicology	3

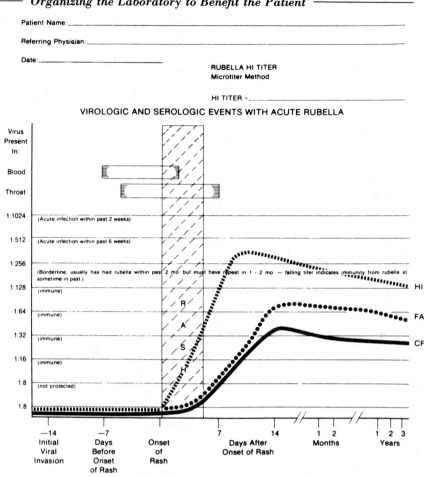

Patient Name:_____

Referring Physician:_____

Date:_____

RUBELLA HI TITER
Microtiter Method

HI TITER =_____

Figure 33–1. Preprinted form for interpretive reporting. Hi = hemagglutination inhibition; CF = complement fixation; FA = fluorescent antibody. (Information courtesy of Emma White, MD, Bakersfield, California.)

3. Such minor monoclonal proteins may be present with clinically evident lymphoproliferative disease (myeloma), evolving lymphoproliferative disease. However, they may also coexist with a variety of nonlymphoproliferative epithelial neoplasms. Finally, in elderly individuals, they may exist as an isolated phenomenon unassociated with disease. If this is found to be the case in this patient, suggest periodic quantitation by electrophoresis. (Courtesy of John C. Neff, MD, Columbus, Ohio)

Fifteen percent used a computer (Figure 33–2 and Table 33–2).

A few respondents sent interpretive reports used in surgical pathology, cytology, and autopsy pathology. Because these reports are conventional in format, they are not included in this chapter.

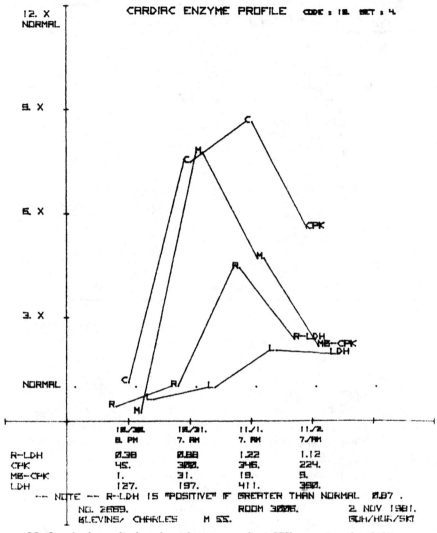

Figure 33–2. Analogue display of serial enzyme studies. CPK = creatine phosphokinase isoenzyme of heart origin; R-LDH = ratio of LDH1 to LDH2. (Information courtesy of Joseph T. Gohmann, MD, Portsmouth, Ohio.)

Comment

It is our impression that many pathologists use interpretive reports. The 146 directors who sent examples of their reports probably represent that smaller group of pathologists who are particularly interested in this approach, who have developed their reports more than others, and who are interested in sharing their work and seeing what others are doing.

The large number of replies from community hospitals and the small num-

---

Table 33—2.

Interpretive Report Generated by a Computer.†

METABOLIC ACIDOSIS, uncompensated
A serious disorder is present with the CO2 content   7. mM
below normal without a compensatory fall in the PCO2. This
suggests that pulmonary disease may also be present. Starvation,
diabetes, renal disease, diarrhea, salicylism, et al, are to be
considered.
  Anion Gap =   18. mEq. [Limit = 14]
  HCO3 DEFICIT =   53. mEq.
    [equivalent to   1.1 amp 8% Na/bicarb OR
    equivalent to   320. ml M/6 Na/Lactate]
  Severe 'K' deficit is calculated at 285. mEq.
  7.28 pH equals a Hydrogen ion concentration [H +] of 48. nEq/l.

Specimen collected at: 3.30 PM, 30 OCT 82

pH	7.28*	Na	138.	OSM	290.	Hosp # 45662
CO2	18.*	K	2.8*	Wt-lbs	140.	g-h-s/SMITH
PvCO2	36.	Cl	102.	TIME: 14:10:03		30-OCT-82

---

†Information courtesy of Joseph T. Gohmann, MD, Portsmouth, Ohio.

---

ber of replies from university hospitals was not unexpected. Clinicians have given these interpretive reports a mixed reception. While it is hazardous to generalize, clinicians in community hospitals tend to welcome these reports, while subspecialists in university centers tend to view these reports as unnecessary because they wish to interpret their own data.

Hobbie and Reece[7] surveyed clinicians regarding computer-generated interpretive reporting of 12-channel chemistry profiles for outpatients and showed that 90% liked it and 80% wanted to see more follow-up suggestions. When this same system was tried in a hospital, it did not work as well and was abandoned after six months. Reasons for failure in the hospital were given as slow turn around time, disinterest by hospital specialists, less interest in diagnostic information than management information, and lack of commitment by laboratory staff. Ashworth and coworkers[8] surveyed clinicians regarding computer-generated interpretive reporting of multitest 20-channel chemistry profiles and thyroid function tests in a hospital setting and showed variable physician acceptance. Many internists were critical of the reports, but the majority of other physicians found them helpful. Sixty-four percent of internists read the interpretive remarks and found the comments helpful in 31% of the cases. Other physicians read the comments 87% of the time and found the comments helpful 58% of the time.

Documentation in the patient's chart of diagnostic possibilities and therapeutic suggestions by the pathologist has caused some clinicians to worry about increased medicolegal liability, especially if an appropriate suggestion is not acted on. The outpatient survey mentioned previously showed one third of the physicians were concerned about medicolegal implications.[7]

The cause of this concern is enigmatic, for attending physicians have the same prerogative of accepting or rejecting the suggestions of the pathologist as they have of any other consultant. Perhaps concern stems from the fact that the pathologist's diagnostic comment is not more conventionally requested, or it may be that the sheer volume of laboratory reports causes an intuitive fear of overlooking something important. Whatever the reason, the problem is real, and pathologists should be aware of it.

One approach is to make an unequivocal diagnosis. An interpretive comment concerning myocardial infarction is as follows:

CPK isoenzyme electrophoresis shows an MB band. LDH isoenzyme electrophoresis shows an elevated fast fraction with LDH-1 greater than LDH-2. This combination is virtually diagnostic of an acute myocardial infarct. No further isoenzyme determinations are necessary to document this diagnosis. (CPK indicates creatine phosphokinase; MB, creatine phosphokinase isoenzyme of heart origin; and LDH, lactic dehydrogenase.) (Courtesy of Henry De Leeuw, MD, Muskegon, Michigan)

Another approach is to define the meaning of the diagnostic terms precisely, eg, "a negative cytology report does not mean that cancer is ruled out with certainty, because false negative reports may be the result of nonrepresentative material."

Another approach is to couch one's comment in terms that do not bind the clinician to a certain course of action, eg, "suggest follow-up liver panel if clinically indicated," or to use a disclaimer indicating that diagnoses based solely on laboratory tests should not be regarded as complete and final, eg, "the list of diagnostic possibilities is incomplete and the order is not necessarily significant."

Interpretive reporting is a problem-directed approach to laboratory studies. A review of interpretive reports encountered in our survey disclosed that many, if not all, were concerned with problem solving. Multiphasic screening was concerned with the general problem of health vs illness. Other reports were directed at the solution of more specific problems, eg, the presence or absence of abnormal function of a particular organ or even the ruling in or out of one specific disease. When the issue of one specific disease is being addressed, interpretive reports can achieve a high degree of certainty. Galen et al[4] have demonstrated this through the high predictive values of serial CPK and LDH isoenzymes in the diagnosis of myocardial infarction.

The laboratory diagnosis of acute myocardial infarction is a good example to illustrate the manner in which reference values, analogue displays, diagnostic lists, and interpretive comments contribute to the information content of an interpretive report. A cardiac injury panel illustrates a basic level of interpretive reporting by providing reference values as follows:

CPK
  Men, 55 to 170 IU/L
  Women, 30 to 135 IU/L

LDH
  Men and women, 71 to 207 IU/L
  (Courtesy of John B. Henry, MD, Syracuse, New York)

Table 33–3.

Diagnostic List for Creatine Phosphokinase (CPK) Isoenzymes.*

Disease	CPK Isograms in Various Diseases†		
	MM CPK$_3$	MB CPK$_2$	BB CPK$_1$
Active myocardial damage, including subendocardial infarct, infarct extension, and cardiac surgery	+ − + + +	Trace- + + +	. . .
Myocardial ischemia	+ − + + +	Trace	. . .
Active skeletal muscle damage, including Duchenne's muscular dystrophy, extensive rhabdomyolysis, polymyositis, early dermatomyositis, myoglobinemia, and severe ischemia of extremities due to vascular disease	+ + − + + + +	0 − +	. . .
Rocky Mountain spotted fever	+ − + +	0 − +	. . .
Reye's syndrome	+ − +	0 − +	. . .
Normal serum	0 − + +	. . .	. . .
Brain injury	0 − + +	. . .	0 − +
Biliary atresia	+ − + +	. . .	0 − +
Malignant tumors (usually with metastases)	+ − + +	O-Trace	0 − + +
Severe shock	+ − + + +	O-Trace	O-Trace
Chronic renal failure	+ − + + +	O-Trace	0 − +

*Information courtesy of Warren B. Helwig, MD, Newport News, Virginia.
†Values indicated occur at peak isoenzyme levels. MM and CPK$_3$ indicate slow electrophoretic CPK isoenzyme; MB and CPK$_2$, intermediate electrophoretic CPK isoenzyme; and BB and CPK$_1$, fast electrophoretic CPK isoenzyme.

Figure 33–2 shows how the information content can be enhanced by a graphic display of serial enzyme studies. Table 33–3 shows the contribution of a diagnostic list for CPK isoenzymes. The interpretive comment concerning myocardial infarction mentioned previously illustrates the most informative manner of interpretive reporting in which a definite diagnosis of acute myocardial infarction has been made.

Interpretive reports should help busy clinicians by providing the information they require to solve clinical problems. They should save time for any medical student, house officer, general practitioner, or specialist who has to page through lists of chemistry, hematology, microbiology, and immunology test results trying to locate, copy, compute, and collate data germane to a particular

problem. Computer-generated interpretive reporting of 20-channel chemistry profiles and thyroid function tests substantially reduced the number of telephone calls
about abnormal results due to age, sex, fasting state, age deterioration of specimen, or hemolysis. In the same manner, the time of the laboratory staff was
conserved by eliminating any need for handwritten, telephoned, or rubber-
stamped comments that were previously required.[8] It has been suggested that the
insertion of problem-directed interpretive reports directly into the progress notes
might further save time for clinicians.

Interpretive reports should benefit patients by closing the gap between the
mere reporting of laboratory test results and their integration into the diagnostic
process. One may argue that simply stating reference values hardly constitutes
interpretive reporting, but without these values interpretation is impossible. Both
the College of American Pathologists through its Inspection and Accreditation
Program and the Joint Commission on the Accreditation of Hospitals insist that
reference values be provided. Furthermore, in recognition of the pitfalls of reporting raw data, these two agencies require the laboratory director or a representative to review patients' laboratory studies to ensure their relevance to patient
care.

A graphic display of data as depicted in Figure 33–2 may have far greater
impact on clinical decision making than numbers alone. And why not include
appropriate diagnostic possibilities that may be useful to patient care? Does not
one first have to think of a diagnosis to make it? Reece[9] found that computer-
generated interpretive reports of 966 abnormal 12-channel chemistry profiles included the right diagnosis in the first five possibilities 67% of the time.

Interpretive reporting is not intended to imply that the pathologist is consistently able to make definitive diagnoses from laboratory results. Rather, it is
meant to highlight the fact that there are many ways in which the information
content and clinical usefulness of laboratory data can be improved. Some of these
are as simple as good form design, inclusion of better reference values, and
graphing or grouping of data in more comprehensible ways. Comments listing
appropriate diagnostic possibilities or recognizing disease processes such as inflammation can also be helpful.

Laboratory directors, particularly pathologists trained broadly in anatomic
and clinical pathology, are in a unique position to contribute to patient care by
interpretive reporting of laboratory data. They are aware, both as a result of individual experience and because of the volumes of data collected by the College
of American Pathologists, of the quantitative aspects of principles relevant to the
use of diagnostic testing (see also Chapter 30). Kassirer and Pauker[10] believe that
these principles, ie, sensitivity and specificity, predictive value, therapeutic
meaning, and cost-effectiveness, particularly in their quantitative aspects, are
grasped by a small minority of physicians. Though the opinion of any consultant
should not be considered absolute, that of the pathologist may be worthwhile. The
pathologist's interpretive reporting should be encouraged because the pathologist

is constantly involved in introduction of new methods, statistical evaluation of analyses, interpretation of multiple studies, and biopsy evaluation, as well as the ultimate quality-control procedure in medicine—the autopsy.

The authors acknowledge the support of Donald A. Senhauser, MD, and the contributions of Kay Cook and Jody Pohl in performing this study.

References

1. Henry JB: Introduction to organ panels, in Henry JB, Giegel JL (eds): *Quality Control in Laboratory Medicine*. New York, Masson Publishing USA Inc, 1976, pp 1–13.
2. Osserman EF, Katz L, Sherman WH, et al: Computer-based case tracing (COMTRAC). *JAMA* 1978;239:1772–1776.
3. Reece RL, Hobbie RK: Computer evaluation of chemistry values: A reporting and diagnostic aid. *Am J Clin Pathol* 1972;57:664–675.
4. Galen RS, Reiffel JA, Gambino R: Diagnosis of acute myocardial infarction: Relative efficiency of serum enzyme and isoenzyme measurements. *JAMA* 1975;232:145–147.
5. Altshuler CH, Bareta J, Cafaro AF, et al: The PALI and SLIC systems. *CRC Crit Rev Clin Lab Sci* 1972;3:379–402.
6. Schecter DS (ed): *American Hospital Association Guide to the Health Care Field*. Chicago, American Hospital Association, 1977.
7. Hobbie RK, Reece RL: A computer reporting and interpretation system: Acceptance and accuracy, in Benson ES, Rubin M (eds): *Logic and Economics of Clinical Laboratory Use*. New York, Elsevier North-Holland Inc, 1978, pp 163–172.
8. Ashworth CT, McConnell TH, Ashworth RD, et al: A computer program for reporting automated chemistry (SMAC) and thyroid function tests with algorithm-derived interpretive comments, in Benson ES, Rubin M (eds): *Logic and Economics of Clinical Laboratory Use*. New York, Elsevier North-Holland Inc, 1978, pp 173–186.
9. Reece RL: Universal unified interpretive reports: Conceivable, believable, and achievable. *Pathologist* 1978;32:343–350.
10. Kassirer JP, Pauker SG: Should diagnostic testing be regulated? *N Engl J Med* 1978;299:947–949.

Chapter 34

Changing Physician Behavior

John M. Eisenberg, MD
Sankey V. Williams, MD

The remarkable increase in overall health care expenditures in the United States is the result of increases both in the price and the utilization of health services. The price of health care, has risen for numerous reasons, including the general inflation in the American economy; because hospitals now pay wages that are competitive with other industries[1]; and because hospitals and physicians now provide a different "product" than was previously available, offering more sophisticated technology to detect and treat disease, new classes of drugs, and new members of the health care team. In addition, the utilization of services has increased for several reasons, including increases in the number of older people, who require more health care[2]; and because the poor and the elderly now have better access to care through Medicaid, Medicare, and other government programs.

Gibson and Mueller[3] have suggested that 52% of the recent increases in health care costs can be attributed to inflation and that 48% can be attributed to increased utilization, including increases in utilization resulting from a larger population. However, not all of the increases in the cost of medical care can be justified by general inflation, increased costs of labor, improved quality of care, an increase in the population, demographic changes, or an increase in the number of those eligible for third-party coverage. Indeed, some of the increases in the utilization of medical services may reflect the cost of services that are not medically necessary.[4–7] These have been attributed to several factors, including patient expectation, increased numbers of physicians,[8] and excessive numbers of hospital beds.[1]

From: Cost Containment and Changing Physicians' Practice Behavior. Can the Fox Learn to Guard the Chicken Coop? *JAMA* 1981;246:2195–2201. Copyright 1981 by the American Medical Association.

Despite the multiple influences on the cost of medical care, the role of physicians is a central one. It has been estimated that between 50% and 80% of health care costs are controlled by physicians.[9] Nevertheless, despite physicians' power and responsibility as the patient's representative in purchasing medical care, few physicians seem to know what it costs. For example, investigators at the Medical College of Ohio, Toledo, found that house staff knew only the approximate cost of 30% of procedures such as laboratory tests and x-ray examinations. Faculty knew the approximate cost of 45% of medical services.[10] At the University of Miami, only 2% of the house staff knew more than 50% of the correct costs, and most physicians tended to underestimate costs.[11] At Cornell Medical Center, NY, both attending physicians and house staff generally knew the approximate cost of a semiprivate room, but less than half the attending physicians and about a fourth of the house staff knew the cost of an electrolyte profile.[12] Finally, Roth[13] found that when 40 physicians in community hospitals were questioned, only 14% of medical care costs were estimated correctly.

In addition to a lack of knowledge about the costs of medical care, several other reasons have been suggested for overuse of medical services by physicians: fear of malpractice charges, peer or supervisor pressure, inexperience, financial incentives, the training and personality of the physician, the type of practice, habit, and a misunderstanding of test results.[14–16] Certainly, costs could be decreased by limiting the size of the medical care "engine," for example, by decreasing the number of hospital beds or controlling the number of expensive technical services. The Health Systems Agencies use this approach when they review the need for new hospitals and new services in existing hospitals. But unless physicians, who control the accelerator and the brake of the medical system, change the speed at which they drive the engine, cost containment will probably not work. If the medical profession is to improve its own performance, if the fox is to be trusted to guard the chicken coop, it is necessary to identify ways to change physician behavior.

The Hospital as Skinner Box: Changing Physician Behavior

In an effort to improve physicians' awareness of the costs of health care and to reduce medical expenditures, six different strategies have been employed: (1) education, (2) peer review with feedback, (3) administrative changes, (4) participation, (5) penalties, and (6) rewards. The remainder of this chapter will review the experience with these approaches to changing physician behavior. This report emphasizes physicians' use of ancillary services such as laboratory tests and x-ray examinations, because more and methodologically better studies have been carried out in this area, but the principles identified here should be applicable to other areas where physician behavior needs to be changed.

Education of Physicians

The most popular approach to changing physician behavior has been to establish education programs. According to the Association of American Medical Colleges, in 1977, 34% of American medical schools had cost-containment education programs for medical students, residents, or both.[17] Programs aimed at medical students may change their attitudes about the cost of medical care and their performance in simulated patient care, but long-term follow-up of their behavior after graduation has not been carried out.[18, 19] In addition, numerous hospitals have initiated educational programs for house staff and attending physicians.[20, 21]

Many educational approaches have been used—discussions, seminars, workshops, case reviews, mortality conferences with emphasis on the cost of care, the employment of cost-containment directors, and newsletters. There are many subjects that can be discussed in these educational programs—the cost and usefulness of laboratory tests and x-ray examinations, drug costs and the use of generic drugs, policies regarding reduced charges for combination requests such as laboratory test panels, discharge planning, preadmission scheduling of tests, and the greater use of other health professionals. Unfortunately, these educational efforts are limited by scanty data regarding the cost-effectiveness of most diagnostic and therapeutic services. In some of these educational programs, evaluation has been carried out to determine how effective they have been.

In an early article, published in 1971, Griner and Liptzin[22] showed that an educational program could reduce the rate of increase in the cost of laboratory testing for several months.[22] One of us (J.M.E.) conducted a study of the Philadelphia Veterans Administration Hospital to reduce overuse of the prothrombin time determination.[23] There were two medical services from two medical schools in the hospital and both had the same high use of the prothrombin time evaluation—85% to 90% of all patients admitted had prothrombin time determinations obtained. With an intensive educational program of posters, conferences, and mailings to the residents on one service, there was a significant decrease in the use of the test, a decrease that did not occur on the other service. When the program was withdrawn, test use returned to its baseline level within six months. Rhyne and Gelbach[24] found similar temporary changes in physicians' ordering of thyroid function profiles. The major lesson to be learned from these studies is that an educational program may have temporary effects, but without a continued program, physicians will probably lapse back into their old habits. The principles of behavior modification would predict such a result, since newly learned behavior generally requires reinforcement to become installed as a regular part of behavior.

Griner[25] has followed his earlier article with a seven-year study showing continued reduction in the use of some tests with an ongoing educational program. Although much of the change was due to a decrease in the use of two tests—the icterus index and the prothrombin time—his group was able to show lower rates of increase than the 13.8% annual increase in hospital laboratory testing found in the rest of the United States at that time.[14]

Several recent educational programs have reported success in altering the use of services by medical residents. Martin and his colleagues[26] at the Brigham and Women's Hospital, Boston, have described success in reducing the use of laboratory tests, but not radiological procedures. Klein et al[27] have induced a change in the use of antibiotics, and Lyle et al[21] have shown changes in several aspects of care. Each of these programs shares a common educational strategy—the preceptorial. In each program a respected physician, senior to the house staff, has conducted individual conferences with the residents. The remarkable success of these individualized programs contrasts with the poorer results of many didactic programs and raises the question: Are these individualized programs more successful at transmitting knowledge or is their success due to the charisma of the respected teacher and acceptance by the resident physicians of an attitude about the value of cost-effective medical care?

Robertson[28] has reported the results of an educational program designed to improve the knowledge of physicians and students regarding the cost of diagnostic tests. After an intensive educational program, there was no improvement in knowledge, and only 40% of the estimates were within 25% of the actual charge. His study casts doubts on the ability of even intensive educational programs to affect knowledge about costs substantially, and suggests that educational programs have other effects. Indeed, Martin et al[26] propose that their effective program may have been dependent on the transmission of new attitudes or a value system to the medical residents.[26]

Numerous studies have been performed regarding education of physicians about the use of prescription drugs, but few of these studies include control groups of physicians and seldom is it possible to draw firm conclusions from the data.

In addition to the potential effect of educational programs specifically designed to reduce overuse, there is evidence that more knowledgeable physicians use laboratory tests more selectively. Internists' scores on the American Board of Internal Medicine's certifying examination are inversely correlated with the number of diagnostic studies they use on patient management problems (G. Webster, MD, oral communication, 1979). At Strong Memorial Hospital, Rochester, NY, Greenland et al[29] showed that the use of diagnostic tests decreased as residents progressed through the three years of graduate medical education, although the investigators were unable to show a clear correlation between test use and knowledge when measured by a questionnaire. It is not known whether formal education of physicians in decision-analysis will enable physicians to make more cost-effective decisions about the use of medical resources.

In addition to these important considerations—use of a variety of educational methods and topics, the need for reinforcement, individualization of education, the impact of improved knowledge, and the relevance of physicians' value systems—the efficacy of educational programs may be influenced by the ability of the educators to address the needs of physicians. It is likely that careful analysis of the strengths and weaknesses of physicians before the educational program will help to focus the intervention and may improve its effectiveness.

In summary, it appears that education may have some effect, albeit temporary, on costs generated by physicians and that the effect of educational programs may not be due to the transmission of information but rather of attitudes about cost-effective medical care. Medical educators have proposed the expansion of these educational programs for students and residents with the assumption that the "child is father to the man" and that knowledge or attitudes learned in training will influence subsequent clinical practice.[30, 31] The success of personalized educational programs may be unique to residency programs and may be costly, but offers a potential method to establish habits of cost-effective use of services early in a physician's career.

Feedback to Physicians

Up to this point, a somewhat narrow definition of education has been used in describing educational programs that are designed to transfer to physicians information about the costs and efficacy of medical care and may have the additional, if unplanned, effect of altering attitudes. A broader definition of education might include feedback to physicians about their patterns of practice. Such a system might show physicians how their utilization compared with that of other physicians or may provide peer review regarding the necessity of the services provided. However, it is important to remember that feedback is more than simply education; it plays on the physician's sense of achievement and desire to excel. Feedback, therefore, inevitably involves a more subtle reinforcement or admonition for current behavior.

There have been several methods used to feed information back to physicians. One popular method is to send physicians copies of the bills of their hospitalized patients and let them know what their care costs. Another is to calculate for physicians their percentile-rank with regard to the use of services by similar physicians. Still another is to conduct chart audits to review the use of laboratory tests, x-ray examinations, or drugs, or to review the management of a particular diagnosis for unnecessary use. However, few hospitals have established explicit criteria for reviewing these charts for overutilization, as has been done for underutilization in the quality assurance audits required by Professional Standards Review Organizations. We propose that quality medical care should include the efficient use of medical resources and that overutilization as well as underutilization should be monitored by the hospital committees.

In theory, one expects feedback programs to be effective. In more than 30 years of research at the Survey Research Center of the University of Michigan, Ann Arbor, Bowers and Franklin[32] have shown that organizational change can be greatly facilitated when data about the system's functioning are collected, fed back to members, and used to provide opportunities for diagnosis and action.

There are several examples of feedback programs in the health services research literature. One of the first was organized at George Washington University, Washington, DC, and showed a 29% decrease in the use of diagnostic services after an audit.[33] Wennberg and his colleagues[34] showed that tonsillectomy rates in Vermont declined 40% during a four-year period following a feedback program that illustrated regional variations for that operation. In Saskatchewan, a review program for hysterectomies was followed by a 33% decrease in hysterectomies performed and a decrease in the proportion of unjustified hysterectomies from 24% to 8%.[35] Craig et al[36] and Counts[37] have described feedback in drug utilization review that was effective in changing physician behavior while Mitchell et al[38] have shown a decrease in the length of stay after cholecystectomy. At the West Virginia University Medical Center, Morgantown, WV, a program providing daily profiles of hospital charges incurred by patients demonstrated a 28% reduction in total hospital charges, including a 30% reduction in laboratory charges.[39] It should be recognized that the educational programs of Martin et al,[26] Klein et al,[27] and Lyle et al[21] were heavily dependent on feedback to change physician behavior and not totally dependent on the physicians' acquiring new knowledge about the cost or efficacy of diagnostic tests. It appears that education with feedback is a more effective strategy than simple education alone, but a controlled trial would be necessary to demonstrate this hypothesis.

At the Hospital of the University of Pennsylvania, Philadelphia,[40] a computer-based feedback system to detect overutilization of laboratory tests by the medical service has been tested. The hospital's computerized laboratory reporting-system provided a daily list of patients who had three or more determinations of a given laboratory test, such as the serum calcium determination, in a short period. A panel of faculty internists established a list of clinical reasons for which multiple determinations would be appropriate. For example, the expert panel thought it to be allowable for a patient with chest pain who was admitted to the coronary care unit to have three determinations of serum lactic dehydrogenase in three days. A chart auditor reviewed the chart of each patient with multiple determinations of the same test to determine whether the criteria for appropriate testing were met. If they were not, a letter was sent to the physicians on the team that ordered the test, including the attending physician, telling them of the audit and inviting them to explain their use of the tests. No personal, individualized education was used. In the first effort to use this program to decrease overutilization, there was no significant change in the ordering of multiple determinations.

Similarly, a clinical information system at Johns Hopkins Hospital, Baltimore, which reported the previous month's utilization by each medical service and by each intern, had no discernible effect on utilization.[41]

One of the largest successful feedback programs was that of the New Mexico Medicaid Program, which operated an Experimental Medical Care Review Organization (EMCRO) between 1971 and 1975. The EMCRO provided feedback to physicians about their use of injectable drugs and, within two years, the use of injections per Medicaid recipient dropped 60%. The program of education and feedback was specifically aimed at physicians whose practice patterns apparently conflicted with guidelines. However, no reduction was demonstrated in the use of other medical services. Claims submitted by the physicians to the Medicaid program were used as the source of data about their practices.[42, 43]

The Professional Services Review Organizations (PSROs) were established in part as an outgrowth of the EMCRO programs. They operate principally as physician feedback systems. Although they are empowered to penalize the physician through fines or expulsion from the Medicare reimbursement program, this is almost never done and therefore has little practical consequence.[4] It is the patient who is notified of personal responsibility for the hospital bill if the PSRO denies third-party payment. However, patients are allowed three days in the hospital after notification, and alternative care can usually be arranged before the patient must begin paying. When alternative care cannot be arranged, it is often because the patient can pay for neither alternative care nor hospital care. Since the hospital is reluctant to press for payment in these circumstances, the patient, like the physician, rarely suffers any real additional financial burden. Therefore, if PSROs work, the reason may be that physicians change their behavior in response to the feedback they receive from their peers in the review process.

Do PSROs work? Although confused by political issues and by some questionable data, the answer is "probably yes." The PSROs probably reduce the number of days of hospital care for Medicare patients by about 2%.[44] There is disagreement about the cost of PSRO reviews and thus disagreement about any net savings that can be attributed to PSROs. Moreover, most activities of PSROs aimed at decreasing overutilization have focused on the necessity for hospitalization and have neglected services provided to those patients who do require hospitalization but may have unnecessary services while in the hospital.

In conclusion, feedback alone may be an effective mechanism for changing physician behavior, but doubts have been raised about its ability to save enough in medical costs to justify the expense of the feedback system. As in the case of educational programs, feedback programs are likely to be most effective if they focus on areas of inappropriate utilization that are perceived to be problems. Physicians and other health care providers can serve as participants in the review process and help to direct the feedback efforts toward potentially remediable utilization patterns. One popular method of identifying problem areas is the generation of practice profiles, which can highlight aberrant styles of practice and focus the review process.

˙Administrative Changes

In addition to education and feedback, some hospitals have used administrative changes to modify physician behavior and contain costs. For example, Strong Memorial Hospital, where Griner also used educational methods, instituted several procedural changes: (1) the hospital eliminated routine chest roentgenograms on admission unless specifically requested by the admitting physician; (2) residents were required to write orders for laboratory tests in the medical order book instead of directly onto a highly structured laboratory requisition form; and (3) third-year residents who, as a group, were known to order tests more appropriately were moved from elective rotations (such as consultation services), where they were not responsible for writing orders, to ward rotations, where they were responsible for day-to-day patient care decisions, while second-year residents were moved to elective rotations. Testing was decreased in association with the combined educational program and administrative changes.[25]

Other programs have used administrative changes to alter the use of diagnostic tests and have been successful. Data from Stanford University Medical Center indicate that when residents were required to fill out their own request forms, laboratory use decreased (K. Marton, MD, written communcation, 1981). Dixon and Laszlo,[45] at the Durham, NC, VA Hospital, limited residents to eight tests per patient per day and showed that laboratory use became more selective and more appropriate with a reduction of testing by 25%. Many hospitals require prior approval of certain drugs and diagnostic tests before they will be administered or performed, but there is inadequate evidence to determine whether the cost of having physicians approve tests or drugs is worth the potential savings. An alternative is to require that certain clinical criteria be met for a test to be done without prior consultation. Numerous policy changes can also be made by the pharmacy to alter physician behavior, most simply by altering the formulary so that a certain drug or a certain preparation of a drug is not available.

Administrative changes to restrict the use of ancillary services also may be instituted by third-party payers. For example, Blue Cross, with the support of the American College of Physicians, has recently suggested that local plans not reimburse hospitals for routine admission testing unless the tests are specifically ordered by a physician. In addition, a number of third-party payers have offered or required second-opinion review prior to surgery and have instituted clerical review of claims prior to payment to assure that laboratory tests can be linked to the patient's medical problems.

Participation by Physicians

While education, feedback, and administrative changes may help to cut costs, an even greater potential for savings exists with physicians' enthusiastic participation in the cost-containment effort. Physicians may participate by helping the hospital to identify potential savings that could be obtained through managerial changes such as the purchase of supplies, energy conservation, or telephone use. But potential for savings also lies in physicians participating in changing their own patterns of practice.

Management theory suggests that with a group of professionals such as physicians, who have highly uncertain tasks requiring extensive problem-solving, member participation in making decisions is the most effective way of changing behavior.[46, 47] In fact, Stoelwinder and Clayton[48] found a reduction in patient stays, a reduced waiting time for emergency services, and a lower rate of increase for admission costs when physicians and other hospital staff jointly addressed problems of better patient care. This is one example of "contingency theory," so-called because the appropriate way to initiate change in an organization is contingent on the work and the people involved.[49] According to contingency theory, neither physicians nor other professionals would be expected to respond favorably to forced change with which they did not agree.

In teaching hospitals, efforts to reduce costs generated by house staff seem to reinforce this conclusion. Several successful efforts to reduce costs in a teaching hospital have used house staff participation—including those at Strong Memorial Hospital,[25] Jackson Memorial Hospital, Miami, and Johns Hopkins Hospital.

Therefore, in addition to involving physicians in the identification of problems for review, they should be active participants in the development of criteria for the appropriateness of services, the planning and implementation of the review process, and the decisions regarding feedback, rewards, and penalties. There is evidence in continuing education programs that physician participation in the development of instructional objectives and needs-assessment, as well as involvement of leaders from the physician community in carrying out the educational program, is associated with changes in physician practice patterns.[50–52]

Financial Rewards and Penalties

While management theorists agree that participation should help to induce change, there is debate about the effectiveness of financial penalties and rewards.[53] Still, there have been a few model efforts to reduce health care costs by imposing penalties for overutilization of outpatient procedures.

Buck and White[54] evaluated the utilization review program of the San Joaquin Foundation for Medical Care and found an association between the number of billing claims adjusted by peer review and subsequent changes in physicians' office practice patterns, most noticeably in their decreased use of office injections. Using similar methods, the New Mexico Medicaid Program found that penalties had little additional impact to that of its program of education and feedback designed to decrease the use of injectable drugs. Whereas the feedback program induced a decrease in injections of 60%, the institution of denials of payment for inappropriate injections was associated with further decreased use of only 15%, for a total reduction of about 75%.[43] It should be noted, however, that physicians were aware that denial of payment might be used if they did not respond to the feedback program, so it cannot be said unequivocally that the 60% decreased utilization was due to feedback alone. It is likely that the threat of denials had some unmeasurable effect even before denials were also implemented. In contrast, Paris et al[55] have reported a decrease in the use of injections, laboratory tests, chest roentgenograms and first billings coincident with the establishment of a claims review and disciplinary program for overutilization in the New York City Medicaid program. Neither of these Medicaid programs used control groups and neither accounted for regression toward the mean, which can be expected with outliers.

There have also been efforts to change physician behavior by offering financial rewards when the physicians exhibit the desired behavior. In 1969 and 1970, the Health Insurance Plan of Greater New York (HIP) offered financial rewards to member physicians in an attempt to reduce patient care costs.[56] More than 40,000 patients were included in the study sample of HIP patients and in the control sample of non-HIP patients matched for age and sex. In the study sample, cost savings were shared between the physician group caring for the patients and the Social Security Administration. During the two years of the study, hospital discharge rates and lengths of hospital stay declined for both the study and control samples, but the changes were proportionately greater for the study sample—7.2% vs 2.4% for discharge rates and 12.1% vs 3.1% for lengths of stay.

Pennsylvania Blue Shield conducted a study in which 91 physicians in ten hospitals agreed to receive a single, lump-sum payment for their services when patients with one of 23 selected diagnoses were admitted to the hospital, regardless of how long the patients stayed or how many services the physicians provided.[57] This is similar to the way surgeons are now paid for many operative procedures. The lum-sum payment was calculated as the mean amount paid for physician services per admission for that diagnosis in the previous year. Patients in the study group had lengths of stay that averaged 3% shorter than those of patients in a control group, a small but statistically significant difference. The appropriate conclusion appears to be that physicians can provide more cost-effective care when the reimbursement system does not include financial rewards that encourage extra services.

Hunt[58] offered psychiatry residents additional money for professional activities such as journals, books, and travel to medical conventions if the residents met guidelines for seeing increased numbers of ambulatory patients during their training program. When compared with the year before the incentive program, the residents dramatically increased the number of patients they saw. Hunt intended the incentives to help residents learn how to manage problems associated with their ambulatory practices following completion of their training programs, but the technique could be used to cut costs by increasing physician efficiency. In contrast, Martin et al[26] found no substantial effect of financial rewards offered to medical residents for reduced use of diagnostic tests.

The most convincing evidence of the effectiveness of financial incentives to change physician behavior comes from studies in which physicians are at risk for both financial penalties and rewards. Health maintenance organizations (HMOs) consistently provide health care that costs 10% to 40% less than care provided comparable populations under the fee-for-service system.[59] In all HMOs, the organization is at risk for losing money if health care costs exceed the premiums paid by patients, but the organization benefits financially when costs in any given year are lower than premiums. Physicians who belong to HMOs admit fewer patients to the hospital, but their patients have comparable lengths of stay and use approximately the same number of ambulatory services as patients in the fee-for-service system.

Similar results have been observed when individual physicians assume the financial risk of their patients' health care. In one such program, patients choose a primary care provider who must refer the patient if specialized care is to be paid by the health plan.[60] The primary care physician authorizes payment from his or her own account for all care provided to patients. The physician shares in any deficit or surplus remaining at the end of the year. The results to date are similar to those of a successful HMO and are substantially better than those of the Blue Cross plan in the area.

An interesting program has been initiated at Johns Hopkins Hospital, where the clinical departments are responsible for their own financial activity, including the inpatient services, and therefore have an incentive to save money, which they apparently have done. With each department operating as a financial responsibility center, the hospital has been reported to have reduced its rate of cost increase by half in three years (*Fortune*, June 18, 1979, pp. 148–154).

Comment

None of these six methods has been shown to reduce costs in all situations when used alone. When education is combined with administrative changes, impressive reductions have been observed in residents' use of diagnostic studies.[25] When peer review and feedback are combined with education, there have been substantial decreases in the number of surgical procedures,[34, 35] decreases in physicians' use of diagnostic procedures,[26, 33] and small decreases in lengths of hospital stay.[44] When financial penalties are combined with education and feedback based on peer review, physicians decrease their use of office injections.[42, 43, 54] When financial rewards are combined with administrative changes, practicing physicians are able to deliver more cost-effective care[56, 57] and residents may increase their productivity.[58] Practicing physicians can deliver still more cost-effective care when administrative changes and participation are combined with both financial penalties and rewards.[59, 60]

This review of the available literature points out several directions for further research. Controlled trials of different interventions should be carried out. Investigators should study the response of physicians in different types of practice settings, including teaching hospitals, community practice, prepaid plans, and government practice. Studies of the efficacy and cost-effectiveness of a number of medical care services will be required before rational efforts can be initiated to contain their costs without compromising quality. Financial support for this type of research is limited at present, but these studies provide the potential for savings greater than the cost of the research if they lead to less costly but effective medical care.

Can the fox learn to guard the chicken coop? Can physicians learn to change their behavior to slow the rapidly rising costs of medical care? We think physicians can control costs. Their self-imposed restraint will turn out to be the most effective force for ensuring rational cost control while preserving the highest possible quality of care. If for no other reason, physicians will recognize that their action in limiting further cost increases is the best alternative available—certainly preferable to heavy-handed regulation.

However, physicians need help from programs such as the ones described in this chapter if they are to develop new patterns of behavior. Medical educators should continue to develop and implement programs to teach students and residents how to take care of patients without wasting resources. Hospital administrators should create new approaches for identifying hospital costs and they should develop innovative strategies for providing their medical staff with the information these physicians need to lower costs. Professional societies should support medical educators in their cost-control efforts, continue to contribute to the peer review process, and expand their involvement with new delivery systems such as the HMO. Third-party payers should identify new reimbursement systems and show that they contribute to cost reduction. Regulators should seek new proposals for controlling costs that engage the cooperation of physicians and thus take advantage of their special knowledge and experience.

While education, feedback, administrative changes, and physician participation may be effective in altering physician behavior, we expect that financial rewards will be one component of the most effective programs. In their absence, financial penalties may be necessary. It is one irony of today's third-party reimbursement system that existing financial incentives do not encourage cost-effective medical care. Indeed, physicians generally are more handsomely rewarded for applying expensive and questionably useful technology to patients' problems than they are for providing personal care. Indeed, they may increase their income several-fold by performing multiple laboratory tests and other diagnostic tests.[61] If this reimbursement system is not realigned, other attempts to induce physicians to contain costs may not be effective.[62, 63]

This study was supported in part by grants from Blue Cross of Greater Philadelphia, the National Fund for Medical Education (sponsored by Prudential Insurance Company of America), and the National Health Care Management Center at the Leonard Davis Institute of Health Economics, University of Pennsylvania (Department of Health, Education, and Welfare grant HSO2577 from the National Center for Health Services Research).

References

1. *Expenditures for Health Care: Federal Programs and Their Effects*, Congressional Budget Office, Government Printing Office, 1977.
2. Kovar MG: Health of the elderly and use of health services. *Public Health Rep* 1977;92:9–19.
3. Gibson R, Mueller M: National health expenditures: Fiscal year 1976. *Soc Secur Bull* April 1977;40:3–22.
4. Eisenberg JM, Rosoff AJ: Physician responsibility for the cost of unnecessary medical services. *N Engl J Med* 1978;299:76–80.
5. Roth JA: The necessity and control of hospitalization. *Soc Sci Med* 1972;6:425–446.
6. Hall FM: Overutilization of radiological examinations. *Radiology* 1976;120:443–448.
7. Kurylo LL: Measuring inappropriate utilization. *Hosp Health Serv Adm* 1976;21:73–89.
8. GMENAC (Graduate Medical Education National Advisory Committee): *Supply and Distribution of Physicians and Physician Extenders*. US Dept of Health, Education, and Welfare publication No. (HRA) 78-11, Bureau of Health Manpower, Division of Medicine, Manpower Supply and Utilization Branch, 1978.
9. Somers AR, Somers HM: A proposed framework for health and health care policies. *Inquiry* 1977;14:115–170.
10. Skipper JK, Smith G, Mulligan JL, et al: Physicians' knowledge of costs: The case of diagnostic tests. *Inquiry* 1976;13:194–198.
11. Dresnick SJ, Roth WI, Linn BS, et al: The physician's role in the cost-containment problem. *JAMA* 1979;241:1606–1609.
12. Nagurney JT, Braham RL, Reader GG: Physician awareness of economic factors in clinical decision-making. *Med Care* 1979;17:727–736.
13. Roth RB: How well do you spend your patients' dollars? *Prism* 1973;1(September):16–17.
14. Fineberg HV: Clinical chemistries: The high cost of low cost technologies, in Altman S, Blendon R (eds): *Medical Technology: The Culprit Behind Health Care Costs?* Proceedings of the Sun Valley Forum on National Health. US Dept of Health, Education, and Welfare publication No. 79-3216, 1979, pp 144–165.
15. Schroeder SA: Variations in physician practice patterns: A review of medical cost implications, in Carels EJ, Neuhauser D, Stason WB (eds): *The Physician and Cost Control*. Cambridge, Mass, Oelgeschlager, Gunn & Hain, Inc, Publishers, 1980, pp 23–50.
16. Hardison JE: Sounding boards: To be complete. *N Engl J Med* 1979;300:193–194.
17. Hudson JI, Braslow JD: Cost containment education efforts in the United States medical schools. *J Med Educ* 1979;54:835–840.

18. Garg ML, Gliebe WA, Kleinberg WM: Student peer review of diagnostic tests at the Medical College of Ohio. *J Med Educ* 1979;54:852–855.

19. Zeleznik C, Gonnella JS: Jefferson Medical College student model utilization review committee. *J Med Educ* 1979;54:848–851.

20. Friedman E: Changing the course of things: Costs enter medical education. *Hospitals* 1979;54:82–85.

21. Lyle CB, Bianchi RF, Harris JH, et al: Teaching cost containment to house officers at Charlotte Memorial Hospital. *J Med Educ* 1979;54:856–862.

22. Griner PF, Liptzin B: Use of the laboratory in a teaching hospital. *Ann Intern Med* 1971;75:157–163.

23. Eisenberg JM: Educational program to modify laboratory use by housestaff. *J Med Educ* 1977;52:578–581.

24. Rhyne RL, Gelbach SH: Effects of an educational feedback strategy on physician utilization of thyroid function panels. *J Fam Pract* 1979;8:1003–1007.

25. Griner PD and Medical Housestaff, Strong Memorial Hospital: Use of laboratory tests in a teaching hospital: Long-term trends. *Ann Intern Med* 1979;90:243–248.

26. Martin AR, Wolf MA, Thibodeau LA, et al: A trial of two strategies to modify the test ordering behavior of medical residents. *N Engl J Med* 1980;303:1330–1336.

27. Klein L, Charache P, Johannes R, et al: Effect of physician tutorials on prescribing patterns and drug cost in ambulatory patients, abstracted. *Clin Res* 1980;28:296.

28. Robertson WO: Costs of diagnostic tests: Estimates by health professionals. *Med Care* 1980;18:556–559.

29. Greenland P, Mushlin AI, Griner PF: Discrepancies between knowledge and use of diagnostic studies in asymptomatic patients. *J Med Educ* 1979;54:863–869.

30. Lawrence RS: The role of physician education in cost containment. *J Med Educ* 1979;54:841–847.

31. Lawrence RS: The role of physician education in cost control, in Carels EJ, Neuhauser D, Stason WB (eds): *The Physician and Cost Control*. Cambridge, Mass, Oelgeschlager, Gunn & Hain Inc, Publishers, 1980, pp 151–159.

32. Bowers DG, Franklin JL: *Survey-Guided Development 1: Data-Based Organizational Change*. La Jolla, Calif, University Associates, 1977.

33. Schroeder SA, Kenders K, Cooper JK, et al: Use of laboratory tests and pharmaceuticals: Variation among physicians and effect of cost audit on subsequent use. *JAMA* 1973;225:969–973.

34. Wennberg JE, Blowers L, Parker R, et al: Changes in tonsillectomy rates associated with feedback and review. *Pediatrics* 1977;59:821–826.

35. Dyck FJ, Murphy FA, Murphy JK, et al: Effect of surveillance on the number of hysterectomies in the province of Saskatchewan. *N Engl J Med* 1977;296:1326–1328.

36. Craig WA, Ulmar SJ, Shaw WR, et al: Hospital use of antimicrobial control program. *Ann Intern Med* 1978;89:793–795.

37. Counts GW: Review and control of antimicrobial usage in hospitalized patients: A recommended collaborative approach. *JAMA* 1977;238:2170–2172.

38. Mitchell JH, Hardacre JM, Wenzel FJ, et al: Cholecystectomy peer review: Measurement of four variables. *Med Care* 1975;13:409–416.

39. Henderson D, D'Alessandri E, Westfall B, et al: Hospital cost containment: A little knowledge helps, abstracted. *Clin Res* 1979;27:279.

40. Eisenberg JM, Williams SV, Garner L, et al: Computer-based audit to detect and correct overutilization of laboratory tests. *Med Care* 1977;15:915–921.

41. Johns RJ, Blum BI: The use of clinical information systems to control costs as well as improve care. *Trans Am Clin Climatol Assoc* 1978;90:140–152.

42. Brook RH, Williams KN: Effect of medical care review on the use of injections: A study of the New Mexico Experimental Medical Care Review Organization. *Ann Intern Med* 1976;85:509–515.

43. Lohr KN, Brook RH, Kaufman MA: Quality of care in the New Mexico Medicaid Program. *Med Care* 1980;18(suppl):1–129.

44. *The Effect of PSROs on Health Care Costs: Current Findings and Future Evaluations*. Congressional Budget Office, Government Printing Office, 1979.

45. Dixon RH, Laszlo J: Utilization of clinical chemistry services by medical housestaff. *Arch Intern Med* 1974;134:1064–1067.

46. Dunn WN, Swierczek FW: Planned organizational change; toward grounded theory. *J Appl Behav Sci* 1977;13:135–137.

47. Weisbord MR, Stoelwinder JU: Linking physicians, hospital management, cost containment and better medical care. *Health Care Mgmt Rev* 1979;4:7–12.

48. Stoelwinder JU, Clayton PS: Hospital organization development: Changing the focus from 'better management' to 'better patient care.' *J Appl Behav Sci* 1978;14:400–414.

49. Morse JJ, Lorsch JW: Beyond Theory Y, in Hampton DR, Summer CF, Webber RA (eds): *Organizational Behavior and the Practice of Management*. Glenview, Ill, Scott Foresman & Co, 1973, pp 650–660.

50. Stross JK, Bole GG: Evaluation of a continuing education program in rheumatoid arthritis. *Arthritis Rheum* 1980;23:846–849.

51. Stross JK, Bole GG: Continuing education in rheumatoid arthritis for the primary care physician. *Arthritis Rheum* 1979;22:787–791.

52. Wang VL, Terry P, Flynn BS, et al: Evaluation of continuing medical education for chronic obstructive pulmonary disease. *J Med Educ* 1979;54:803–811.

53. Hampton DR, Summer LE, Webber RA (eds): *Organizational Behavior and the Practice of Management*. Glenview, Ill, Scott Foresman & Co, 1973, pp 609–614.

54. Buck CR Jr, White KL: Peer review: Impact of a system based on billing claims. *N Engl J Med* 1974;291:877–883.

55. Paris M, McNamara J, Schwartz M: Monitoring ambulatory care: Impact of a surveillance program on clinical practice patterns in New York City. *Am J Public Health* 1980;70:783–788.

56. Jones E, Densen PM, Altman I, et al: HIP incentive reimbursement experiment: Utilization and costs of medical care, 1969 and 1970. *Soc Security Bill* 1974; 37:3–21.

57. Markel GA: Per case reimbursement for Medicaid services. National Center for Health Services Research Summary Series, NCHSR-US Dept of Health, Education, and Welfare publication No. PHS 79–3230, 1978.

58. Hunt DD: Effects of incentives on economic behavior and productivity of psychiatric residents. *J Psych Educ* 1980;4:4–13.

59. Luft HS: How do health-maintenance organizations achieve their 'savings'? *N Engl J Med* 1978;298:1336–1343.

60. Moore S: Cost containment through risk–sharing by primary care physicians. *N Engl J Med* 1979;300:1359–1362.

61. Schroeder SA, Showstack JA: Financial incentives to perform medical procedures and laboratory tests: Illustrative models of office practice. *Med Care* 1978;16: 289–298.
62. *A Manpower Policy for Primary Health Care*. Washington, DC, National Academy of Science, Institute of Medicine, 1978.
63. Peterson ML: The Institute of Medicine report 'A Manpower Policy for Primary Health Care': A commentary from the American College of Physicians. *Ann Intern Med* 1980;92:843–851.

Chapter 35

Shared Clinical Laboratories

Elias Amador, MD

Physicians use the clinical laboratory to obtain more information each year. The kinds of laboratory tests available have grown steadily for the past 30 years (Figure 35–1). Even more strikingly, the total tests produced by the clinical laboratory have grown exponentially (Figure 35–2) at a compound rate of about 13% per year (Table 35–1).

Most of these tests are done in local clinical laboratories, which, however, are not equipped to perform all the various types of tests needed by the physicians in a given region. In order to solve this problem, one solution would be to do nonemergency tests in a central laboratory, with each clinical facility retaining a small laboratory for emergency service.[1] Such a shared laboratory system could perform most tests, including the more complex ones, in an acceptable time, and the high volume would lower the cost per test.[2–6]

The time elapsed between the request of a test and the result being reported to the physician, ie, the turnaround time (TAT), is critical to a test's usefulness.[7] Some test results are needed as soon as possible, eg, blood glucose in decompensated diabetes, whereas the physician can wait for hours or even days for many other test results. One way to establish the appropriate TAT for each test is by a committee composed of test users and providers. The tests can be grouped as requiring a TAT of one hour or less, four hours, eight hours, and 24 hours. This grouping can be the basis for planning the laboratory resources and for allocation of tests between the on-site laboratory and the central laboratory, based on the patient's needs.

From: Shared Clinical Laboratories. *JAMA* 1976;236:1162–1165. Copyright 1976 by the American Medical Association.

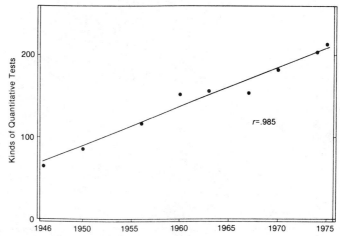

Figure 35–1. Growth of kinds of quantitative and semiquantitative laboratory tests in common use (based on Tables of Normal Laboratory Values published at intervals, since 1946, by the New England Journal of Medicine). Slope indicates that tests listed have grown steadily in linear fashion. Numbers will be proportionately larger if qualitative tests (microbial cultures, immunohematology, cytology, and other tests) are included, but historical data were not available to author.

Laboratory Sharing

The configuration of a shared or a central laboratory system can vary greatly. Regionalization is already widespread for blood banking through regional blood banks run by the American Red Cross or groups of hospitals.[8] Highly specialized laboratories for genetic screening also function as regional referral centers.[9] The following are some of the configurations.

Central Shared Laboratories

Currently, certain groups of pathologists in the United States have formed laboratory networks, each with a central laboratory. Each participating hospital also has an on-site laboratory staffed by a pathologist. The Clinical Laboratory Medical Group, located in Los Angeles County,[10] has local laboratories in seven hospitals and specimen pickup stations in five medical buildings. The central laboratory operates a messenger service to bring in the specimens from the peripheral laboratories. The results are reported to each participant as they are obtained by means of computer-driven teletypewriters. The central laboratory performs all automated and nonemergency manual chemical assays, endocrine tests, immunologic, serologic, bacteriologic, cytologic, and histologic tests. The automated analytical equipment is connected on-line to a small computer that prepares a punched tape and drives a teletypewriter. The tape from the small computer

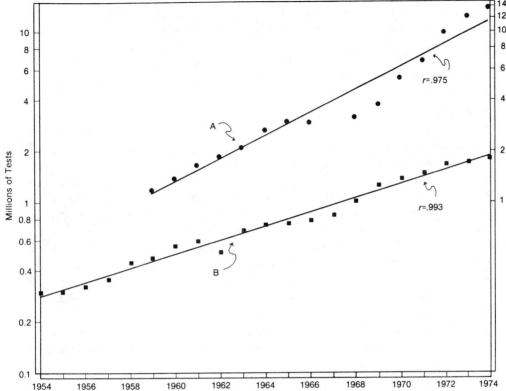

Figure 35–2. Laboratory workload over 20-year period, plotted semilogarithmically. Workload has increased exponentially in two widely separated, large general hospitals; A, Los Angeles County/University of Southern California Medical Center, and B, University Hospitals of Cleveland. In hospital A, number of tests that could be ordered by physician from 1960 to 1969 was limited by ration stamps and other types of restrictions accounting for fluctuations in growth rate. Exponential slope is very similar to that of hospital B.

Table 35–1.		
Growth of Workload in Two Separate Hospital Laboratories.		
Laboratory*	Doubling Time, yr	Compound Annual Growth Rate, %
A	4.2	18
B	7.2	10
Mean	5.7	13

*Laboratory A, Los Angeles County/University of Southern California Medical Center, 1959–1974. Laboratory B (tests for adult patients), University Hospitals of Cleveland, Ohio, 1954–1974.

together with all requisitions and manual results are merged into a larger computer that maintains and updates all files. This computer, in turn, drives teletypewriters located in the satellite laboratories so that results are available on a short turnaround basis. Each hospital's laboratory is near the emergency ward. It provides a blood bank, around-the-clock blood typing and cross-matching, emergency blood-gas determinations, chemical assays, blood cell counting, and blood clotting tests.

A laboratory system composed of many clinics, seven hospitals with their laboratories, and two central laboratories is used by the Southern California Permanente Medical Group to service its clinic outpatients and hospital inpatients. The area served is centered around Los Angeles, extending as far south as San Diego and as far west as Hawaii. The laboratory network performs some 30 million tests annually, 9 million of which are done centrally. About 80% of the specimens processed in a central laboratory come from outpatients, and the remainder come from hospitalized patients. The transportation service is divided into seven geographic regions; within each region the specimens from the local clinics are taken to the closest hospital. A separate messenger vehicle collects the appropriate specimens from each hospital for processing in one of the central laboratories. Test results are reported on the same day as ordered for inpatients and no later than 24 hours for outpatients. The transportation system is coordinated by the director of the central laboratories in order that the messengers adhere closely to their schedules.

Within the central laboratories, groups of technologists are permanently assigned to process all specimens from a specific region or hospital and to handle telephone inquiries about these tests. Using this method, almost no specimens or finished results have been lost. In addition, they report minimal telephone interruptions and very low personnel turnover.

The types of tests performed at each laboratory site are determined according to need, and each test methodology is standardized throughout the system. Thus, if a given test is done in the peripheral and central laboratories, the same method is used at all test sites. Similarly, methods for quality control are identical throughout the system. All reagents and culture media are prepared centrally. A central maintenance shop services all instruments and stocks replacement units. Significant savings are said to result from this practice. The clinicians interviewed by the author were well satisfied with the laboratory service they received.

Significant defects in the Permanente systems are the absence of teaching programs for residents and student technologists and the total absence of research. Conversely, from the viewpoint of service and economy, the Permanente laboratory system appears to be outstanding.

Of these two centralized laboratory systems, one uses electronic computers extensively for data acquisition, collection, and reporting,[10] whereas in the other system, these functions are performed manually. This author observed no significant differences in the quality of service provided by these systems attributable to the presence or absence of computers.

Partial Centralization

A centralized chemistry laboratory has been used since 1967 by the five hospitals of the University of Pittsburgh School of Medicine.[2] The laboratory is located in a three-story building that houses routine and special chemistry, microchemistry, instrument repair and maintenance, teaching programs, and research.

The laboratory is controlled by a committee of administrators from the participating hospitals. This committee meets monthly. One hospital acts as administrative agent and provides all supporting services. The pathology chiefs of each hospital act as a professional advisory committee. Income is provided by each user on a cost-for-service rendered. A similar arrangement is used by the Hospital-Pathologist Central Laboratory of Orange County, California,[4] where 15 hospitals, some as large as 500 beds, have joined to form a central chemistry laboratory. This is housed in its own building, and performs automated and manual chemistry, endocrine tests, toxicology, and therapeutic drug tests. Service is on a seven-day-per-week basis, and some emergency work is done. Specimens are picked up and results are delivered three times a day. The management is similar to that already described.

Cooperative Laboratory Systems

This system, an example of which is located in Chicago, is built around the laboratories of four hospitals, each having less than 250 beds.[5] Each participating hospital has one, main, specialized laboratory plus an on-site frozen blood section, blood banking, hematology, and emergency chemical assays facilities. Hospital A laboratory is specialized in histopathology and radioimmunoassay, hospital B in biochemistry, hospital C in microbiology, and hospital D in immunology and serology. The four hospitals are linked by a messenger-driven automobile, with three pickup circuits each day (Figure 35–3). Eisenstaedt,[5] who described this system,[5] has shown that despite inflation, the cost per test for chemistry, histopathology, serology, and microbiology has remained stable over several years. Conversely, a marked increase in productivity and versatility has resulted. The TAT for tests that are requested on a stat basis is two hours. Each hospital pays on a direct monthly cost-per-test basis, which is agreed to by third-party payers.

Regional Laboratories

In large geographic regions with a low population, a regional laboratory can service a large number of participating hospitals. In Oklahoma,[11] a central

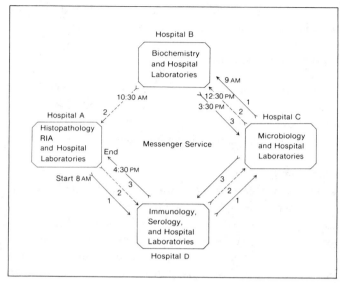

Figure 35–3. System of cooperative hospital laboratories described by Eisenstaedt.[3] Each hospital has one specialized laboratory plus its own frozen section, blood bank, hematology, and emergency chemistry facilities. Messenger uses one automobile and follows three daily routes shown by arrows. RIA = radioimmunoassay laboratory.

laboratory is associated with 63 participating hospitals, each of which also maintains its own laboratory. The central laboratory provides specimen transportation mainly during the night so that specimens arrive at the regional laboratory by 5 AM. The TAT is 12 to 18 hours. All results are telephoned to the participating laboratory over a WATS line, followed by a written follow-up. The central laboratory provides each participating hospital laboratory with quality control samples, bacteriological environmental surveys, calibration standards, reagents, and consummable supplies. Frozen sections are performed on-site by a visiting pathologist. Biopsy specimens, surgical specimens, and histologic autopsy specimens are processed in the central laboratory within 24 hours. Such a regional laboratory may serve participating hospitals as well as physicians in private practice by processing the specimens on appropriate schedules.

Regional Specialty Laboratories

Certain tests are sufficiently specialized and of relatively low demand so that a single specialized laboratory may serve a very large population. Examples include testing for rare bleeding disorders, genetic screening, chromosome analyses, and tissue typing for transplant compatibility, as well as testing for drugs of abuse or toxic compounds.[12] In the Los Angeles County hospital system, such a concept has been implemented in part in the areas of toxicology, drugs of abuse, hematopathology, and genetic screening.

Functional Considerations: Structure and Management

The basic professional requirements for laboratory medicine are identical, regardless of whether the laboratory is located in a large hospital or a regional facility. First, the staff in charge must be able to exercise authority commensurate with its responsibility and have the ability to implement decisions, to choose and reward staff, and to control the laboratory budget. An advantage of such management is that adequate professional staff may be maintained, and research resources may be provided from the generated income to further the intellectual development of laboratory medicine through programs of teaching and research.

Second, the success of a shared laboratory system requires the continued confidence and interest in the well-being of the participating institutions. One way this can be done is by having a board of directors composed of at least one pathologist and one administrator from each institutional member. A representative of the major clinical services might also be a board member. Such a board would guarantee that the physicians, laboratory PhDs, and other staff from participating institutions will have a voice in the policies and practices of the laboratory.[2, 4]

Third, essential to the success of a shared laboratory system is a smoothly functioning system for specimen collection, transportation, and result reporting. All of these functions must be effectively controlled by the director of the laboratory system. An effective method for keeping track of the specimens is essential. (A positive audit trail is necessary to locate lost or allegedly lost specimens.) Reporting of results must be in writing but can be supplemented by prior notification of results over the telephone and must be backed up by a reliable system for the retrieval of previous results. This backup system can be on a computer, microfilm, or paper and must be kept up to date so that telephone inquiries may be promptly answered.

Fourth, the rapid growth of laboratory medicine requires varied and intensive teaching programs for the laboratory personnel. These programs are difficult to establish and maintain in small laboratories. A regional teaching facility would allow efficient use of teaching personnel and facilities. A centralized pool of teaching personnel and audiovisual facilities could be available, and special equipment and space could be justified by the large number of students. Moreover, a centralized teaching facility could easily offer seminars and postgraduate courses in recent advances in laboratory medicine to the professional public.

Comment

The development of laboratory medicine is favored by the need for rapid test TAT, physician and personnel convenience, and test accuracy at an acceptable cost. The published experience seems to indicate that these needs may be satisfied by sharing or centralization of most laboratory services. Uniformity in test methods and reporting nomenclature, normal ranges, and other factors would also result from such an approach. Such a system could make available rapid, accurate, and sophisticated laboratory support for physicians practicing in smaller hospitals, rural areas, and ghetto communities. This sharing of expensive facilities is also in accord with current trends in health care. The clinical experience with shared clinical laboratories so far has been favorable,[3] and further use and refinement of shared laboratories seems to be warranted as a rational and economical way to satisfy the rapidly growing clinical needs for more laboratory data.

References

1. Clinical diagnostic chemicals become big business. *Chem Eng News* 1975;53:8–9.
2. Amenta JS, Luebs HW: Centralized chemistry laboratory. *Hospitals* 1967;41:58–62.
3. Astolfi AA, Matti LB: Survey profiles shared services. *Hospitals* 1972;46:61–65.
4. Dahlgren TE: Six hospitals share a central laboratory and save money. *Mod Hosp* 1969;112:92–93.
5. Eisenstaedt WF: A cooperative laboratory a must for the future. *Lab Med* 1974; 5:16–19.
6. Benson ES, Brown PA, Dorsey DB, et al: Will consolidated clinical laboratories supplant individual hospital laboratories? *Hum Pathol* 1973;4:437–448.
7. Lundberg GD: *Managing the Patient Focused Laboratory*. Oradell, NJ, Medical Economics, Inc, 1975.
8. Schmidt PJ: Regional blood transfusion system. *Pathologist* 1973;27:219–220.
9. Lynch HT: *International Directory of Genetic Services*, ed 3. White Plains, NY, The National Foundation—March of Dimes, White Plains, NY, 1971.
10. Poletti BJ, Zack JF Jr, Mueller TJ: Computer control in the clinical laboratory. *Am J Clin Pathol* 1970;53:731–738.
11. Hain RF, Stephenson JM: Spreading the wealth. *Med Lab Observer*, 1970, pp 43–47.
12. Lundberg GD, Walberg CB, Gupta RC: Patient-focused approach to organization of a clinical toxicology laboratory. *Lab Med* 1972;3:14–16.

Index

Numbers in italics refer to pages in the text containing figures.